Treatment Outcomes in Older Adults with Cancer

Treatment Outcomes in Older Adults with Cancer

Guest Editor

Mackenzi Pergolotti

MDPI

Basel • Beijing • Wuhan • Barcelona • Belgrade • Novi Sad • Cluj • Manchester

Guest Editor
Mackenzi Pergolotti
Outcomes and Research
Select Medical
Mechanicsburg
USA

Editorial Office
MDPI AG
Grosspeteranlage 5
4052 Basel, Switzerland

This is a reprint of the Special Issue, published open access by the journal *Cancers* (ISSN 2072-6694), freely accessible at: https://www.mdpi.com/journal/cancers/special_issues/929L6X424C.

For citation purposes, cite each article independently as indicated on the article page online and as indicated below:

Lastname, A.A.; Lastname, B.B. Article Title. *Journal Name* **Year**, *Volume Number*, Page Range.

ISBN 978-3-7258-7969-4 (Hbk)
ISBN 978-3-7258-7970-0 (PDF)
https://doi.org/10.3390/books978-3-7258-7970-0

Contents

About the Editor

Mackenzi Pergolotti

Mackenzi Pergolotti, PhD, MS, OTR/L, FACRM is Vice President of Outcomes and Research for the Outpatient Division at Select Medical, where she leads strategy and oversight for outcomes measurement, registry development, and rehabilitation research across a national network of outpatient clinics. She earned her PhD in Occupational Science from the University of North Carolina at Chapel Hill and holds an academic appointment with the University of North Carolina at Chapel Hill, Division of Occupational Science and Occupational Therapy.

Dr. Pergolotti's scholarly work focuses on cancer rehabilitation and geriatric oncology, with particular emphasis on functional outcomes, patient reported outcomes, and the implementation of evidence based rehabilitation models within oncology care. Her research spans the cancer continuum and addresses the integration of rehabilitation into clinical practice to improve function, quality of life, and care delivery for individuals living with and beyond cancer.

She has authored an extensive body of peer reviewed publications, abstracts, and book chapters, and has served as a principal investigator, co investigator, and consultant on federally funded research. Dr. Pergolotti is a Fellow of the American Congress of Rehabilitation Medicine and serves on the Editorial Board of the *Journal of Geriatric Oncology*. She is actively involved in national and international efforts to advance rehabilitation research, practice, and policy in oncology.

cancers

MDPI

Article

Implementing a Geriatric Assessment-Guided Rehabilitation Care Model in Community Oncology Care: Feasibility and Impact on Patient-Reported and Performance-Based Outcomes †

Mackenzi Pergolotti [1,2,3,*], Kelley C. Wood [1], Mary Hidde [1,4], Tiffany D. Kendig [1], Deanna Meehan [5], Katie Hutzayluk [5], Alaina M. Newell [1,6], Jessica Bertram [7], Ashley Lightner [1], Stacye Mayo [1], Alina Hedaya [1,5], Smith Giri [8,9] and Grant R. Williams [8,9]

1 ReVital Cancer Rehabilitation, Select Medical, Mechanicsburg, PA 17055, USA; kecwood@selectmedical.com (K.C.W.); mchidde@gmail.com (M.H.); tkendig@selectmedical.com (T.D.K.); amnewell@selectmedical.com (A.M.N.); anlightner@bswrehab.com (A.L.); smayo@selectmedical.com (S.M.)
2 Department of Occupational Therapy, University of North Carolina, Chapel Hill, NC 27599, USA
3 Department of Occupational Therapy, Colorado State University, Fort Collins, CO 80523, USA
4 Medpace, Inc., Denver, CO 80202, USA
5 Kessler Rehabilitation Center, Kessler Institute for Rehabilitation, Select Medical, Chester, NJ 07930, USA; dmeehan@kessler-rehab.com (D.M.); khutzayluk@kessler-rehab.com (K.H.)
6 Department of Physical Therapy, South College, Knoxville, TN 37909, USA
7 Outpatient Division, Baylor Scott and White Institute for Rehabilitation, Dallas, TX 75246, USA; jbertram@bswrehab.com
8 Institute for Cancer Outcomes and Survivorship, University of Alabama at Birmingham, Birmingham, AL 35233, USA; smithgiri@uabmc.edu (S.G.); grwilliams@uabmc.edu (G.R.W.)
9 Lewis and Faye Manderson Cancer Center, Tuscaloosa, AL 35401, USA
* Correspondence: mpergolotti@selectmedical.com

† This paper is an extension of a conference paper. Kendig, T.; Wood, K.C.; Bertram, J.; Hidde, M.; Ronnen, E.A.; Lightner, A.N.; Mayo, S.; Hedaya, A.; Newell, A.M.; Meehan, D.; Hutzayluk, K.; Carroll, R.; Williams, G.R.; Pergolotti, M. Using an electronic capture geriatric assessment to guide rehabilitation triage for adults with cancer during systemic therapy. *J. Clin. Oncol.* **2023**, *19*, 474–474. https://doi.org/10.1200/OP.2023.19.11_SUPPL.474.

Simple Summary: This study assessed the feasibility of conducting an online monthly geriatric assessment (GA) to identify frailty in adults with cancer who were about to begin a new treatment at a community oncology practice. The GA classified patients into three categories: frail, pre-frail, or robust. Patients identified as frail or pre-frail were referred to outpatient cancer rehabilitation services, including physical and occupational therapy. Feedback from participants indicated that this approach was both feasible and well received. Furthermore, those who attended rehabilitation experienced significant improvements in quality of life, mobility, fitness, and strength.

Abstract: Background: Adults with cancer who are pre-frail or frail are at risk of poor outcomes. Geriatric assessment (GA) is recommended to assess and manage vulnerability and risk of frailty in older adults with cancer (≥65) and to inform referrals in supportive services, including rehabilitation. Yet, adoption of the GA in community oncology practice lags, and frailty among adults younger than 65 often goes undetected and/or unaddressed. We evaluated the feasibility of a GA-guided rehabilitation care model and assessed changes in patient-reported and performance-based outcomes after rehabilitation. Methods: Adults (≥18 years) starting systemic therapy at a community oncology practice enrolled in the study. The GA was administered online and monthly for one year. Frailty/pre-frailty was identified using a previously validated 44-item index. The oncology team was notified of frail/pre-frail patients and then made referrals to outpatient rehabilitation. Feasibility outcomes (recruitment, retention, fidelity) and participant acceptability [7 items, 0–5 Likert scale] were analyzed descriptively. Patient-reported and performance-based outcomes

 https://doi.org/10.3390/cancers17193274

were examined using the paired t-test. Results: 48% of eligible patients enrolled (N = 141), and 83% completed at least one GA. Frailty/pre-frailty was identified in 40% of the GAs, resulting in 282 referrals to rehabilitation (99% fidelity). Acceptability scores ranged from 3.5 ± 1.7 to 4.7 ± 0.6. Participants who attended rehabilitation (52%) improved significantly in outcomes measuring health-related quality of life, mobility, aerobic capacity, and strength (all $p < 0.05$). Conclusion: Implementing a GA-guided rehabilitation care model was feasible and acceptable to patients receiving systemic treatment. Those who attended rehabilitation experienced significant improvement in patient-reported and performance-based outcomes.

Keywords: neoplasms; geriatric assessment; rehabilitation; triage; health services evaluation; patient reported outcome measures

1. Introduction

Systemic cancer treatments are associated with high levels of cancer-related burden and frailty. Frailty is characterized by an increasing vulnerability to stressors, related to the accumulation of deficits, which decreases a patient's physiologic reserve and resilience to stressors. In cancer, systemic treatment is associated with an increase in risk of frailty, which increases one's risk of poor tolerability of cancer treatment, of unplanned hospitalization, long-term functional disability, poor quality of life, and early mortality [1–5]. Therefore, detecting and addressing frailty early is critical to a patient's care experience and long-term well-being.

Recent guidelines from the American Society of Clinical Oncology (ASCO) recommend routine use of a geriatric assessment (GA) to identify vulnerability and risk of frailty and to provide targeted supportive care interventions, including rehabilitation (physical, occupational, and speech therapy [PT/OT/ST]), to treat GA impairments among older adults (65 and older) [6]. Adoption of these guidelines has the potential to enhance patient experience and reduce the risk of poor treatment tolerability and survival outcomes. However, integration of the GA and GA-guided care pathways into community oncology practice, although possible [7], remains a challenge due to a lack of access to a geriatrician and other supportive care services in the community [8]. Instead, researchers recommend a focus on self-administered geriatric assessments, with direct referrals to needed services, yet this has not been tested in a community-based setting.

While traditionally associated with older adults, frailty and GA impairments are increasingly recognized as issues across the age spectrum [9–11]. Emerging evidence highlights that accelerated aging and geriatric syndromes, including frailty, are not exclusively tied to chronological age [8,9]. The functional and economic burdens associated with cancer in working-age adults underscore the need for routine screening and early interventions to address impairments that may affect treatment outcomes and quality of life [12]. Furthermore, functional components of frailty, such as falls, difficulty with daily activities, and other impairments amendable to rehabilitation, were more common among younger adults. These findings challenge traditional assumptions that frailty and GA impairments primarily affect older adults and underscore the need to expand GA use to adults younger than 65.

To address these gaps, we conducted a prospective, pragmatic, single-arm, clinical trial integrating a GA-guided rehabilitation (defined here as physical, occupational, and speech therapy) care pathway in community oncology care for both older and younger adults initiating systemic treatment. We aimed to evaluate the feasibility of a GA-guided rehabilitation care model (only) and assess the impact of cancer-specialized outpatient rehabilitation services on health-related quality of life (HRQOL) and functional outcomes. We focused on HRQOL and functional outcomes due to their association with the ability to tolerate systemic treatment [13], unplanned hospitalization [14,15], chemotherapy-induced peripheral neuropathy severity [16], and mortality [7,10], although the literature supports the benefits of rehabilitation on these outcomes [16]. To support the broader adoption of GA-guided care and inform future research, we also report implementation strategies in alignment with the Exploration, Preparation, Implementation, Sustainment (EPIS) framework [17].

2. Materials and Methods

2.1. Study Design

This is a prospective pragmatic feasibility study conducted to evaluate the feasibility, acceptability, and impacts of the GA-guided rehabilitation care model for adults with cancer initiating a new line of systemic therapy. Study design and intervention reporting were guided by the Consolidated Standards of Reporting Trials (CONSORT) extension guidelines for feasibility and pilot studies [18] and the template for the intervention description and replication (TIDieR) checklist [19]. The study was approved by the Kessler Foundation Institutional Review Board (E-1132-20) and registered as a clinical trial (NCT04852575).

2.2. Study Population

English-speaking adults with cancer (18 years or older) initiating a new line of systemic cancer treatment (chemotherapy, immunotherapy, or hormonal therapy) at a multi-site community oncology private practice in East Brunswick, NJ, USA (Astera Cancer Care) were eligible. Astera is a physician-owned, community oncology practice with eleven medical oncology clinics, eight radiation clinics and three breast surgery locations. The care team at Astera includes medical oncology, radiation oncology, breast surgery, advanced practice providers, pharmacists, social workers, palliative care, and research. Individuals with no valid email address, had been referred for hospice care, or had self-reported inability (technical or cognitive) to complete online questionnaires were excluded.

2.3. Recruitment and Enrollment

From January to 31 December 2021, eligible patients were recruited during a pre-chemotherapy education session with an oncology advanced practice provider (APP) and were provided an additional opportunity to enroll if they elected to attend a pre-chemotherapy rehabilitation evaluation. As part of the pre-chemotherapy education session, APPs were trained to educate patients on the study and, when doing so in person, provide the study flyer. In addition, a reminder was added to the visit note in the electronic medical record (EMR) to support the APP's ability to remember to introduce the study and to record patients' interests. Those who agreed to contact the study coordinator were identified daily by the study team using an EMR-generated report, from which the study coordinator would call eligible patients within 48 h. Informed consent was obtained verbally in accordance with the ethical standards of the institutional review board. Once consented, each participant was enrolled in a REDCap (Research Electronic Data Capture) database [20,21] designed for this study. Throughout the follow-up period, the study coordinator routinely reviewed the EMR and removed study participants who had begun hospice services or passed away.

2.4. Data Collection

All GA data was collected using REDCap [20]. GAs were administered automatically at the time of enrollment (time point one), and monthly for 12 months (total of thirteen time periods over 12 months). Up to two weekly reminder emails and one telephone reminder were sent. Demographic (age, sex, race, ethnicity) and clinical characteristics (cancer type, stage, treatment regimen, etc.) were extracted from the oncology EMR for all participants. We did not estimate a target sample size for this study; instead, we worked towards the goals of a one-year collection and evaluating the feasibility of the process.

2.5. Intervention

The GA-guided rehabilitation care model included routine screening using a patient-reported GA, which was used to detect frailty and coordinate triage processes among the rehabilitation and oncology care teams. Participants referred to rehabilitation received individualized services provided by licensed physical and occupational therapists who had completed a cancer-specialized certification program provided by the ReVital Cancer Rehabilitation (Select Medical) and could elect to attend services at home (via synchronous telemedicine) or at an outpatient, in-community (as opposed to cancer center or hospital) clinic location. Physical therapy (PT) focused on improving range of motion, strength, and endurance. The goal of the visits was to maintain or improve cardiovascular capacity, physical health, and fitness. The therapy included 4 components: (1) cardiovascular, (2) strength training, (3) balance training, and (4) flexibility training. Occupational therapy (OT) focused on improving patients' functioning in performing activities of daily living (ADL) such as bathing, food preparation, and managing medications, all and instrumental activities of daily living (IADL) such as upper extremity function, pain interference and social and vocational participation (i.e., the ability to return to work). Speech therapy (ST) focused on speech, swallowing, and language impairments. All PT/OT/ST interventions were tailored to the individual and their needs.

GA Tool and Administration. Monthly, participants were emailed a link to complete the online GA via REDCap. The GA used in this study, the Cancer and Aging Resilience Evaluation (CARE) GA, has been previously validated [22] and aligns with the GA recommended by ASCO [6]. Details of the CARE GA are provided in Supplement S1. The GA measures the following domains of frailty, each having been described previously [22,23]: the ability to complete daily activities, health-related quality of life, treatment side effects, and comorbid conditions.

Frailty identification and triage. GAs were scored by REDCap 11.0.0 software using a previously validated 44-item deficit accumulation model [9,24,25]. The frailty index score was calculated, and then scores were categorized as robust (0–0.2), pre-frail (0.21–0.35), or frail (>0.35) [24]. The study coordinator emailed a list of newly identified participants with pre-frail/frail status to the oncology team daily for review and, if appropriate, referral to cancer-specialized outpatient rehabilitation services. Referrals were placed by the oncology team using order sets available in their EMRs.

2.6. Implementation Strategies

Implementation strategies were selected by the study team a priori and iterated during each phase of the trial to create an iterative learning environment, maximizing implementation. In the exploration phase, strategies were focused on engaging and obtaining buy-ins from key stakeholders in the oncology and rehabilitation practice. In the planning phase, strategies were focused on identifying barriers and facilitators to the proposed intervention, developing educational materials, quality monitoring, and feedback systems to support implementation. During the implementation phase, additional strategies were employed to audit progress and provide feedback to key members of the oncology and rehabilitation teams, to centralize technical support, and to implement rounding calls regarding patients' needs and operational challenges. In the sustainability phase, strategies were used to grow and adapt the program to meet demand—for example, expanding rehabilitation services to additional outpatient locations, therapists, and specialties (e.g., lymphedema and speech therapy), and improving systems to efficiently relay clinical data between the oncology and rehabilitation teams to optimize patient care and experience.

Strategies and examples are described in Supplement S2 according to the phase of implementation within the Exploration, Preparation, Implementation, Sustainment (EPIS) framework [17].

2.7. Feasibility Outcomes

Feasibility outcomes included: recruitment rate, retention rate, and fidelity. The recruitment rate was measured as the proportion of eligible patients who enrolled during the 1-year recruitment period. Retention rate was measured in three ways: (1) the proportion of enrolled participants who completed at least one GA during the 1-year follow-up period; (2) the proportion of enrolled participants who completed the GA in the months M1, M3, M6, and M12; and (3) the average number of GAs completed by each participant who completed at least 1 GA (possible range from 1 to 13). Common benchmarks for recruitment rates in similar feasibility studies are between 50 and 75% [26] and median recruitment rate is 38% [27]. Fidelity was measured as oncology clinician compliance to rehabilitation referrals and the proportion of referred participants who attended rehabilitation (conversion).

2.8. Acceptability Outcomes

As part of the month 12 GA, participants completed an 8-item acceptability survey that included seven six-point Likert scale items (0- completely disagree to 5- completely agree) and the average amount of time it took them to complete the GA (in mins).

2.9. Patient-Reported and Performance-Based Outcomes

Patient Reported Outcomes Measurement Information System (PROMIS®) health-related quality of life (HRQOL) outcomes included: Global Health (10 items, scored into global physical health (GPH), global mental health (GMH)), Physical Function (PF, 4-item), and Ability to Participate in Social Roles and Activities (SRA, 4-item). Each measure was scored using the appropriate T-score [28]. PROMIS measures have been developed and validated by the National Institutes of Health (NIH) [28], shown to be reliable and useful in oncology care and rehabilitation [29–31], and have been associated with cancer treatment and survival outcomes [9,15]. Higher T-scores indicate more of the domain being measured and have been shown to be sensitive and specific to capture improvement or decline in HRQOL during or following cancer treatment [32]. The established within-group minimal important change (MIC) is two points on the T-score scale, any change at or above this threshold is considered a clinically significant improvement [33].

Performance-based outcomes included: strength (handgrip strength [lbs.], 5-time sit-to-stand test [repetitions performed], and 30 s sit-to-stand test [repetitions performed]) [34–36], aerobic capacity (6-min walk test [distance, feet], and 2-min step test [repetitions performed]) [30,32], and mobility Timed Up-and-Go test [time, seconds]) [35].

2.10. Statistical Analyses

Feasibility endpoints were analyzed descriptively. Continuous scores are presented as mean with standard deviation or median with interquartile range (IQR). Categorical scores are presented as frequencies. Independent *t*-tests, Chi-squared or Fisher's exact test were used to examine differences in characteristics between participants who enrolled versus those who completed at least one GA. Paired samples *t*-test (1-sided) were used to examine improvements in patient-reported and performance-based measures from initial evaluation to discharge. One-sided *t*-tests were used to evaluate pre-post differences because the primary hypothesis was that rehabilitation would result in improvement in

HRQOL and functional outcomes. As a sensitivity analysis, we also examined two-sided tests and confirmed that the direction and significance of results remained consistent. Significance was determined a priori as $p < 0.05$. All analyses were performed using IBM SPSS Statistics (Version 27).

3. Results

3.1. Feasibility

The recruitment rate was 48%; 141 of 245 eligible participants who were contacted enrolled in the study. Recruitment and enrollment details are provided in Figure 1 using the CONSORT extension for pilot and feasibility trials [37]. Of the enrolled patients, 51.9% were aged 64 years or younger, whereas 48.1% were aged 65 or older. Out of all the participants, 82% completed at least one GA (n = 116), and their characteristics are reported in Table 1. There were no significant differences among those who completed at least one GA and those who completed none. The monthly GA completion rate ranged from 35.9% (M9) to 69.5% (BL; Figure 2). Participants completed a median of three GAs (IQR = 1–10).

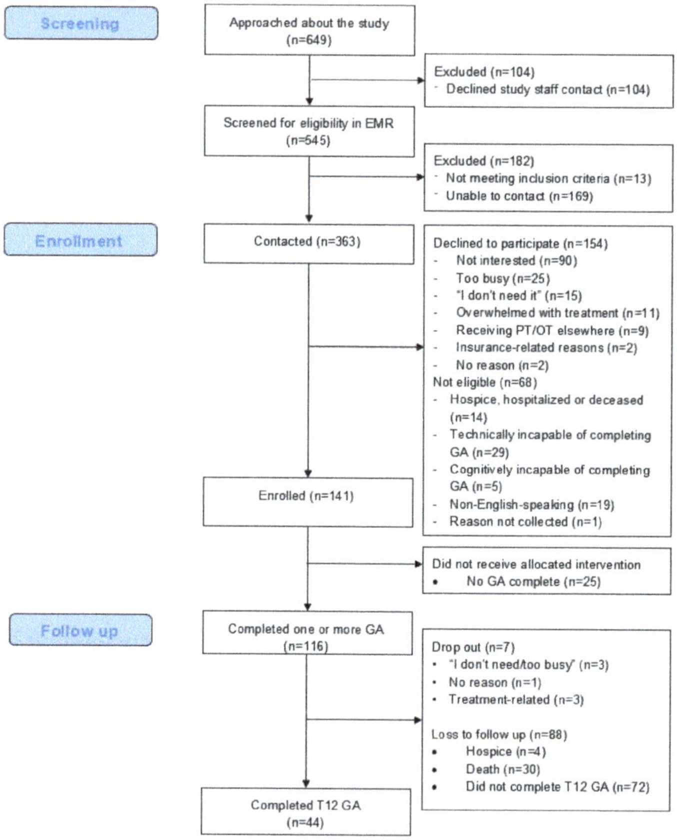

Figure 1. Participant screening, enrollment, and retention.

Table 1. Participant characteristics: all enrolled versus completed at least 1 geriatric assessment (GA).

	All Enrolled (n = 141)	Completed at Least 1 GA (n = 116)	p-Value
Demographics			
Age	63.64 ± 10.81	64.15 ± 10.83	0.227
Sex			0.416
Male	52, 36.9%	41, 35.3%	
Female	89, 63.1%	75, 64.7%	
Race			0.871
White	88, 62.4%	77, 66.4%	
Black	14, 9.9%	12, 10.3%	
Asian	6, 4.26%	5, 4.3%	
Other	9, 6.38%	7, 6.0%	
Unknown or missing	24, 17.0%	15, 12.9%	
Ethnicity (Hispanic/Latino)	8, 5.7%	7, 7.1%	0.947
Cancer diagnosis			
Cancer type			0.179
Breast	49, 34.8%	43, 37.1%	
Head and neck	4, 2.8%	3, 2.6%	
Hematologic	25, 17.7%	20, 17.2%	
Gynecologic	9, 6.4%	7, 6.0%	
Genitourinary	7, 5.0%	7, 6.0%	
Gastrointestinal	28, 19.9%	22, 9.0%	
Lung	16, 11.3%	13, 11.2%	
Other	3, 2.1%	0, 0%	
Stage			0.646
0 to 2	44, 31.2%	38, 32.76	
3 to 4	37, 26.2%	61, 52.59%	
Unknown	23, 16.3%	14.66%	
Recurrence (at time of recruitment)	24, 17.0%	21, 18.3%	0.452
Treatment information			
First line therapy (Yes)	101, 71.6%	82, 70.7%	0.593
Number of cycles planned	11.66 ± 7.72	11.70 ± 7.88	0.892
Completed all cycles	58, 41.1%	47, 40.5%	0.748
Started new therapy during study	75, 53.2%	59, 50.9%	0.324

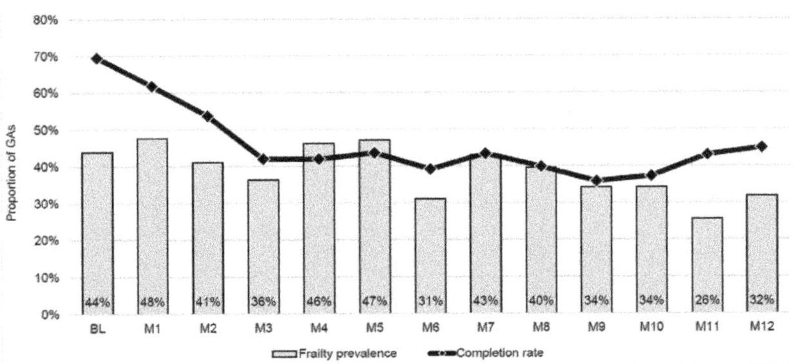

Figure 2. Monthly geriatric assessment completion rate and prevalence of frailty.

Frailty, or pre-frailty status, was identified in 40% of all completed GAs (n = 285). The monthly prevalence of frailty ranged from 26.6% (M11) to 47.6% (M1; Figure 2). Results of frailty by age and differences in reasons for frailty were published previously [23]. Twelve cases were not identified due to a technical issue in GA scoring in REDcap. Compliance with rehabilitation referrals by the oncology team was 99% (282/285 referrals). Cases not referred to rehabilitation were not eligible due to hospitalization or starting hospice. Of those referred, an additional 38 cases (13.6%) were not eligible for rehabilitation due to the following reasons: receiving home therapy (25.6%), insurance not accepted (23.1%), hospitalized (20.5%), inpatient rehabilitation (12.8%), disease progression or discontinuing treatment (7.7%), recently deceased (5%), receiving hospice care (2.6%) or moved to another state (2.6%). Conversion to rehabilitation was 51.7%. Reasons for non-conversion included not interested/do not need (74.6%), not feeling well from treatment or illness (9.1%), and receiving rehab elsewhere (9.1%). Characteristics regarding the use of rehabilitation services are reported in Table 2. No adverse events were reported due to completing GA or attending rehabilitation.

Table 2. Rehabilitation utilization characteristics, n = 46.

	n, % or Median (IQR)
Service type	
Physical therapy (PT)	39, 84.8%
Occupational therapy (OT)	1, 2.2%
Multidiscipline (PT/OT)	5, 10.9%
Speech	1, 2.2%
Insurance type	
Private	27 (57.4%)
Medicare/Medicaid/Medicare Advantage	19 (41.3%)
Rehabilitation needs [a]	
Falls	27, 21.6%
Mobility	20, 16.0%
Pain	18, 14.4%
Weakness	16, 12.8%
Fatigue	12, 9.6%
Limited ROM	12, 9.6%
ADL limitation	10, 8.0%
Neuropathy	5, 4.0%
Other	3, 2.4%
Lymphedema	2, 1.6%
Length of stay	17.84 (5.96 to 20.71)
Visits attended	12.00 (5.50 to 25.25)
Discharge reason	
Program complete/goals met	15, 32.6%
Patient choice	11, 23.9%
Hospitalized	7, 15.2%
Surgery	3, 6.0%
Hospice	3, 6.0%
Physician discretion due to disease progression	1, 2.0%
Unknown	6, 13%

[a] Identified from International Classification of Diseases (ICD-10) codes applied by the treating therapist; up to four codes applied per case.

3.2. Participant Acceptability

Participant acceptability survey scores are reported in Table 3. The median time to complete the GA was 10 min (IQR: 5 to 10 min). Most respondents agreed the GA was simple to complete (98%), took an appropriate amount of time (95%), was helpful to monitor for treatment side effects (86%), was an added benefit to their care (81%), and that they would recommend it to peers (89%).

Table 3. Patient experience survey items and responses, n = 44.

Question	Average Rating (SD)	% "Agreed"
The monthly evaluation was simple to complete online	4.70 ± 0.63	97.73%
The amount of time it took me to complete the online monthly evaluation was appropriate	4.57 ± 0.97	95.45%
The online monthly evaluation was helpful to monitor for potential side effects of cancer treatment	4.16 ± 1.24	86.36%
I feel the online monthly evaluation helped me to have access to multidisciplinary care when I needed it	3.50 ± 1.72	72.72%
I would recommend the online monthly evaluation to others who are starting a new cancer treatment	4.16 ± 1.31	88.64%
The online monthly evaluation was an added benefit of receiving my care	4.07 ± 1.45	81.82%
I feel that my therapist(s) used my monthly evaluation to individualize my care *	3.79 ± 1.38	87.50%

Likert scale: (0) completely disagree, (5) completely agree. "Agreed" defined as rating ≥3 out of 5. * Answered only by those who attended rehabilitation.

3.3. Rehabilitation Outcomes

Pre/post outcomes (any measure was included, either patient-reported or performance-based) were available for 91.3% of those who attended rehabilitation (n = 42), 31 had patient-reported outcomes, and 37 had performance-based outcomes. Statistically and clinically significant improvement, unadjusted, was observed in each patient-reported outcome (Table 4) and performance-based outcome, except for hand grip strength (Table 5). Improvement in handgrip strength was not significant ($p = 0.183$) and did not reach the MIC of 3.53 lbs. (mean change: +2.52, 11.86 lbs., CI: −8.237 to 3.195).

Table 4. PROMIS® Health-related quality of life outcomes of frail or pre-frail participants before and after rehabilitation.

	Specific Domains Measured	Initial Evaluation Mean, SD	Final Evaluation Mean, SD	Change Mean, SD	Change T-Score	Percent Achieving MIC
Global physical health	Overall health, ability to perform daily activities, fatigue, pain.	39.38, 7.12	43.30, 7.48	+3.92, 6.86	3.18 *	58.10%
Global mental health	Mood, ability to think, feelings of anxiety or depression, satisfaction with social activities and relationships.	45.76, 7.98	49.03, 7.17	+3.27, 7.89	2.31 *	54.80%
Physical function	Ability to do household chores, walk up/down stairs, walk at least 15 min, and run errands.	37.73, 8.35	40.79, 8.00	+3.06, 7.12	2.40 *	54.80%
Ability to participate in social roles and activities	Ability to do leisure and family activities, work, and activities with friends.	45.18, 8.11	47.49, 7.47	+2.31, 6.82	1.89 *	41.90%

n = 31. * Significant improvement in T-score from initial to final evaluation, one-sided $p < 0.05$. MIC = Minimal important change indicating clinically significant improvement (2 points) [33].

Table 5. Performance-based outcomes of frail or pre-frail participants before and after rehabilitation.

	n	Initial Evaluation Mean, SD	Discharge Mean, SD	Change Mean, SD	Change T-Score	MIC Value	Percent Achieving MIC
Mobility							
Timed Up-and-Go (seconds)	27	15.16, 6.23	12.81, 5.31	−2.34, 4.15	2.93 *	−1 s [35]	48.1%
Aerobic capacity							
Six-minute walk test (feet)	9	641.67, 375.77	863.44, 347.61	+221.78, 235.5	2.83 *	+65.6 feet [35]	88.9%
Two-minute step test (step repetitions)	5	57.00, 20.25	67.80, 19.72	+10.80, 5.45	4.43 *	+9.61 [38]	100%
Strength							
Handgrip strength (lbs.)	19	45.00, 12.31	47.52, 13.64	+2.52, 11.86^	0.93	+3.53 lbs [34]	47.4%
Five times sit-to-stand (seconds)	19	18.26, 5.67	15.44, 6.33	−2.82, 3.3	3.72 *	−2.3 s [35]	63.2%
30 s sit-to-stand (repetitions)	12	10.00, 4.49	12.50, 4.93	2.50, 4.81	1.80 *	+2 repetitions [36]	58.3%

* Significant improvement from initial to final evaluation, one-sided $p < 0.05$.

4. Discussion

Pragmatic feasibility studies are essential to test GA-guided care models recommended by the ASCO guidelines and understand how to implement them successfully. In our study, we found a non-age-restricted GA-guided rehabilitation care model was feasible and acceptable during systemic treatment in a community oncology setting with a recruitment rate of 48%, high retention rates among enrolled participants, and 99% referral compliance by the oncology team. Those who attended rehabilitation improved significantly in patient-reported and performance-based outcomes previously associated with increased chemotherapy toxicity, hospitalization, and mortality [9,14,15]. Our study adds to the growing body of literature on the integration of GA into oncology practice by testing implementation in a community oncology practice, and by focusing on integrating rehabilitation intervention. Furthermore, by not restricting participation based on age, we provide additional evidence that younger adults may also benefit from this GA-guided pathway.

GA-guided management interventions have been associated with improved chemotherapy completion [39,40], fewer grade three to five toxicities [41,42], improved patient satisfaction with patient–provider communication [43], and lower risk of short-term mortality [44]. However, connecting patients to rehabilitation continues to be a challenge [45–47]. Barriers have been well documented, including resource constraints, knowledge of services (when/who to refer), perceived value of services, and organizational challenges, including referring outside of a healthcare system and maintaining connection/communication with outside providers [48,49]. The GA-based EMR-integrated rehabilitation referral pathway used in this study may be a solution to previously described barriers by creating a bridge between the oncology team and cancer-specialized rehabilitation clinicians.

Building the bridge between oncology and supportive care in the real world is challenging. Our findings demonstrate the importance of the partnership between non-co located community oncology and rehabilitation services, and the potential value-add of the successful partnership between these teams in a patient's cancer journey [50]. In addition, by reporting implementation strategies and how we used them to create an iterative learning process, we hope that the findings of this study will be helpful in informing future efforts to implement similar models of care. The partnership between the oncology and rehabilitation teams in this study was integral to success. In preparation for the study, members of the oncology and rehabilitation team worked together to design the EMR-integrated referral pathway, educational materials for patients, and reminder systems for clinicians. During the study, the rehabilitation study and oncology advanced practice provider teams communicated daily via email regarding triaged patients. The clinical rehabilitation team communicated as needed with the oncology team regarding patients' progress or needs. The ability of the therapists and the oncology providers to communicate often, we believe, was key to helping patients feel supported and for patients to view their therapist as an extension of the oncology team.

This study also provides pragmatic evidence to understand the value of rehabilitation services during systemic treatment. Although previous randomized studies including rehabilitation and exercise interventions have shown enhanced outcomes during systemic treatment [50,51], less than 20% of patients access these services in the real world [48,49]. Due to low use, there is limited data available to truly understand the value-add of integrating these services into routine oncology care as recommended by practice guidelines and standards [52–56]. At baseline, participants in this study reported significant needs, one standard deviation below the norm, in terms of global physical health and physical function. This is significant due to the range of ages and types of cancer in the sample, and further demonstrates the critical need for rehabilitation during treatment. Upon discharge from rehabilitation services, patients achieved significant improvements in patient-reported outcomes of HRQOL and physical performance-based outcomes previously associated with the ability to tolerate systemic treatment [14], unplanned hospitalization [14,15], chemotherapy-induced peripheral neuropathy severity [16], and even mortality [13,14]. Interestingly, these improvements were observed despite 30% of participants being discharged from rehabilitation to hospitalization, hospice, or disease progression. Although underpowered and lacking a non-rehabilitation comparison group, when considered against the findings of previous randomized studies and longitudinal studies showing declines during treatment [57–59], the findings of this study provide preliminary evidence that clinically significant improvements may occur for patients who are frail/pre-frail and attending rehabilitation during systemic treatment. Interestingly, seven cases who participated in this study but were not identified as frail or pre-frail in the GA also attended rehabilitation during the 12-month follow-up period, suggesting that those considered "robust" may also have needs for and interest in receiving rehabilitation services.

Limitations and Future Directions

While our study provides valuable insights into the feasibility and potential impact of a GA-guided rehabilitation pathway in community oncology practice, several limitations warrant consideration. Firstly, our recruitment rate of 48% may introduce selection bias, potentially influencing the generalizability of our findings. Future studies could enhance the recruitment rate by administering the GA directly from the oncology EMR or patient portal, as compared to REDcap used in this study. Secondly, although conversion to rehabilitation in this study (51.7%) was higher than in previous reports [45,47], continuing to build trusting partnerships between oncology and rehabilitation through clear communication of the value-add is needed to enhance conversion and adherence. Thirdly, this study focused solely on cancer rehabilitation needs and did not directly address other significant impairments and potential needs of patients undergoing systemic treatments, including but not limited to exercise physiology, nutrition, social support, spiritual/emotional care, financial toxicity resources, and neuropsychology, among others. We strongly recommend that future work include the expansion of the team and services beyond cancer rehabilitation as defined in this study. Finally, although improvement in rehabilitation outcomes was observed in this study, this is a small, single group study designed to evaluate feasibility. Therefore, risk for confounding and selection bias are possible in the pre/post analysis, causality cannot be determined, and generalizability may be limited. Larger adequately powered studies including a comparison or control group are needed to better understand the effects of rehabilitation for frail populations receiving cancer treatment. In the current study, the sample size was too small to account for covariates including patient age in the analysis, which has been associated with rehabilitation effects in other studies. Notably, there were insignificant differences in age between those who did (M = 62.18) and did not receive rehabilitation (M = 64.06, $p = 0.480$). Future studies should also investigate the direct effects of attending rehabilitation on additional outcomes key to healthcare quality, including unplanned hospitalization, the ability to tolerate treatment, costs, and mortality. In addition, this study informed next steps in clinical care, including creating a "prehabilitation" referral pathway for patients before chemotherapy, similar to how a prehab program would be designed before surgery, to prevent severe declines in function and potential for late- and long-lasting impairments.

5. Conclusions

The integration of rehabilitation services into GA-guided care models may be a practical solution to optimize patient experience and quality of life by addressing functional needs. Our study adds to the growing evidence supporting the feasibility and acceptability of integrating rehabilitation services into GA-guided clinical pathways for individuals with cancer. Future research should continue to refine implementation strategies, assess long-term outcomes, and explore the generalizability of GA-guided care models in diverse patient populations and settings. By integrating geriatric-assessment-guided rehabilitation pathways into clinical practice, oncology clinicians can optimize outcomes and improve the quality of life for individuals with cancer across the lifespan.

Supplementary Materials: The following supporting information can be downloaded at: https://www.mdpi.com/article/10.3390/cancers17193274/s1, Supplement S1: Cancer and Aging Resiliency Evaluation (CARE), Supplement S2: Implementation strategies used to implement a GA-guided rehabilitation referral pathway.

Author Contributions: M.P., T.D.K., and K.C.W. conceptualized the study. M.H. and K.C.W. managed study enrollment and data collection. D.M. and K.H. delivered rehabilitation care. A.M.N. led education of the rehabilitation therapists. A.L. and S.M. supported operations and workflows. A.H. managed the rehabilitation program. J.B. supported data extraction and management. K.C.W. led data extraction, analysis, and initial manuscript preparation with support from M.P., S.G., and G.R.W. All authors have read and agreed to the published version of the manuscript.

Funding: Author Giri reports research funding from Janssen and Sanofi and consulting fees from Janssen, Sanofi; Speakers Bureau: Sanofi. Author Williams reports Speakers Bureau for Takeda.

Institutional Review Board Statement: The study was conducted in accordance with the Declaration of Helsinki and approved by the Kessler Institutional Review Board for the Protection of Human Subjects (IRB #: E-1132-20, 7/13/21) for studies involving humans.

Informed Consent Statement: Informed consent was obtained from all subjects involved in the study, and to publish this paper.

Data Availability Statement: Data and materials are available upon request from the corresponding author.

Acknowledgments: Adults with cancer who participated in therapy and Select Medical leadership and therapists in the following divisions/markets: Kessler Rehabilitation and NovaCare Rehabilitation centers. Oncology providers and administrative staff at Astera Cancer who assisted with the trial, including Ellen Ronnen, Rachel Carroll, and Lauren Kiley.

Conflicts of Interest: Authors Mackenzi Pergolotti, Kelley C. Wood, Tiffany D. Kendig, Deanna Meehan, Katie Hutzayluk, Jessica Bertram, Alaina M. Newell, Ashley Lightner, Stacye Mayo, and Alina Hedaya receive salaries from Select Medical. Mary Hidde was receiving wages from Select Medical at the time of the study. M. Hidde is a current employee of Medpace, Inc. Grant R. Williams is the president of the International Society of Geriatric Oncology (SIOG). The remaining authors have no relevant financial or non-financial interests to disclose. The content is solely the responsibility of the authors and does not necessarily represent the official views of Select Medical.

References

1. Goede, V. Frailty and cancer: Current perspectives on assessment and monitoring. *Clin. Interv. Aging* **2023**, *18*, 505–521. [CrossRef]
2. Williams, G.R.; Deal, A.M.; Sanoff, H.K.; Nyrop, K.A.; Guerard, E.J.; Pergolotti, M.; Shachar, S.S.; Reeve, B.B.; Bensen, J.T.; Choi, S.K.; et al. Frailty and health-related quality of life in older women with breast cancer. *Support. Care Cancer* **2019**, *27*, 2693–2698. [CrossRef] [PubMed]
3. Han, C.J.; Rosko, A.E.; Spakowicz, D.J.; Hammer, M.J.; Von Ah, D. Associations of frailty with symptoms, and HRQOL in older cancer survivors after cancer treatments: A systematic review and meta-analyses. *Qual. Life Res.* **2024**, *33*, 583–598. [CrossRef]
4. Mozessohn, L.; Li, Q.; Liu, N.; Leber, B.; Khalaf, D.; Sabloff, M.; Christou, G.; Yee, K.; Chodirker, L.; Parmentier, A.; et al. Impact of Frailty on Health Care Resource Utilization and Costs of Care in Myelodysplastic Syndromes. *JCO Oncol. Pract.* **2023**, *19*, e559–e569. [CrossRef]
5. Min, G.J.; Cho, B.S.; Park, S.-S.; Park, S.; Jeon, Y.-W.; Shin, S.H.; Yahng, S.A.; Yoon, J.H.; Lee, S.E.; Eom, K.S.; et al. Physical and Psychological Impairments as Practical Frailty Markers in Elderly AML Fit for Intensive Chemotherapy; Interim Data of a Prospective Cohort Study. *Blood* **2019**, *134*, 3831. [CrossRef]

6. Dale, W.; Klepin, H.D.; Williams, G.R.; Alibhai, S.M.H.; Bergerot, C.; Brintzenhofeszoc, K.; Hopkins, J.O.; Jhawer, M.P.; Katheria, V.; Loh, K.P.; et al. Practical Assessment and Management of Vulnerabilities in Older Patients Receiving Systemic Cancer Therapy: ASCO Guideline Update. *J. Clin. Oncol.* **2023**, *41*, 4293–4312. [CrossRef]
7. Williams, G.R.; Deal, A.M.; Jolly, T.A.; Alston, S.M.; Gordon, B.B.E.; Olajide, O.A.; Taylor, W.C.; Messino, M.J.; Muss, H.B. Feasibility of geriatric assessment in community oncology clinics. *J. Geriatr. Oncol.* **2014**, *5*, 245–251. [CrossRef]
8. Williams, G.R.; Weaver, K.E.; Lesser, G.J.; Dressler, E.; Winkfield, K.M.; Neuman, H.B.; Kazak, A.E.; Carlos, R.; Gansauer, L.J.; Kamen, C.S.; et al. Capacity to provide geriatric specialty care for older adults in community oncology practices. *Oncologist* **2020**, *25*, 1032–1038. [CrossRef]
9. Giri, S.; Mir, N.; Al-Obaidi, M.; Clark, D.; Kenzik, K.M.; McDonald, A.; Young-Smith, C.; Paluri, R.; Nandagopal, L.; Gbolahan, O.; et al. Use of Single-Item Self-Rated Health Measure to Identify Frailty and Geriatric Assessment-Identified Impairments Among Older Adults with Cancer. *Oncologist* **2022**, *27*, e45–e52. [CrossRef]
10. Giri, S.; Al-Obaidi, M.; Weaver, A.; Kenzik, K.M.; McDonald, A.; Clark, D.; Young-Smith, C.; Paluri, R.; Nandagopal, L.; Gbolahan, O.; et al. Association Between Chronologic Age and Geriatric Assessment-Identified Impairments: Findings from the CARE Registry. *J. Natl. Compr. Cancer Netw.* **2021**, *19*, 922–927. [CrossRef] [PubMed]
11. Segaux, L.; Broussier, A.; Oubaya, N.; Leissing-Desprez, C.; Laurent, M.; Naga, H.; Fromentin, I.; David, J.P.; Bastuji-Garin, S. Several frailty parameters highly prevalent in middle age (50–65) are independent predictors of adverse events. *Sci. Rep.* **2021**, *11*, 8774. [CrossRef]
12. Park, J.; Look, K.A. Health Care Expenditure Burden of Cancer Care in the United States. *Inquiry* **2019**, *56*, 0046958019880696. [CrossRef]
13. Al Obaidi, M.; Giri, S.; Mir, N.; Kenzik, K.; McDonald, A.M.; Smith, C.Y.; Gbolahan, O.B.; Paluri, R.K.; Bhatia, S.; Williams, G.R. Use of self-rated health to identify frailty and predict mortality in older adults with cancer. Results from the care study. *J. Clin. Oncol.* **2020**, *38*, 12046. [CrossRef]
14. van Abbema, D.L.; van den Akker, M.; Janssen-Heijnen, M.L.; van den Berkmortel, F.; Hoeben, A.; de Vos-Geelen, J.; Buntinx, F.; Kleijnen, J.; Tjan-Heijnen, V.C.G. Patient- and tumor-related predictors of chemotherapy intolerance in older patients with cancer: A systematic review. *J. Geriatr. Oncol.* **2019**, *10*, 31–41. [CrossRef]
15. Sikorskii, A.; Tam, S.; Given, B.; Given, C.W.; Adjei Boakye, E.; Zatirka, T.; Nair, M.; Su, W.-T.K.; Jogunoori, S.; Watson, P.; et al. Thresholds in PROMIS scores anchored to subsequent unscheduled health service use among people diagnosed with cancer. *JCO Oncol. Pract.* **2024**, *20*, 1391–1400. [CrossRef]
16. Lin, K.-Y.; Shun, S.-C.; Lai, Y.-H.; Liang, J.-T.; Tsauo, J.-Y. Comparison of the Effects of a Supervised Exercise Program and Usual Care in Patients with Colorectal Cancer Undergoing Chemotherapy. *Cancer Nurs.* **2014**, *37*, E21–E29. [CrossRef] [PubMed]
17. Moullin, J.C.; Dickson, K.S.; Stadnick, N.A.; Rabin, B.; Aarons, G.A. Systematic review of the Exploration, Preparation, Implementation, Sustainment (EPIS) framework. *Implement. Sci.* **2019**, *14*, 1. [CrossRef]
18. Eldridge, S.M.; Chan, C.L.; Campbell, M.J.; Rabin, B.; Aarons, G.A. CONSORT 2010 statement: Extension to randomised pilot and feasibility trials. *BMJ* **2016**, *355*, i5239. [CrossRef]
19. Hoffmann, T.C.; Glasziou, P.P.; Boutron, I.; Rabin, B.; Aarons, G.A. Better reporting of interventions: Template for intervention description and replication (TIDieR) checklist and guide. *BMJ* **2014**, *348*, g1687. [CrossRef] [PubMed]
20. Harris, P.A.; Taylor, R.; Thielke, R.; Payne, J.; Gonzalez, N.; Conde, J.G. Research electronic data capture (REDCap)—A metadata-driven methodology and workflow process for providing translational research informatics support. *J. Biomed. Inform.* **2009**, *42*, 377–381. [CrossRef] [PubMed]
21. Harris, P.A.; Taylor, R.; Minor, B.L.; Elliott, V.; Fernandez, M.; O'Neal, L.; McLeod, L.; Delacqua, G.; Delacqua, F.; Kirby, J.; et al. The REDCap consortium: Building an international community of software partners. *J. Biomed. Inform.* **2019**, *95*, 103208. [CrossRef]
22. Williams, G.R.; Kenzik, K.M.; Parman, M.; Al-Obaidi, M.; Francisco, L.; Rocque, G.B.; McDonald, A.; Paluri, R.; Navari, R.M.; Nandagopal, L.; et al. Integrating geriatric assessment into routine gastrointestinal (GI) consultation: The Cancer and Aging Resilience Evaluation (CARE). *J. Geriatr. Oncol.* **2019**, *11*, 270–273. [CrossRef]
23. Pergolotti, M.; Wood, K.C.; Hidde, M.; Tendig, T.D.; Ronnen, E.A.; Giri, S.; Williams, G.R. Geriatric assessment-identified impairments and frailty in adults with cancer younger than 65: An opportunity to optimize oncology care. *J. Geriatr. Oncol.* **2024**, *15*, 101751. [CrossRef]
24. Guerard, E.J.; Deal, A.M.; Williams, G.R.; Jolly, T.A.; Wood, W.A.; Muss, H.B. Construction of a frailty index for older adults with cancer using a geriatric assessment. *J. Clin. Oncol.* **2015**, *33*, 9535. [CrossRef]
25. Giri, S.; Al-Obaidi, M.; Harmon, C.; Clark, D.; Ubersax, C.; Dai, C.; Young-Smith, C.; Outlaw, D.; Gbolahan, O.; Khushman, M.; et al. Patient-reported geriatric assessment-based frailty index among older adults with gastrointestinal malignancies. *J. Am. Geriatr. Soc.* **2023**, *71*, 136–144. [CrossRef]
26. Harris, L.K.; Skou, S.T.; Juhl, C.B.; Jäger, M.; Bricca, A. Recruitment and retention rates in randomised controlled trials of exercise therapy in people with multimorbidity: A systematic review and meta-analysis. *Trials* **2021**, *22*, 396. [CrossRef]

27. Reynolds, S.A.; O'Connor, L.; McGee, A.; Kilcoyne, A.Q.; Connolly, A.; Mockler, D.; Guinan, E.; O'Neill, L. Recruitment rates and strategies in exercise trials in cancer survivorship: A systematic review. *J. Cancer Surviv.* **2024**, *18*, 1233–1242. [CrossRef]
28. Cella, D.; Riley, W.; Stone, A.; Rothrock, N.; Reeve, B.; Yount, S.; Amtmann, D.; Bode, R.; Buysse, D.; Choi, S.; et al. The Patient-Reported Outcomes Measurement Information System (PROMIS) developed and tested its first wave of adult self-reported health outcome item banks: 2005–2008. *J. Clin. Epidemiol.* **2010**, *63*, 1179–1194. [CrossRef]
29. Pergolotti, M.; Wood, K.; Kendig, T. Pragmatic test-retest and concurrent reliability of three PROMIS® measures in breast cancer rehabilitation. *Arch. Phys. Med. Rehabil.* **2024**, *105*, e63. [CrossRef]
30. Pergolotti, M.; Wood, K.C.; Kendig, T.D.; Mayo, S. Impact of Real-World Outpatient Cancer Rehabilitation Services on Health-Related Quality of Life of Cancer Survivors across 12 Diagnosis Types in the United States. *Cancers* **2024**, *16*, 1927. [CrossRef] [PubMed]
31. Tran, T.X.M.; Park, J.; Lee, J.; Jung, Y.-S.; Chang, Y.; Cho, H. Utility of the Patient-Reported Outcomes Measurement Information System (PROMIS) to measure primary health outcomes in cancer patients: A systematic review. *Support. Care Cancer* **2020**, *29*, 1723–1739. [CrossRef]
32. Jensen, R.E.; Moinpour, C.M.; Potosky, A.L.; Lobo, T.; Hahn, E.A.; Hays, R.D.; Cella, D.; Smith, A.W.; Wu, X.C.; Keegan, T.H.M.; et al. Responsiveness of 8 PROMIS® Measures in a Large, Community-Based Cancer Study Cohort. *Cancer* **2017**, *123*, 327. [CrossRef]
33. Terwee, C.B.; Peipert, J.D.; Chapman, R.; Lai, J.S.; Terluin, B.; Cella, D.; Griffith, P.; Mokkink, L.B. Minimal important change (MIC): A conceptual clarification and systematic review of MIC estimates of PROMIS measures. *Qual. Life Res.* **2021**, *30*, 2729–2754. [CrossRef]
34. Labott, B.K.; Bucht, H.; Morat, M.; Morat, T.; Donath, L. Effects of Exercise Training on Handgrip Strength in Older Adults: A Meta-Analytical Review. *Gerontology* **2019**, *65*, 686–698. [CrossRef]
35. Fisher, M.I.; Lee, J.; Davies, C.C.; Geyer, H.; Colon, G.; Pfalzer, L. Oncology section EDGE task force on breast cancer outcomes: A systematic review of outcome measures for functional mobility. *Rehabil. Oncol.* **2015**, *33*, 19–31. [CrossRef]
36. Zanini, A.; Crisafulli, E.; D'Andria, M.; Gregorini, C.; Cherubino, F.; Zampogna, E.; Azzola, A.; Spanevello, A.; Chetta, A. Minimal clinically important difference in 30 second sit-to-stand test after pulmonary rehabilitation in patients with COPD. *Eur. Respir. J.* **2018**, *52*, OA5199. [CrossRef]
37. Abbade, L.P.F.; Abbade, J.F.; Thabane, L. Introducing the CONSORT extension to pilot trials: Enhancing the design, conduct and reporting of pilot or feasibility trials. *J. Venom. Anim. Toxins Incl. Trop. Dis.* **2018**, *24*, 4. [CrossRef] [PubMed]
38. Nogueira, M.A.; Almeida, T.D.N.; Andrade, G.S.; Ribeiro, A.S.; Rêgo, A.S.; da Silva Dias, R.; Ferreira, P.R.; Penha, L.R.L.N.; de Oliveira Pires, F.; Dibai-Filho, A.V.; et al. Reliability and Accuracy of 2-Minute Step Test in Active and Sedentary Lean Adults. *J. Manip. Physiol. Ther.* **2021**, *44*, 120–127. [CrossRef]
39. Lund, C.M.; Vistisen, K.K.; Olsen, A.P.; Bardal, P.; Schultz, M.; Dolin, T.G.; Rønholt, F.; Johansen, J.S.; Nielsen, D.L. The effect of geriatric intervention in frail older patients receiving chemotherapy for colorectal cancer: A randomised trial (GERICO). *Clin. Study Br. J. Cancer* **2021**, *124*, 1949–1958. [CrossRef]
40. Ørum, M.; Eriksen, S.V.; Gregersen, M.; Jensen, A.R.; Jensen, K.; Meldgaard, P.; Nordsmark, M.; Damsgaard, E.M. The impact of a tailored follow-up intervention on comprehensive geriatric assessment in older patients with cancer—A randomised controlled trial. *J. Geriatr. Oncol.* **2021**, *12*, 41–48. [CrossRef]
41. Li, D.; Sun, C.L.; Kim, H.; Soto-Perez-De-Celis, E.; Chung, V.; Koczywas, M.; Fakih, M.; Chao, J.; Cabrera Chien, L.; Charles, K.; et al. Geriatric Assessment-Driven Intervention (GAIN) on Chemotherapy-Related Toxic Effects in Older Adults with Cancer: A Randomized Clinical Trial. *JAMA Oncol.* **2021**, *7*, e214158. [CrossRef]
42. Mohile, S.G.; Mohamed, M.R.; Xu, H.; Culakova, E.; Loh, K.P.; Magnuson, A.; Flannery, M.A.; Obrecht, S.; Gilmore, N.; Ramsdale, E.; et al. Evaluation of geriatric assessment and management on the toxic effects of cancer treatment (GAP70+): A cluster-randomised study. *Lancet* **2021**, *398*, 1894–1904. [CrossRef]
43. Mohile, S.G.; Epstein, R.M.; Hurria, A.; Heckler, C.E.; Canin, B.; Culakova, E.; Duberstein, P.; Gilmore, N.; Xu, H.; Plumb, S.; et al. Communication with Older Patients with Cancer Using Geriatric Assessment: A Cluster-Randomized Clinical Trial from the National Cancer Institute Community Oncology Research Program. *JAMA Oncol.* **2020**, *6*, 196. [CrossRef]
44. Ørum, M.; Jensen, K.; Gregersen, M.; Meldgaard, P.; Damsgaard, E.M. Impact of comprehensive geriatric assessment on short-term mortality in older patients with cancer-a follow-up study. *Eur. J. Cancer* **2019**, *116*, 27–34. [CrossRef]
45. Brick, R.; Natori, A.; Moreno, P.I.; Molinares, D.; Koru-Sengul, T.; Penedo, F.J. Predictors of cancer rehabilitation medicine referral and utilization based on the Moving Through Cancer physical activity screening assessment. *Support. Care Cancer* **2023**, *31*, 216. [CrossRef] [PubMed]
46. Pergolotti, M.; Alfano, C.M.; Cernich, A.N.; Yabroff, K.R.; Manning, P.R.; de Moor, J.S.; Hahn, E.E.; Cheville, A.L.; Mohile, S.G. A health services research agenda to fully integrate cancer rehabilitation into oncology care. *Cancer* **2019**, *125*, 3908–3916. [CrossRef] [PubMed]

47. Pergolotti, M.; Deal, A.M.; Lavery, J.; Reeve, B.B.; Muss, H.B. The prevalence of potentially modifiable functional deficits and the subsequent use of occupational and physical therapy by older adults with cancer. *J. Geriatr. Oncol.* **2015**, *6*, 194–201. [CrossRef]
48. Dale, W.; Williams, G.R.; RMacKenzie, A.; Soto-Perez-de-Celis, E.; Maggiore, R.J.; Merrill, J.K.; Katta, S.; Smith, K.T.; Klepin, H.D. How Is Geriatric Assessment Used in Clinical Practice for Older Adults with Cancer? A Survey of Cancer Providers by the American Society of Clinical Oncology. *JCO Oncol. Pract.* **2021**, *17*, 336–344. [CrossRef]
49. Sum, G.; Nicholas, S.O.; Nai, Z.L.; Ding, Y.Y.; Tan, W.S. Health outcomes and implementation barriers and facilitators of comprehensive geriatric assessment in community settings: A systematic integrative review. *BMC Geriatr.* **2022**, *22*, 379. [CrossRef] [PubMed]
50. Pergolotti, M.; Deal, A.M.; Williams, G.R.; Bryant, A.L.; McCarthy, L.; Nyrop, K.A.; Covington, K.R.; Reeve, B.B.; Basch, E.; Muss, H.B. A randomized controlled trial of outpatient CAncer REhabilitation for older adults: The CARE Program. *Contemp. Clin. Trials* **2015**, *44*, 89–94. [CrossRef]
51. Penna, G.B.; Otto, D.M.; da Silva, T.C.; Pedroni, A.S.; Macagnan, F.E. Physical rehabilitation for the management of cancer-related fatigue during cytotoxic treatment: A systematic review with meta-analysis. *Support. Care Cancer* **2023**, *31*, 129. [CrossRef]
52. Brick, R.; Lyons, K.D.; Bender, C.; Eilers, R.; Ferguson, R.; Pergolotti, M.; Toto, P.; Skidmore, E.; Leland, N.E. Factors influencing utilization of cancer rehabilitation services among older breast cancer survivors in the USA: A qualitative study. *Support. Care Cancer* **2022**, *30*, 2397–2405. [CrossRef] [PubMed]
53. Stout, N.L.; Santa Mina, D.; Lyons, K.D.; Robb, K.; Silver, J.K. A systematic review of rehabilitation and exercise recommendations in oncology guidelines. *CA Cancer J. Clin.* **2020**, *71*, 149–175. [CrossRef] [PubMed]
54. Ligibel, J.A.; Bohlke, K.; Alfano, C.M. Exercise, Diet, and Weight Management During Cancer Treatment: ASCO Guideline Summary and Q&A. *JCO Oncol. Pract.* **2022**, *18*, OP2200277. [CrossRef]
55. National Accreditation for Breast Centers (NAPBC). *Optimal Resources for Breast Cancer: 2024 Standards*; NAPBC: Chicago, IL, USA, 2024.
56. American College of Surgeons. *Optimal Resources for Cancer Care: 2020 Standards*; American College of Surgeons: Chicago, IL, USA, 2020.
57. Lin, K.Y.; Cheng, H.C.; Yen, C.J.; Hung, C.H.; Haung, Y.T.; Yang, H.L.; Cheng, W.T.; Tsai, K.L. Effects of Exercise in Patients Undergoing Chemotherapy for Head and Neck Cancer: A Pilot Randomized Controlled Trial. *Int. J. Environ. Res. Public Health* **2021**, *18*, 1291. [CrossRef]
58. Cespedes Feliciano, E.M.; Vasan, S.; Luo, J.; Binder, A.M.; Rowan, S.; Chlebowski, T.; Quesenberry, C.; Banack, H.R.; Caan, B.J.; Paskett, E.D.; et al. Long-term Trajectories of Physical Function Decline in Women with and Without Cancer. *JAMA Oncol.* **2023**, *9*, 395–403. [CrossRef] [PubMed]
59. Hurria, A.; Soto-Perez-de-Celis, E.; Allred, J.B.; Cohen, H.J.; Arsenyan, A.; Ballman, K.; Le-Rademacher, J.; Jatoi, A.; Filo, J.; Mandelblatt, J.; et al. Functional Decline and Resilience in Older Women Receiving Adjuvant Chemotherapy for Breast Cancer. *J. Am. Geriatr. Soc.* **2019**, *67*, 920–927. [CrossRef]

cancers

Article

SBRT in the Very Elderly: A Viable Option for Pulmonary Oligometastases?

Samuel M. Vorbach *, Meinhard Nevinny-Stickel, Ute Ganswindt and Thomas Seppi

Department of Radiation Oncology, Medical University of Innsbruck, 6020 Innsbruck, Austria
* Correspondence: samuel.vorbach@i-med.ac.at; Tel.: +43-512-504-23142

Simple Summary: The population of individuals aged $\geq$ 80 years is rapidly increasing, leading to more cancer diagnoses in this group. Stereotactic body radiotherapy (SBRT) is an established treatment for pulmonary oligometastases, but data for the very elderly are limited. We retrospectively analysed 34 patients aged $\geq$ 80 years (median 83) with 46 histologically confirmed pulmonary oligometastases treated with SBRT (median BED10: 112.5 Gy). Median follow-up was 22.6 months. One-, two-, and three-year local control rates were 95.2%, 95.2%, and 90.2%. Median overall survival was 46.6 months; 3-year cancer-specific survival was 70.9%. No grade $\geq$ 3 toxicities occurred; grade 2 pneumonitis and dermatitis were rare (2.9% each) and manageable. No significant predictors for local control or survival were identified. SBRT is safe, effective, and well-tolerated in patients aged $\geq$ 80 years with pulmonary oligometastases, supporting its use as a curative-intent option in this growing demographic.

Abstract: Background/Objectives: The global population of individuals aged $\geq$ 80 years is rapidly growing, leading to an increasing incidence of cancer diagnoses in this age group. While stereotactic body radiotherapy (SBRT) has proven effective in treating pulmonary oligometastases, patients over 80 remain underrepresented in clinical analyses. This study aimed to evaluate clinical outcomes and toxicity of SBRT for pulmonary oligometastases in octogenarians. Methods: This retrospective, single-centre analysis included 34 patients aged $\geq$ 80 years treated with SBRT for histologically confirmed pulmonary oligometastases between 2010 and 2024. Results: A total of 46 pulmonary metastases were treated with curative intent using fractionation schemes of 3 $\times$ 15 Gy, 6 $\times$ 8 Gy, or 10 $\times$ 6 Gy. Median biologically effective dose (BED10) was 112.5 Gy. Follow-up included regular CT imaging and toxicity assessment according to CTCAE. With a median follow-up of 22.6 months, 1-, 2-, and 3-year local control (LC) rates were 95.2%, 95.2%, and 90.2%, respectively. Median overall survival (OS) was 46.6 months, with 1-, 2-, and 3-year OS rates of 78.4%, 71.4%, and 59.5%. Progression-free survival (PFS) at 1, 2, and 3 years was 63.4%, 51.6%, and 47.3%, respectively. No grade $\geq$ 3 toxicities were observed. Grade 2 pneumonitis and dermatitis occurred in 2.9% each and were well managed. Asymptomatic rib fractures were detected in 5.9% of patients. No significant predictors for LC, PFS, or OS were identified in univariate analysis. Conclusions: SBRT for pulmonary oligometastases in patients $\geq$ 80 years is feasible, safe, and effective. High local control, favourable cancer-specific survival, and minimal toxicity support its use as a curative-intent treatment in this growing patient population. These findings contribute important site- and age-specific evidence and support the inclusion of very elderly patients in future prospective SBRT trials.

Keywords: pulmonary oligometastases; stereotactic body radiotherapy; very elderly; radiotherapy

 https://doi.org/10.3390/cancers17152512

1. Introduction

The global population is ageing rapidly, with individuals aged 80 years and over representing an increasingly important demographic group: it is estimated that there will be 265 million people aged 80 years and over by the mid-2030s [1], and the global population aged 80 years and older is expected to triple by 2050 [2]. This demographic shift has profound implications for healthcare systems worldwide, particularly for cancer care, as age remains the most important risk factor for developing cancer [3,4].

The number of cancer patients in the very elderly demographic group is increasing rapidly. In 2022, an estimated 2.6 million new cancer cases across all disease stages (14% of all diagnoses) and 2.1 million cancer deaths (22% of all cancer deaths) occurred in adults aged 80 and older [2]. This proportion is expected to increase dramatically, with estimates suggesting that by 2050, about 6.9 million new cancers will be diagnosed in adults aged 80 years and over, accounting for 20.5% of all cancer cases [5].

Despite the growing burden of cancer in the very elderly patients, this population remains severely underrepresented in the clinical trials that drive treatment guidelines. For example, while people aged 70 and older make up about 42% of the overall cancer population, they represent only about 24% of the participants in clinical trials submitted to the FDA, and less than 10% of patients aged 70 years and older are enrolled in National Cancer Institute trials [6]. Another analysis of 302 randomised clinical trials found that across all oncological diseases, trial participants were significantly younger than the general patient population, with a median age difference of 6.49 years [7]. Even when included, these elderly trial participants tend to be fitter than the average older patient, with fewer comorbidities or impairments [8]. This underrepresentation means that the evidence that guides modern cancer treatment is largely based on younger, healthier populations and may not be fully generalisable to frail older patients. There is a clear need for studies focused on the very elderly to provide the best possible treatment decisions for this growing cohort.

Several recent studies have aimed to better characterise the barriers contributing to the exclusion of older adults from cancer research and treatment. Ludmir et al. [9] analysed 742 oncological randomised controlled trials comprising 449,720 participants and found that 10.1% included an upper age limit, with a median cut-off of 72 years (interquartile range 70–80), thereby explicitly restricting access for older patients. Tang et al. [10] conducted a population-based study of 677 individuals aged $\geq$ 65 years with metastatic lung cancer (median age 84) and found that 53.4% would typically be excluded from trials, most commonly due to poor performance status, cardiac disease, or a history of prior malignancy. Patel et al. [11] conducted a comprehensive analysis of modern phase III oncological randomised controlled trials to evaluate the incidence and factors associated with exclusion criteria related to prior malignancy within the past five years (PMEC-5). PMEC-5 criteria were identified in 41% of trials, occurring more frequently in industry-sponsored studies and those assessing targeted therapies. The presence of PMEC-5 was independently associated with increased age disparities. Their findings suggest that PMEC-5 criteria likely contribute significantly to age-related disparities in cancer trial enrolment.

Beyond trial design, older patients also face disparities in real-world treatment. In a systematic review of 102 observational studies, Bastiaannet and Pilleron [12] found that adults aged $\geq$ 60, particularly those over 80, were significantly less likely to receive standard therapies such as surgery, chemotherapy, and radiotherapy, irrespective of cancer type or care setting. However, when treated, fit older adults experienced outcomes comparable to younger patients, suggesting they can benefit from standard therapies when appropriately assessed. These considerations are equally relevant in the management of metastatic disease in older adults, where the evidence supporting local therapies remains scarce.

The lung is one of the most common sites of metastatic disease in cancer patients. Autopsy studies have shown that up to half of patients who die from extrathoracic malignancies have pulmonary metastases (PMs) [13,14]. Common primary tumours that metastasise to the lung include breast, colorectal, renal, head and neck cancer, and sarcomas [14,15]. Specifically, the diagnosis of oligometastatic disease is becoming more common, largely driven by advances in imaging technologies and more effective systemic therapies that extend the survival of cancer patients [16]. The term 'oligometastatic disease' was first introduced by Hellman and Weichselbaum [17] in 1995, and refers to an intermediate state between localised cancer and advanced disease. It is currently most commonly characterised by the presence of five or fewer metastatic lesions that are amenable to targeted local therapies. The clinical rationale for treating such lesions with local therapies is based on the hypothesis that managing oligometastatic disease can delay progression, prolong survival, and possibly lead to long-term remission in carefully selected patients [18]. Among these approaches, stereotactic body radiotherapy (SBRT), also known as stereotactic ablative body radiotherapy (SABR), has become a widely used, non-invasive treatment option. SBRT achieves excellent local control rates of over 90% for lung metastases and is generally well tolerated, with grade 3 or higher toxicities reported in approximately 5% of patients in several studies [19,20].

The potential for curative treatment in selected patients with oligometastatic disease has been strongly supported by the landmark SABR-COMET trial [21], a randomised, multicentre phase II trial that compared standard palliative treatment with SBRT to all known metastatic sites in patients with a controlled primary tumour and 1–5 metastases. SBRT significantly improved overall survival (OS), with median survival increasing from 28 to 41 months, and a significant proportion of patients remained progression-free at long-term follow-up [22].

However, it is important to recognise that the SABR-COMET trial, like many pivotal oncology trials, included relatively few very elderly patients. The oldest patient enrolled was 75 years old. Therefore, the applicability of these trial findings to patients aged 80 years and older remains somewhat uncertain. In real-world clinical practice, this very elderly population is often discussed in multidisciplinary tumour boards (MDTs) and often deemed ineligible for systemic therapy or pulmonary metastasectomy due to frailty, comorbidities, or poor performance status [23]. In these cases, SBRT may be a uniquely suitable alternative due to its non-invasive nature and limited treatment burden. However, robust data on the outcomes and toxicity of SBRT specifically in octogenarians with pulmonary oligometastases remain limited. Two retrospective studies included patients aged 65 years and older [24] and 70 years and older [25], respectively. While one study has focused exclusively on patients aged 80 years and older [26], all three studies have one common limitation: the inclusion of patients with metastatic lesions to multiple anatomical sites, which limits the site-specific interpretation of toxicity and outcome data for lung SBRT.

The aim of the present study was to report the outcomes and toxicities of SBRT for lung oligometastases in patients aged over 80 years.

2. Materials and Methods

2.1. Study Population

Between January 2010 and January 2024, 34 patients aged 80 years or older with histologically confirmed pulmonary oligometastases were treated with SBRT at the Department of Radiation Oncology, Medical University of Innsbruck, Austria. Oligometastatic disease was defined as the presence of up to five lesions suitable for local treatment, and was classified according to ESTRO and EORTC consensus [27].

All cases were reviewed by an institutional multidisciplinary tumour board. All patients had undergone curative-intent standard-of-care treatment of their primary tumour prior to developing lung metastases. Following the detection of lung metastases, CT-guided or bronchoscopic biopsy was routinely performed for histological verification of lung lesions. Patients were subsequently reassessed by the tumour board based on histological findings and assigned to SBRT. All pulmonary metastases were treated with curative intent.

Data were collected on the type of primary tumour, initial treatment, systemic therapy received before or after SBRT, and the time from diagnosis of the primary tumour to the appearance of pulmonary metastases. Demographic data were also collected before an SBRT course. The Charlson Comorbidity Index [28] was calculated to more precisely assess the burden of comorbidities. A SBRT course was defined as all SBRT treatments given within one month.

The study was approved by the ethics committee of the institutional review board of the Medical University of Innsbruck (EC No. approval: 1343/2024). All procedures conducted in this study involving human participants are in accordance with the ethical standards of the institutional review board, as well as with the Helsinki Declaration (1964) and its later amendments or equivalent ethical standards.

2.2. Techniques of Radiotherapy

Patients were immobilised in the supine position using the Elekta BodyFIX system. A four-dimensional CT scan was performed to assess tumour location and respiratory motion over time. For target volume delineation, the gross tumour volume (GTV) was defined as the radiologically evident disease and contoured, incorporating co-registered imaging when available. An internal target volume (ITV) was defined to account for respiratory motion effects on the GTV. The planning target volume (PTV) was generated by uniformly expanding the ITV by 5 mm in all directions. Organs at risk (such as the lungs, spinal cord, trachea, bronchial tree, oesophagus, chest wall, and blood vessels) were delineated to minimise radiation exposure. Tumours were classified as central [29] or ultra-central [30] as previously described. Dose prescriptions varied according to the location of the lesion, and the proximity of the lesion to critical structures, with the following regimens applied: 60 Gy in 10 fractions, 48 Gy in 6 fractions, or 45 Gy in 3 fractions. The corresponding dose prescription modalities included the 65% isodose, the 80% isodose, or the 100% isodose. Treatment planning was performed using precisePLAN (Elekta AB, Stockholm, Sweden) until 2013, and subsequently with Pinnacle Software (most recent version V14; Philips Medical, Fitchburg, MA, USA) until the end of the study. SBRT plans were generated to maximise target volume coverage while minimising dose to surrounding organs at risk. Coverage ranged from 0.88 to 1.00 (mean 0.98, 95% CI: 0.97 to 0.99). A conformity index, defined as the ratio of the absolute volume enclosed by the prescribed isodose to the absolute volume of the PTV, was allowed up to 1.6, with a median value of 1.39 and a range from 1.12 to 1.60. Patients were treated with three-dimensional conformal radiotherapy (3D-CRT) or VMAT using an Elekta Synergy linear accelerator until 2013, and a Versa HD linear accelerator thereafter (both from Elekta AB, Stockholm, Sweden). Daily cone beam CT scans were used to verify and, if necessary, adjust patient positioning to ensure metastasis coverage within the PTV.

2.3. Follow-Up

After completion of SBRT, follow-up radiological imaging (usually CT scan, PET-CT if necessary) was performed every 3 months for 1.5 years and then every 6 months thereafter. Any equivocal findings were evaluated by the multidisciplinary tumour board and, if necessary, a short-term follow-up including CT scan was initiated. Tumour response was classified according to the Response Evaluation Criteria in Solid Tumours (RECIST) [31], and in the case of metabolic imaging, according to the PET Response Evaluation Criteria in Solid Tumours (PERCIST) [32].

Local control was defined as the absence of progression in the treated lesion and measured as the time from the end of SBRT to either progression or the last imaging follow-up. PFS was defined as the time from the end of SBRT to disease progression, either within or outside the treatment, death from any cause, or the last imaging. For patients with sequential oligometastatic disease who underwent an additional SBRT course, a second PFS was defined as the interval from the end of the second SBRT course to progression. Systemic treatment-free survival was defined as the time from the end of SBRT to initiation of systemic treatment or to death from any cause. OS was measured from the completion of SBRT to death from any cause or the date of the last follow-up. Cancer-specific survival (CSS) was defined as the time from completion of SBRT to death attributable to cancer or the date of the last follow-up. Follow-up time was calculated from the date of completion of SBRT to the date of the last available CT scan. Toxicity was assessed by medical history, physical examination, laboratory tests, and medical imaging and graded according to the Common Terminology Criteria for Adverse Events (CTCAE).

2.4. Statistical Analysis

Descriptive analysis was used to summarise relevant patient and treatment characteristics. LC, PFS, systemic treatment-free survival, CSS, and OS were assessed using the Kaplan–Meier method. Univariate and multivariate analyses of potential prognostic factors for clinical outcomes were performed using the Cox proportional hazards model. Multivariate analysis was performed by using the rule of stepwise backward elimination of non-significant factors. p values < 0.05 were considered to be significant. The linear quadratic model was used to calculate the respective biologically effective doses (BEDs) for all radiotherapy prescription doses, assuming an alpha/beta ratio of 10 (BED10). All statistical analyses were performed using SPSS Statistics (V26, IBM Cooperation, Armonk, NY, USA).

3. Results

3.1. Patient Population

This study included 34 patients with a total of 46 pulmonary oligometastases treated with SBRT. The median follow-up time was 22.6 months (range, 2.6–86.1 months). The median time from diagnosis of pulmonary oligometastases to SBRT was 36 days (range, 8–78 days).

Patient demographics, characteristics of lung metastases, and treatment details are summarised in Table 1. The median age at the start of SBRT was 83 years (range, 80–92 years), and the majority of patients were male (70.6%). Most patients had an ECOG performance score of 0–1 (84.2%) and a Charlson Comorbidity Index of 0–2 (76.3%).

Table 1. Patient, lesion, and treatment characteristics.

Characteristic		**Value or No (%)**
Total no. of patients		34
Total no. of metastases		46
Sex	Male	24 (70.6%)
	Female	10 (29.4%)
Age at start of SBRT	Median	83
	Range	80–92
ECOG performance status at SBRT	0	12 (31.6%)
	1	20 (52.6%)
	2	6 (15.8%)
CCI at SBRT	0–2	29 (76.3%)
	3–5	9 (23.7)
Primary tumour	Colorectal	14 (41.2%)
	Head and neck	4 (11.8%)
	NSCLC	3 (8.8%)
	Gynaecological	3 (8.8%)
	Other	10 (29.4%)
Time between diagnosis of the primary tumour and diagnosis of PM (months)	Median	27.5
	Range	1–245
Systemic therapy prior to SBRT	Yes	7 (19.4%)
	No	29 (80.6%)
Oligometastatic classification at the time of PM diagnosis	Synchronous oligometastatic	6 (15.8%)
	Metachronous oligorecurrence	25 (65.8%)
	Repeat oligorecurrence	7 (18.4%)
SBRT courses per patient	1 course	30 (88.2%)
	2 courses	4 (11.8%)
PMs treated per SBRT course	Total number of patients (PMs)	38 (=46 PMs; 100%)
	Patients with 1 PM per SBRT course	31 (=31 PMs; 67.4%)
	Patients with 2 PMs per SBRT course	6 (=12 PMs; 26.1%)
	Patients with 3 PMs per SBRT course	1 (=3 PMs; 6.5%)
Diameter PM (mm)	Median	13
	Range	6–42
PM Location	Right upper lobe	11 (23.9%)
	Right middle lobe	3 (6.5%)
	Right lower lobe	12 (26.1%)
	Left upper lobe	9 (19.6%)
	Lingula	2 (4.3%)
	Left lower lobe	9 (19.6%)

Table 1. *Cont.*

Characteristic		Value or No (%)
PM Location	Peripheral Central Ultra-central	37 (80.4%) 7 (15.2%) 2 (4.3%)
PTV (cm^3)	Median Range	16.0 4.5–97.8
Single dose prescribed (PTV encompassing, Gy)	Median Range	15 6–15
Total dose prescribed (PTV encompassing, Gy)	Median Range	45 45–60
BED10 at PTV periphery (Gy)	Median Range	112.5 86.4–112.5

SBRT: stereotactic body radiotherapy; ECOG: Eastern Cooperative Oncology Group; CCI: Charlson Comorbidity Index; PM: pulmonary metastasis; PTV: planning target volume; BED: biologically effective dose.

Primary tumours were predominantly colorectal (41.2%), followed by head and neck (11.8%), non-small cell lung cancer (8.8%), gynaecological (8.8%), and various other types (29.4%). The median interval between diagnosis of the primary tumour and diagnosis of lung metastases was 27.5 months (range, 1–245 months). Most patients (80.6%) had received no systemic therapy prior to SBRT. At the time of SBRT, no patients received concomitant systemic therapy.

Of the 46 metastases treated, 31 (67.4%) were present as single metastases at the time of SBRT, while the remaining 15 metastases (32.6%) were treated simultaneously in groups of 2 or 3. Lesions had a median diameter of 13 mm (range, 6–42 mm) with common locations in the right lower lobe (26.1%) and right upper lobe (23.9%). Most metastases were peripheral (80.4%), with few central (15.2%) or ultra-central (4.3%) lesions.

The median PTV was 16.0 cm^3 (range, 4.5–97.8 cm^3). Dose prescriptions included 3×15 Gy (n = 28, 60.9%), 10×6 Gy (n = 5, 10.9%) and 6×8 Gy (n = 13, 28.3%), resulting in a median biologically BED10 at the PTV periphery of 112.5 Gy (range, 86.4–112.5 Gy).

3.2. Outcomes

Among all patients who underwent SBRT, the LC rate at one, two, and three years was 95.2% (95% CI: 82.0 to 98.8%), 95.2% (82.0 to 98.8%), and 90.2% (70.4 to 97.0%), respectively (see Figure 1). On univariate analysis, none of the factors examined—primary tumour type, BED10, or the status of oligometastatic disease—were identified as significant predictors of local control in SBRT-treated pulmonary oligometastases (see Table 2).

Table 2. Univariate analysis of factors related to local control.

Factor	HR (CI 95%)	*p* Value
Primary tumour		
CRC	1 (reference)	
Other	0.52 (0.05–5.94)	0.602
BED10		
<100	1 (reference)	
>100	0.28 (0.03–3.12)	0.302
PTV size in ml		
≤16	1 (reference)	
>16	0.54 (0.05–6.04)	0.620

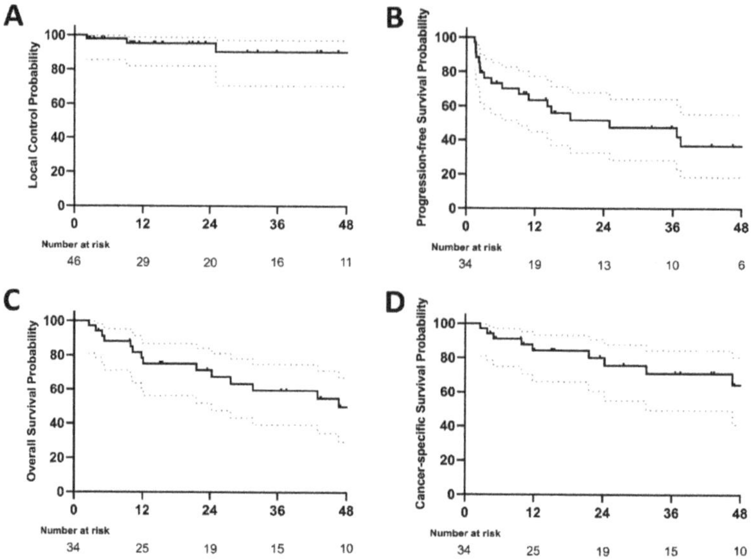

Figure 1. Kaplan–Meier plots showing (**A**) local control (46 treated pulmonary metastases), (**B**) progression-free survival, (**C**) overall survival, and (**D**) cancer-specific survival of 34 patients aged ≥ 80 years (dotted grey lines indicate 95% confidence interval).

One-, two-, and three-year progression-free survival rates were 63.4% (44.5 to 77.4%), 51.6% (32.4 to 67.8%), and 47.3% (28.3 to 64.1%), respectively. Univariate analysis did not identify any of the factors studied as significant predictors of progression-free survival (Table 3). Four patients (11.8%) developed sequential oligometastatic disease following SBRT treatment of their initial pulmonary oligometastases. Each of these patients subsequently received a second course of SBRT, resulting in a second median progression-free survival (PFS) of 8.5 months (range 2.5–54.9 months). A total of seven patients (20.6%) received systemic therapy after SBRT due to further disease progression. The median time to initiation of systemic treatment was 9.4 months (range 2.9–78.1). Systemic treatment-free survival was 62.3% (43.2 to 76.6%) at one year, 62.3% (43.2 to 76.6%) at two years, and 46.9% (30.6 to 67.5%) at three years.

Table 3. Univariate analysis of factors related to PFS and OS.

	Univariate Hazard Ratio for PFS		**Univariate Hazard Ratio for OS**	
Factor	**HR (CI 95%)**	***p* Value**	**HR (CI95%)**	***p* Value**
Sex				
Male	1 (reference)		1 (reference)	
Female	1.27 (0.48–3.35)	0.636	1.38 (0.55–3.46)	0.491
CCI				
0	1 (reference)		1 (reference)	
≥1	0.99 (0.40–2.45)	0.987	0.80 (0.32–1.96)	0.618
Primary tumour				
CRC	1 (reference)		1 (reference)	
Other	1.24 (0.50–3.12)	0.639	0.88 (0.37–2.11)	0.771
Number of PM				
1	1 (reference)		1 (reference)	
>1	1.56 (0.58–4.23)	0.379	1.19 (0.46–3.12)	0.721
Systemic therapy prior to SBRT				
No	1 (reference)		1 (reference)	
Yes	1.90 (0.71–5.07)	0.198	0.77 (0.25–2.31)	0.638

Median OS was 46.6 months. OS at one, two, and three years was 78.4% (59.9 to 89.1%), 71.4% (52.0 to 84.1%), and 59.5% (39.3 to 74.9%), respectively. Univariate analysis did not identify any significant predictors of overall survival (Table 3). A total of 21 patients died during follow-up, of whom 13 had progressive tumour disease. The remaining eight patients died of causes unrelated to their oligometastatic cancer: three died of cardiovascular disease, three of infections, and two of unknown causes but with no evidence of tumour progression before death. Accordingly, cancer-specific survival was 84.3% (66.2% to 93.2%) at one year, 80.1% (60.5% to 90.7%) at two years, and 70.9% (49.3% to 84.6%) at three years.

3.3. Toxicities

SBRT was well tolerated in this clinically fragile cohort, with no grade 3 or higher toxicities observed. All patients completed the treatment without interruption. One patient (2.9%) developed grade 2 pneumonitis, which was effectively treated with corticosteroids; the patient subsequently returned to baseline activity levels and reported no increase in his pre-existing dyspnoea. One patient (2.9%) developed grade 2 radiation dermatitis, which was adequately controlled with topical therapy.

During follow-up, three patients (8.8%) reported a subjective increase in pre-existing dyspnoea, all of whom had underlying chronic obstructive pulmonary disease. Conversely, two patients (5.9%) with baseline dyspnoea experienced symptomatic improvement after SBRT. Asymptomatic rib fractures were detected in two patients (5.9%) on routine follow-up CT imaging, both of which were already consolidated at the time of diagnosis, and neither patient reported pain or required clinical management. No patients reported persistent or severe fatigue during the follow-up.

4. Discussion

This retrospective single-centre analysis offers valuable real-world evidence on the role of stereotactic body radiotherapy in a highly specific and understudied population: patients aged 80 years and older with histologically confirmed pulmonary oligometastases. Our findings demonstrate excellent 3-year local control (90.2%), favourable cancer-specific survival (70.9%), and a remarkably low toxicity profile, with no observed grade ≥ 2 adverse events. These results provide strong support for the safety, efficacy, and feasibility of SBRT in a very elderly cohort traditionally underrepresented in clinical trials.

Our outcomes align with and extend previous research across different studies. In evidence, Scorsetti et al. [25] reported 1- and 2-year LC rates of 86.8% and 76.3% in elderly patients with mixed metastatic sites (median age 79), alongside a 2-year OS of 72.0% and minimal toxicity. Compared to our study, which focuses exclusively on lung metastases and includes an older cohort (median age 83), we observed similarly favourable survival and an even more favourable safety profile. This difference may be partially attributable to the anatomical focus and consistently high BED10 values in our protocol (median 112.5 Gy).

The report of Cuccia et al. [26] represents one of the few studies to exclusively examine SBRT in octogenarians; however, only 30% of their patients have the lung as the treatment site. With 61 patients aged ≥ 80, they reported LC rates of 98.8% and 88.2% at 1 and 2 years and no grade ≥ 2 toxicity. Our results echo this efficacy and tolerability, although with slightly lower 1-year LC (95.2%) but longer median OS (46.6 months vs. 20 months). Our exclusive focus on pulmonary lesions and uniform multidisciplinary assessment may have contributed to more durable outcomes.

Lancia et al. [24] examined SBRT in elderly patients with isolated metastases (median age 75) and highlighted the feasibility of short-course "blitzkrieg" regimens, showing 2- and 3-year LC of 87% with manageable toxicity. Our study confirms that even older cohorts can benefit from these stereotactic strategies.

Landmark studies such as SABR-COMET [22] have established SBRT as an effective strategy in selected oligometastatic patients, but have largely excluded those aged ≥ 80. In contrast, our work bridges this gap by offering site-specific, age-specific data, complementing broader trials while addressing their limitations in geriatric representation. On the other hand, our data is supported by the SABR-COMET trial, also demonstrating that a substantial number of patients can actually be treated curatively with SBRT, because they show progression-freedom still after years post-SBRT of the lung.

Together, these comparisons highlight several important topics. First, across all known studies, chronological age alone does not preclude patients from benefiting from ablative local therapy since there is growing evidence of prolonged PFS and OS at moderate toxicity risk. Second, the toxicity profile of SBRT remains favourable even in the oldest-old, supporting its consideration over more invasive or systemic options. Third, while data from mixed anatomical sites are informative, our study's focus on pulmonary lesions enables a clearer interpretation of lung-specific side effects—key for clinical decision-making in thoracic oncology.

Importantly, our study also adds nuance to the discussion around treatment sequencing. We observed that 20.6% of patients eventually required systemic therapy, but with a median delay of 9.4 months. This underlines the potential of SBRT to defer systemic treatment, preserving quality of life and limiting toxicity—an aspect of particular relevance in elderly care.

Nonetheless, limitations remain. The retrospective nature and small sample size introduce possible selection biases, and our findings, while compelling, would benefit from validation in prospective trials incorporating geriatric assessment tools and quality-of-life metrics. In addition, the median follow-up in our cohort may be insufficient to fully capture all late toxicities. However, given the advanced age and limited life expectancy of this patient cohort, long-term follow-up is inherently constrained.

5. Conclusions

Our study demonstrates that SBRT is a safe, effective, and durable treatment option for pulmonary oligometastases in patients aged ≥ 80 years. SBRT offers a curative-intent modality in a population often considered ineligible for systemic therapy. These findings, placed alongside a growing body of literature, strongly advocate for the inclusion of octogenarians in future SBRT trials and for a paradigm shift toward individualised local therapies in geriatric oncology.

Author Contributions: Conceptualisation, S.M.V. and T.S.; methodology, S.M.V., U.G. and T.S.; validation, S.M.V.; formal analysis, S.M.V.; investigation, S.M.V.; data curation, S.M.V. and M.N.-S.; writing—original draft preparation, S.M.V. and T.S.; writing—review and editing, S.M.V., M.N.-S., U.G. and T.S.; visualisation, S.M.V.; supervision, U.G. and T.S. All authors have read and agreed to the published version of the manuscript.

Funding: This research received no external funding.

Institutional Review Board Statement: The study was conducted in accordance with the Declaration of Helsinki and was approved by the Ethics Committee of the Medical University of Innsbruck (1343/2024) on 6 December 2024.

Informed Consent Statement: Patient consent was waived due to the retrospective study design.

Data Availability Statement: The data presented in this study are available upon reasonable request from the corresponding author.

Conflicts of Interest: The authors declare no conflicts of interest.

References

1. Vollset, S.E.; Goren, E.; Yuan, C.-W.; Cao, J.; Smith, A.E.; Hsiao, T.; Bisignano, C.; Azhar, G.S.; Castro, E.; Chalek, J.; et al. Fertility, mortality, migration, and population scenarios for 195 countries and territories from 2017 to 2100: A forecasting analysis for the global burden of disease study. *Lancet* **2020**, *396*, 1285–1306. [CrossRef]
2. Shah, R.; Battisti, N.M.L.; Brain, E.; Gnangnon, F.H.; Kanesvaran, R.; Mohile, S.; Noronha, V.; Puts, M.; Soto-Perez-De-Celis, E.; Pilleron, S. Updated cancer burden in oldest old: A population-based study using 2022 Globocan estimates. *Cancer Epidemiol.* **2025**, *95*, 102716. [CrossRef]
3. Soerjomataram, I.; Bray, F. Planning for tomorrow: Global cancer incidence and the role of prevention 2020–2070. *Nat. Rev. Clin. Oncol.* **2021**, *18*, 663–672. [CrossRef]
4. Laconi, E.; Marongiu, F.; DeGregori, J. Cancer as a disease of old age: Changing mutational and microenvironmental landscapes. *Br. J. Cancer* **2020**, *122*, 943–952. [CrossRef]
5. Pilleron, S.; Soto-Perez-de-Celis, E.; Vignat, J.; Ferlay, J.; Soerjomataram, I.; Bray, F.; Sarfati, D. Estimated global cancer incidence in the oldest adults in 2018 and projections to 2050. *Int. J. Cancer* **2021**, *148*, 601–608. [CrossRef]
6. Sedrak, M.S.; Freedman, R.A.; Cohen, H.J.; Muss, H.B.; Jatoi, A.; Klepin, H.D.; Wildes, T.M.; Le-Rademacher, J.G.; Kimmick, G.G.; Tew, W.P.; et al. Older adult participation in cancer clinical trials: A systematic review of barriers and interventions. *CA A Cancer J. Clin.* **2021**, *71*, 78–92. [CrossRef] [PubMed]
7. Ludmir, E.B.; Mainwaring, W.; Lin, T.A.; Miller, A.B.; Jethanandani, A.; Espinoza, A.F.; Mandel, J.J.; Lin, S.H.; Smith, B.D.; Smith, G.L.; et al. Factors associated with age disparities among cancer clinical trial participants. *JAMA Oncol.* **2019**, *5*, 1769–1773. [CrossRef] [PubMed]
8. Sedrak, M.S.; Mohile, S.G.; Sun, V.; Sun, C.-L.; Chen, B.T.; Li, D.; Wong, A.R.; George, K.; Padam, S.; Liu, J.; et al. Barriers to clinical trial enrollment of older adults with cancer: A qualitative study of the perceptions of community and academic oncologists. *J. Geriatr. Oncol.* **2020**, *11*, 327–334. [CrossRef] [PubMed]
9. Ludmir, E.B.; Subbiah, I.M.; Mainwaring, W.; Miller, A.B.; Lin, T.A.; Jethanandani, A.; Espinoza, A.F.; Mandel, J.J.; Fang, P.; Smith, B.D.; et al. Decreasing incidence of upper age restriction enrollment criteria among cancer clinical trials. *J. Geriatr. Oncol.* **2020**, *11*, 451–454. [CrossRef] [PubMed]
10. Tang, M.; Pearson, S.-A.; Schaffer, A.L.; Lewis, C.R.; John, T.; Simes, R.J.; Lee, C.K. Are clinical trial eligibility criteria representative of older patients with lung cancer? A population-based data linkage study. *J. Geriatr. Oncol.* **2021**, *12*, 930–936. [CrossRef]
11. Patel, R.R.; Parisi, R.; Verma, V.; Kouzy, R.; Jaoude, J.A.; Lin, T.A.; Fuller, C.D.; VanderWalde, N.A.; Jagsi, R.; Smith, B.D.; et al. Association between prior malignancy exclusion criteria and age disparities in cancer clinical trials. *Cancers* **2022**, *14*, 1048. [CrossRef]
12. Bastiaannet, E.; Pilleron, S. Epidemiology of cancer in older adults: A systematic review of age-related differences in solid malignancies treatment. *Curr. Oncol. Rep.* **2025**, *27*, 290–311. [CrossRef] [PubMed]
13. Prisciandaro, E.; Ceulemans, L.J.; Van Raemdonck, D.E.; Decaluwé, H.; De Leyn, P.; Bertolaccini, L. Impact of the extent of lung resection on postoperative outcomes of pulmonary metastasectomy for colorectal cancer metastases: An exploratory systematic review. *J. Thorac. Dis.* **2022**, *14*, 2677–2688. [CrossRef] [PubMed]
14. Gerull, W.D.; Puri, V.; Kozower, B.D. The epidemiology and biology of pulmonary metastases. *J. Thorac. Dis.* **2021**, *13*, 2585–2589. [CrossRef] [PubMed]
15. Chen, H.; Stoltzfus, K.C.; Lehrer, E.J.; Horn, S.R.; Siva, S.; Trifiletti, D.M.; Meng, M.-B.; Verma, V.; Louie, A.V.; Zaorsky, N.G. The epidemiology of lung metastases. *Front. Med.* **2021**, *8*, 723396. [CrossRef]
16. Reyes, D.K.; Pienta, K.J. The biology and treatment of oligometastatic cancer. *Oncotarget* **2015**, *6*, 8491–8524. [CrossRef]
17. Hellman, S.; Weichselbaum, R.R. Oligometastases. *J. Clin. Oncol.* **1995**, *13*, 8–10. [CrossRef]
18. Hafez, N.; Gettinger, S. Oligometastatic disease and local therapies: A medical oncology perspective. *Cancer J.* **2020**, *26*, 144–148. [CrossRef]
19. Lo, S.S.; Fakiris, A.J.; Chang, E.L.; Mayr, N.A.; Wang, J.Z.; Papiez, L.; Teh, B.S.; McGarry, R.C.; Cardenes, H.R.; Timmerman, R.D. Stereotactic body radiation therapy: A novel treatment modality. *Nat. Rev. Clin. Oncol.* **2010**, *7*, 44–54. [CrossRef]
20. Vorbach, S.M.; Mangesius, J.; Dejaco, D.; Seppi, T.; Santer, M.; Nedden, S.Z.; Sarcletti, M.P.; Pointner, M.J.; Hart, T.J.; Riechelmann, H.; et al. Survival, treatment outcome, and safety of multiple and repeated courses of stereotactic body radiotherapy for pulmonary oligometastases of head and neck squamous cell carcinoma. *Cancers* **2023**, *15*, 5253. [CrossRef] [PubMed]
21. Palma, D.A.; Olson, R.; Harrow, S.; Gaede, S.; Louie, A.V.; Haasbeek, C.; Mulroy, L.; Lock, M.; Rodrigues, P.G.B.; Yaremko, B.P.; et al. Stereotactic ablative radiotherapy versus standard of care palliative treatment in patients with oligometastatic cancers (sabr-comet): A randomised, phase 2, open-label trial. *Lancet* **2019**, *393*, 2051–2058. [CrossRef]
22. Harrow, S.; Palma, D.A.; Olson, R.; Gaede, S.; Louie, A.V.; Haasbeek, C.; Mulroy, L.; Lock, M.; Rodrigues, G.B.; Yaremko, B.P.; et al. Stereotactic radiation for the comprehensive treatment of oligometastases (sabr-comet): Extended long-term outcomes. *Int. J. Radiat. Oncol. Biol. Phys.* **2022**, *114*, 611–616. [CrossRef]

23. Puts, M.T.; Hardt, J.; Monette, J.; Girre, V.; Springall, E.; Alibhai, S.M. Use of geriatric assessment for older adults in the oncology setting: A systematic review. *JNCI J. Natl. Cancer Inst.* **2012**, *104*, 1134–1164. [CrossRef]
24. Lancia, A.; Ingrosso, G.; Carosi, A.; Bottero, M.; Cancelli, A.; Turturici, I.; Ponti, E.; Santoni, R. Oligometastatic cancer in elderly patients: The "Blitzkrieg" Radiotherapy approach: Sbrt in oligometastatic elderly patients. *Aging Clin. Exp. Res.* **2019**, *31*, 109–114. [CrossRef]
25. Scorsetti, M.; Clerici, E.; Navarria, P.; D'Agostino, G.; Piergallini, L.; De Rose, F.; Ascolese, A.; Tozzi, A.; Iftode, C.; Villa, E.; et al. The role of stereotactic body radiation therapy (sbrt) in the treatment of oligometastatic disease in the elderly. *Br. J. Radiol.* **2015**, *88*, 20150111. [CrossRef] [PubMed]
26. Cuccia, F.; Mazzola, R.; Pastorello, E.; Figlia, V.; Giaj-Levra, N.; Nicosia, L.; Ricchetti, F.; Rigo, M.; Attinà, G.; Vitale, C.; et al. Sbrt for elderly oligometastatic patients as a feasible, safe and effective treatment opportunity. *Clin. Exp. Metastasis* **2021**, *38*, 475–481. [CrossRef] [PubMed]
27. Guckenberger, M.; Lievens, Y.; Bouma, A.B.; Collette, L.; Dekker, A.; deSouza, N.M.; Dingemans, A.-M.C.; Fournier, B.; Hurkmans, C.; Lecouvet, F.E.; et al. Characterisation and classification of oligometastatic disease: A european society for radiotherapy and oncology and european organisation for research and treatment of cancer consensus recommendation. *Lancet Oncol.* **2020**, *21*, e18–e28. [CrossRef]
28. Charlson, M.E.; Pompei, P.; Ales, K.L.; MacKenzie, C.R. A new method of classifying prognostic comorbidity in longitudinal studies: Development and validation. *J. Chronic Dis.* **1987**, *40*, 373–383. [CrossRef] [PubMed]
29. Chang, J.Y.; Bezjak, A.; Mornex, F.; IASLC Advanced Radiation Technology Committee. Stereotactic ablative radiotherapy for centrally located early stage non–small-cell lung cancer: What we have learned. *J. Thorac. Oncol.* **2015**, *10*, 577–585. [CrossRef]
30. Giuliani, M.E.; Filion, E.; Faria, S.; Kundapur, V.; Toni Vu, T.T.T.; Lok, B.H.; Raman, S.; Bahig, H.; Laba, J.M.; Lang, P.; et al. Stereotactic radiation for ultra-central non-small cell lung cancer: A safety and efficacy trial (sunset). *Int. J. Radiat. Oncol.* **2024**, *120*, 669–677. [CrossRef]
31. Eisenhauer, E.A.; Therasse, P.; Bogaerts, J.; Schwartz, L.H.; Sargent, D.; Ford, R.; Dancey, J.; Arbuck, S.; Gwyther, S.; Mooney, M.; et al. New response evaluation criteria in solid tumours: Revised recist guideline (version 1.1). *Eur. J. Cancer* **2009**, *45*, 228–247. [CrossRef] [PubMed]
32. O, J.H.; Lodge, M.A.; Wahl, R.L. Practical percist: A simplified guide to pet response criteria in solid tumors 1.0. *Radiology* **2016**, *280*, 576–584. [CrossRef] [PubMed]

cancers

MDPI

Article

Characteristics, Treatment and Outcomes of Stage I to III Colorectal Cancer in Patients Aged over 80 Years Old

Melissa R. Yeo [1] and Ioannis A. Voutsadakis [2,3,*]

1 Northern Ontario School of Medicine, Sudbury, ON P3E 2C6, Canada; meyeo@nosm.ca
2 Algoma District Cancer Program, Sault Area Hospital, Sault Ste. Marie, ON P6B 0A8, Canada
3 Section of Internal Medicine, Division of Clinical Sciences, Northern Ontario School of Medicine, Sudbury, ON P3E 2C6, Canada
* Correspondence: ivoutsadakis@yahoo.com or ivoutsadakis@nosm.ca

Simple Summary: Colorectal cancer is the most common gastrointestinal neoplasm and affects older patients aged over 80 years old in about 10% of cases. The treatment of these patients is more complicated than the treatment of younger patients due to their comorbidities and frailty. This research examines a cohort of older colorectal cancer patients to identify characteristics and treatment strategies used in their management and compares them with those in younger colorectal cancer patients.

Abstract: Background: Colorectal cancer primarily affects older adults and poses treatment challenges due to age-related comorbidities and frailty, which hinder surgical and chemotherapy options for many elderly patients. This study aims to analyze treatment and disease patterns in elderly colorectal cancer patients, aged over 80 years old, to inform personalized therapies that accommodate their unique clinical needs and improve their outcomes. Patients and Methods: The medical records of all patients aged 80 years old and above, and those aged 65 to 75 years old, who were diagnosed with colorectal cancer at a cancer center in Canada over a seven year period, were retrospectively reviewed. Results: No significant differences in the initial presentation, location, grade or stage at colorectal cancer diagnosis were observed between age groups. Patients aged 80 years old and above were less likely to receive neoadjuvant and adjuvant chemotherapy treatments for stage II disease (19.2% versus. 58.6%, $p = 0.002$; 7.9% versus. 40.0%, $p = 0.002$). There were also differences in the intensity of chemotherapy received and the frequency of dose reductions (76.0% vs. 10.0%, $p = 0.0001$), neoadjuvant and adjuvant radiation therapy (34.6% vs. 65.5%, $p = 0.02$) and surgical management (83.7% vs. 95.3%, $p = 0.006$). Despite these differences in treatments, recurrence rates were not statistically significant between the two groups. However, overall survival was reduced in the older age group. Conclusions: Treatment plans for patients aged 80 years old and above should be tailored to the patient's colorectal cancer presentation, comorbidity status and life expectancy, weighing the impact of cancer treatments on the patient's short- and long-term outcomes.

Keywords: colorectal cancer; octogenarians; geriatric patients; chemotherapy; radiation therapy; adjuvant

1. Introduction

Colorectal cancer is the most prevalent gastrointestinal malignancy and affects about 2 million people worldwide [1]. It ranks third in incidence after lung and breast cancers and second in mortality after lung cancer globally. Therefore, colorectal cancer remains a prominent public health concern, despite progress in developing treatments that have improved survival outcomes for patients with metastatic disease [2]. Despite the introduction and availability of novel targeted therapies and immunotherapy for a sub-set of colorectal cancer patients, most patients rely still on cytotoxic chemotherapy, both in early and metastatic settings. Although colorectal cancer diagnosis in younger persons has been increasing in recent years, the incidence in older populations is the highest, increasing with age [3–5]. The incidence of colorectal cancer per 100,000 population increases from 66.1 in those between 55 and 60 years old, to 214.7 for those 80 to 85 years old, and 234.7 for people above 85 years old [5]. In addition, the older population has frequent comorbidities and frailty that make oncologic treatments for these cancers more toxic and difficult to administer [6]. Given their frailty, older patients are often considered poor surgical candidates and many clinicians are also reluctant to treat this population of older adults with cytotoxic chemotherapies [6].

Early localized colorectal cancer may be cured with surgical resection [7]. More advanced localized cancers with deep penetration into the colonic wall or with extension to regional mesenteric lymph nodes carry a higher risk of recurrence after surgical resection, reaching 50% to 60% for lymph node-positive cancers, and require adjuvant chemotherapy to decrease this risk and improve the chance of a cure [2]. As a result, many patients with localized colorectal cancers have an oncologic indication for adjuvant fluoropyrimidine-based chemotherapy. Older patients tend to undergo screening for colorectal cancer less often, and are frequently diagnosed with symptomatic disease, which is more often of a more advanced stage [8]. Therefore, a combination of more advanced disease and an inability to receive, or reluctance to administer, adjuvant treatment in older colorectal cancer patients may lead to inferior outcomes. On the other hand, toxic treatments may carry an unacceptably high risk of adverse effects in older patients, especially those with significantly reduced organ reserves, and in these cases toxic treatments with the potential for serious harm should be avoided, even when a high recurrence risk is present [9]. Unfortunately, in such cases, elderly patients are left only with palliative options, and suffer short survivals and decreased quality of life due to progressive cancer symptoms.

In this report, we present the characteristics, treatments and outcomes of patients older than 80 years old diagnosed with localized colorectal cancer in our center, and compare them with patients of younger age presenting with the same disease, with the aim of better understanding the differences that characterize the disease in younger and older patients and optimizing outcomes.

2. Patients and Methods

Patients' electronic records were retrospectively reviewed, and patients over 80 years old who had been treated for colorectal cancer in our cancer center between 2016 and 2023 were identified for inclusion in the study. The length of the reviewed period of medical records for the study was based on the prevalence of octogenarians in populations of colorectal cancer patients in the literature, with the aim of obtaining a sample size of more than 100 patients. This number of patients (and a similar number of controls) was considered sufficient for revealing major clinically relevant differences between the groups. The records of included patients were assessed, and demographic, cancer and outcome characteristics were extracted and documented in the study database. Data for a control cohort of younger colorectal cancer patients aged 65 to 75 treated during the same time period, matched by date of diagnosis, were extracted and reviewed. Information of interest that was recorded in the study database included the location, grade and stage of tumors, laboratory parameters, tumor markers, such as Carcinoembryonic Antigen (CEA), initial patient presentation and comorbidities. Comorbidities were assessed through reviewing medical notes, laboratory studies and the pharmacologic therapies that patients were receiving. Data on patient treatments and outcomes, including surgical treatment, neoadjuvant and adjuvant chemotherapy, dose of chemotherapy and adverse effects, and radiation therapy, were also extracted from electronic medical records. Adverse effects from treatments were evaluated from medical records, and, in cases in which the adverse effect was not directly attributed to treatment, the timing of occurrence and plausibility of relatedness were considered in attributing the side effects to the treatment. Overall survival was calculated as the time from diagnosis to the patient's death, or censored to the time of the last follow-up. Progression-free survival was calculated as the time from diagnosis to the time of disease recurrence, or was censored to the time of the last follow-up without recurrence.

The primary data recorded in the study database were used to calculate descriptive statistics, including means and medians, standard deviation and range. Differences between the older and younger colorectal cancer group in the clinical and biologic parameters of interest were statistically compared with the χ^2 test or Fisher's exact test. Kaplan–Meier survival curves were constructed for the visual evaluation of the overall survival (OS) and progression-free survival (PFS) of the two groups of patients. The Log Rank test was employed for the statistical comparison of the PFS and OS curves. All the resulting p values were considered to be significant at the level of $p < 0.05$. Statistical calculations were performed using GraphPad (GraphPad Software, Boston, MA, USA, www.graphpad.com/quickcalcs/) (URL last accessed on 10 November 2024). The Kaplan–Meier curves and Log Rank test were performed using an online tool based on R (statskingdom.com/Kaplan–Meier.html) (URL last accessed on 11 November 2024). The protocol of the research was approved by the Research Ethics Board of the hospital (Research Ethics Board number 2021-05-01).

3. Results

One hundred and four patients aged 80 years old and older (older group) were diagnosed with non-metastatic colorectal cancer and treated in a single cancer center between 2016 and 2023. A similar group of one hundred and six patients aged 65–75 (younger group) were diagnosed and treated during the same time period, and were included as controls. The mean age of the older group was 85 years old (range: 80–95). The mean age of the younger group was 71 years old (range: 65–75) (Table 1). There was no significant difference between male versus female sex in each group. Patients in the younger group more frequently had a family history of various cancers other than colorectal cancer (65.1%) when compared to the older group (53.1%), with this difference approaching statistical significance ($p = 0.08$, Table 1); however, no significant difference was observed regarding family history of colorectal cancer between the two groups. Colorectal cancer in the younger group was numerically more frequently diagnosed on screening compared to the older group (older group: 25.0%, younger group: 39.8%, $p = 0.1$). Conversely, initial presentation with symptoms of colorectal cancer was more frequent in the older group (bleeding or anemia: older group: 61.5%, younger group: 48.5%; bowel changes or obstruction: older group: 13.5%, younger group: 11.7%). Localized colorectal tumors also presented at similar anatomic locations between each group, with right-sided colon cancers being the most common site of tumor development (older group: 61.2%, younger group: 53.8%), followed by rectosigmoid and rectal tumors (older group: 25.2%, younger group: 27.3%) and then left-sided tumors (older group: 13.6%, younger group: 18.9%) (Table 1). No significant difference was observed between the older group and the younger group regarding the stage and grade of the cancer at initial diagnosis. In the older group, localized tumors were most commonly diagnosed as stage II malignancies (31.2%), whereas in the younger group, patients were more likely to be diagnosed with stage III malignancies (42.6%), although these differences were not statistically significant. Grade 3 tumors were the most common in both age groups (older group: 51.3%, younger group: 49.4%) (Table 1).

Table 1. Patient and disease characteristics in colorectal cancer patients aged over 80 years old versus patients aged 65–75 years old.

Characteristic	All (%) (n = 210)	Group > 80 Years Old (%) (n = 104)	Group 65–75 Years Old (%) (n = 106)	p
Mean Age (Range)		85 (80–95)	71 (65–75)	
Gender				
Male	116 (55.2%)	53 (51.0%)	63 (59.4%)	0.21
Female	94 (44.8%)	51 (49.0%)	43 (40.6%)	
Family History of Colon Cancer				
Yes	44 (21.6%)	22 (22.4%)	22 (20.8%)	0.77
No	160 (78.4%)	76 (77.6%)	84 (79.2%)	
N/A	6	6	0	
Family History of Other Cancers				
Yes	121 (59.3%)	52 (53.1%)	69 (65.1%)	0.08
No	83 (40.7%)	46 (46.9%)	37 (34.9%)	
N/A	6	6	0	
Presentation of Disease				
Incidental/Screening	67 (32.4%)	26 (25.0%)	41 (39.8%)	0.10
Anemia/Bleeding	114 (55.1%)	64 (61.5%)	50 (48.5%)	
Bowel Changes/Obstruction	26 (12.5%)	14 (13.5%)	12 (11.7%)	
N/A	3	0	3	
Location of Tumor				
Right	120 (57.4%)	63 (61.2%)	57 (53.8%)	0.48
Left	34 (16.3%)	14 (13.6%)	20 (18.9%)	
Rectal/Rectosigmoid	55 (26.3%)	26 (25.2%)	29 (27.3%)	
N/A	1	1	0	
Stage at Diagnosis				
I	40 (21.3%)	17 (19.5%)	23 (22.7%)	0.45
II	73 (38.8%)	38 (43.7%)	35 (34.7%)	
III	75 (39.9%)	32 (36.8%)	43 (42.6%)	
N/A	22	17	5	
Grade of Tumor				
1	24 (14.2%)	14 (17.5%)	10 (11.2%)	0.37
2	60 (35.5%)	25 (31.2%)	35 (39.4%)	
3	85 (50.3%)	41 (51.3%)	44 (49.4%)	
N/A	41	24	17	

In examining the laboratory values at initial diagnosis between the older and younger group, no significant differences were observed in CEA levels, lactate dehydrogenase (LDH), albumin levels, platelet counts or random glucose levels between the older and younger study participants (Table 2). Elevated creatinine levels were found to be significantly more frequent in the older age group (15.4%) compared to the younger group (3.8%, $p = 0.004$) (Table 2).

Table 2. Laboratory values at initial presentation in patients with localized colorectal cancer aged over 80 years old versus patients aged 65 to 75 years old.

	All (%) (n = 210)	**Group > 80 Years Old (n = 104)**	**Group 65–75 Years Old (n = 106)**	p
CEA				
≤4.7 µg/L	129 (70.5%)	66 (72.5%)	63 (68.5%)	0.55
>4.7 µg/L	54 (29.5%)	25 (27.5%)	29 (31.5%)	
N/A	27	13	14	
LDH				
≤210 U/L	181 (90.0%)	90 (90.9%)	91 (89.2%)	0.69
>210 U/L	20 (10.0%)	9 (9.1%)	11 (10.8%)	
N/A	9	5	4	
Albumin				
<35 g/L	59 (29.2%)	33 (33.0%)	26 (25.5%)	0.24
≥35 g/L	143 (70.8%)	67 (67.0%)	76 (74.5%)	
N/A	8	4	4	
Platelets				
≤400 × 10^9/L	185 (88.9%)	93 (90.3%)	92 (87.6%)	0.54
>400 × 10^9/L	23 (11.1%)	10 (9.7%)	13 (12.4%)	
N/A	2	1	1	
Glucose				
≤7 mmol/L	87 (52.4%)	45 (97.6%)	42 (50.0%)	0.53
>7 mmol/L	79 (47.6%)	37 (2.4%)	42 (50.0%)	
N/A	44	22	22	
Creatinine				
≤130 µmol/L	189 (90.4%)	88 (84.6%)	101 (96.2%)	0.004
>130 µmol/L	20 (9.6%)	16 (15.4%)	4 (3.8%)	
N/A	1	0	1	

Patients in the older age group were significantly less likely to receive neoadjuvant chemotherapy for rectosigmoid and rectal cancers (older group: 19.2%, younger group: 58.6%, $p = 0.002$), and adjuvant chemotherapy for stage II tumors (older group: 7.9%, younger group: 40.0%, $p = 0.002$), compared to their younger counterparts (Table 3). No significant difference was noted overall in adjuvant chemotherapy treatment for stage III tumors. In the older cohort who received adjuvant chemotherapy, a significant number of patients received reduced or modified doses of treatment (76.0%, $p = 0.0001$), compared to the younger cohort (10.0%). There was also a significant difference in the types of adjuvant chemotherapy used to treat stage II and III cancers between each age group ($p = 0.00002$). In the older cohort, monotherapy with Capecitabine was most commonly used (60.0%), followed by FOLFOX (5-FU/Folinic acid/Oxaliplatin) or CAPOX (Capecitabine/Oxaliplatin) (28.0%), and FOLFIRI (5-FU/Folinic acid/Irinotecan)/Bevacizumab) (12.0%). Combination therapy with FOLFOX or CAPOX was the most common treatment used in the younger cohort (82.0%), followed by Capecitabine (12.0%) and FOLFIRI/Bevacizumab (6.0%) (Table 3). Both neoadjuvant and adjuvant radiation therapy for rectosigmoid and rectal tumors were used significantly less in the older age group (older group: 34.6%, younger group: 65.5%, $p = 0.02$), whereas palliative radiation was significantly more common in the older cohort, although it was required in few cases in both groups (older group: 10.6%, younger group: 1.9%, $p = 0.01$). Older patients were also significantly less likely to undergo surgery for treatment of their colorectal cancer, compared to their younger counterparts (older group: 83.7%, younger group: 95.3%, $p = 0.006$) (Table 3).

Table 3. Cancer treatments in patients with colorectal cancer aged over 80 years old versus patients aged 65 to 75 years old.

Treatment	All (%)	Group > 80 Years Old (%)	Group 65–75 Years Old (%)	p
Neoadjuvant chemotherapy (rectosigmoid/rectal)				
Yes	22 (40.0%)	5 (19.2%)	17 (58.6%)	0.002
No	33 (60.0%)	21 (80.7%)	12 (41.4%)	
Adjuvant chemotherapy (stage II)				
Yes	17 (23.3%)	3 (7.9%)	14 (40.0%)	0.002
No	56 (76.7%)	35 (92.1%)	21 (60.0%)	
Adjuvant chemotherapy (stage III)				
Yes	58 (77.3%)	22 (68.7%)	36 (83.7%)	0.13
No	17 (22.7%)	10 (31.3%)	7 (16.3%)	
Type of adjuvant chemotherapy (stage II and III)				
Capecitabine	21 (28.0%)	15 (60.0%)	6 (12.0%)	0.00002
FOLFOX or CAPOX	48 (64.0%)	7 (28.0%)	41 (82.0%)	
FOLFIRI/Bevacizumab	6 (8.0%)	3 (12.0%)	3 (6.0%)	
Adjuvant chemotherapy dose reduction				
Yes	24 (32.0%)	19 (76.0%)	5 (10.0%)	0.0001
No	51 (68.0%)	6 (24.0%)	45 (90.0%)	
Neoadjuvant/adjuvant radiation (rectosigmoid/rectal)				
Yes	28 (50.9%)	9 (34.6%)	19 (65.5%)	0.02
No	27 (49.1%)	17 (65.4%)	10 (34.5%)	
Palliative radiation				
Yes	13 (6.2%)	11 (10.6%)	2 (1.9%)	0.01
No	197 (93.8%)	93 (89.4%)	104 (98.1%)	
Surgery				
Yes	188 (89.5%)	87 (83.7%)	101 (95.3%)	0.006
No	22 (10.5%)	17 (16.3%)	5 (4.7%)	

In those patients who received chemotherapy, adverse effects were analyzed. Common adverse effects reported in both age groups included fatigue, neutropenia, peripheral neuropathy, hand–foot syndrome and cutaneous toxicities, bowel habit changes (constipation, diarrhea), nausea/vomiting, mucositis and others, including dehydration, visual changes, bleeding and dizziness (Table 4). Peripheral neuropathy was significantly more common in the younger age group (37.3%, $p = 0.01$), whereas other adverse effects (dehydration, bleeding) were reported significantly more often in the older age group (28.1%, $p = 0.04$) (Table 4).

Table 4. Chemotherapy-associated adverse effects in patients with colorectal cancer aged over 80 years old versus patients aged 65–75 years old.

Adverse Effect	All (%) (n = 91)	Group > 80 Years Old (%) (n = 32)	Group 65–75 Years Old (%) (n = 59)	p
Fatigue				
Yes	19 (20.9%)	7 (21.9%)	12 (20.3%)	1.00
No	72 (79.1%)	25 (78.1%)	47 (79.7%)	
Neutropenia (grade 4)				
Yes	4 (4.4%)	0 (0.00%)	4 (6.8%)	0.3
No	87 (95.6%)	32 (100.00%)	55 (93.2%)	
Peripheral neuropathy				
Yes	25 (27.5%)	3 (9.4%)	22 (37.3%)	0.01
No	66 (72.5%)	29 (90.6%)	37 (62.7%)	
Hand–foot syndrome/skin changes				
Yes	19 (20.9%)	10 (31.3%)	9 (15.2%)	0.10
No	72 (79.1%)	22 (68.7%)	50 (84.8%)	
Bowel changes (diarrhea, constipation)				
Yes	34 (37.4%)	12 (37.5%)	22 (37.3%)	1.00
No	57 (62.6%)	20 (62.5%)	37 (62.7%)	
Nausea/vomiting				
Yes	18 (19.8%)	5 (15.6%)	13 (22.0%)	0.59
No	73 (80.2%)	27 (84.4%)	46 (78.0%)	
Mucositis				
Yes	7 (7.7%)	3 (9.4%)	4 (6.8%)	0.69
No	84 (92.3%)	29 (90.6%)	55 (93.2%)	
Other (dehydration, vision changes, bleeding, dizziness)				
Yes	15 (16.5%)	9 (28.1%)	6 (10.2%)	0.04
No	76 (83.5%)	23 (71.9%)	53 (89.8%)	

Regarding comorbidities in each age group, some differences were also noticed. In the younger age group, the rate of obesity (BMI > 30) was significantly higher (older group: 28.8%, younger group: 46.2%, $p = 0.01$) (Table 5). In the older age group, hypertension, cardiovascular/neurovascular diseases and dyslipidemia were significantly more common. In contrast, the prevalence of diabetes was not different between patients of the two age groups (Table 5). Patients in the older group with cardiovascular/neurovascular comorbidities were less likely to have received combination chemotherapy (6.3% of cases) than patients in the older group without such comorbidities (17.1% of cases), although this difference did not reach statistical significance ($p = 0.08$).

Table 5. Comorbidities in patients with colorectal cancer aged over 80 years old versus patients aged 65–75 years old.

Comorbidities	All (%) (*n* = 210)	Group > 80 Years Old (%) (*n* = 104)	Group 65–75 Years Old (%) (*n* = 106)	*p*
Obesity (*n* = 210)				
BMI > 30	79 (37.6%)	30 (28.8%)	49 (46.2%)	0.01
BMI ≤ 30	131 (62.4%)	74 (71.2%)	57 (53.8)	
Diabetes (*n* = 209)				
Yes	67 (31.9%)	36 (34.6%)	31 (29.2%)	0.43
No	142 (67.6%)	68 (65.4%)	74 (69.8%)	
Hypertension (*n* = 209)				
Yes	158 (75.2%)	87 (83.7%)	71 (66.9%)	0.007
No	51 (24.8%)	17 (16.3%)	34 (32.1%)	
Cardiovascular/neurovascular disease (*n* = 209)				
Yes	99 (47.1%)	68 (65.4%)	31 (29.2%)	0.0001
No	110 (52.4%)	36 (34.6%)	74 (69.8%)	
Dyslipidemia (*n* = 209)				
Yes	108 (51.4%)	62 (59.6%)	46 (43.4%)	0.02
No	101 (48.6%)	42 (40.4%)	59 (55.7%)	

The median progression-free survival in the older age group was 16.0 months (range, 0.3 months–8.9 months), and the median progression-free survival in the younger age group was 27.4 months (0.2 months–101.1 months). There was no statistically significant difference in progression-free survival between the two age groups (Log Rank $p = 0.31$) (Figure 1). The median overall survival (OS) in the older group was 26.3 months (range, 0.3 months–96.2 months), and the median overall survival in the younger age group was 39.7 months (range, 1.5 months–172.5 months) (Log Rank $p = 0.00001$) (Figure 2).

Table 6 shows the major differences in the presentation, comorbidities, treatments and adverse effects between the older and younger colorectal cancer patients, as observed in the cohorts of the study.

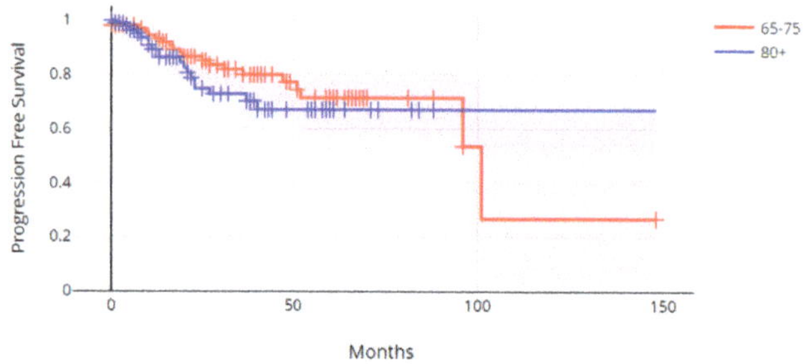

Figure 1. Progression-free survival of patients with colorectal cancer aged over 80 years old versus patients aged 65 to 75 years old. Log Rank test $p = 0.3$.

Table 6. The main differences between the older (aged over 80 years old) and younger (aged 65 to 75 years old) colorectal cancer patients observed in this study.

Characteristic	Comparison	p Value
Demographics		
Family history of other cancers besides colorectal cancer	Trend of higher prevalence in younger group	0.08
Presentation of disease	Trend of more frequent presentation with anemia or bleeding in older group	0.1
Laboratory evaluation		
Creatinine	Older group more frequently (15.4% of cases) had elevated values than younger group (3.8% of patients)	0.004
Treatments		
Neoadjuvant chemotherapy in patients with rectal/rectosigmoid cancer	More commonly administered in younger group (58.6% of patients) than in older patients (19.2%)	0.002
Adjuvant chemotherapy	More frequent use of adjuvant chemotherapy for stage II cancers in younger group (40% versus 7.9% of older patients), but no difference in use of adjuvant chemotherapy for stage III patients	0.002
Type of adjuvant chemotherapy	More frequent use of adjuvant capecitabine monotherapy in older group (60% versus 12% in younger group)	0.00002
Adjuvant chemotherapy dose reduction	More frequently performed in older group (76% versus 10% in younger group)	0.0001
Neoadjuvant/adjuvant radiation in patients with rectal/rectosigmoid cancer	More frequently given in younger patients (65.5% of patients versus 34.6% of patients in older group)	0.02
Surgery	Fewer patients in older age group were treated surgically (83.7% versus 95.3% in younger group)	0.006
Adverse effects		
Peripheral neuropathy	More frequent in younger patients (37.3%) than in older patients (9.4%), consistent with more frequent use of oxaliplatin in this group	0.01
Hand–foot syndrome	Trend for higher incidence in older group (31.3% versus 15.2% of patients in younger group)	0.10
Comorbidities		
Obesity	Higher prevalence in younger group (46.2%) than in older patients (28.8%)	0.01
Hypertension, cardiovascular disease and dyslipidemia	More prevalent in younger patients	0.007, 0.0001, 0.02

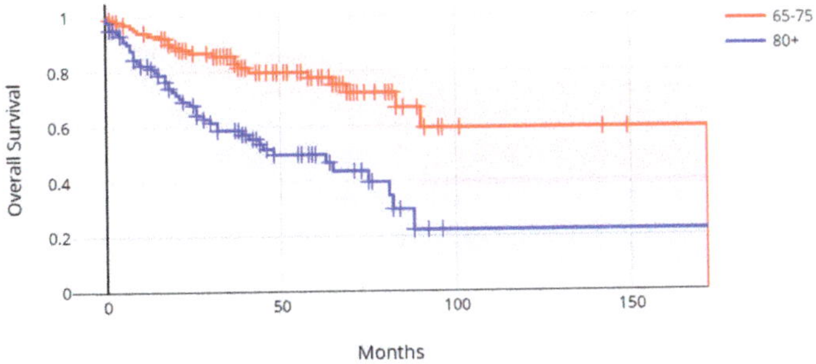

Figure 2. Overall survival of patients with colorectal cancer aged over 80 years old versus patients aged 65 to 75 years old. Log Rank test $p = 0.00001$.

4. Discussion

Several of the most frequent cancers are more prevalent in older patients, and this trend is expected to increase with the aging of the population in western countries. About one in six adults are diagnosed with cancer at an age older than 80 years old [10]. Patients in this age group tend to receive treatments according to the standard of care for their specific type and stage of cancer less often, due to a perception of futility or excessive toxicity of treatments in the elderly. For example, a study from Canada showed that more than one-third fewer patients aged 80 or older were seen in surgical consultation for their cancer compared to cancer patients aged 65 years old and younger [10]. In addition, older patients were also less likely to be seen in medical and radiation oncology consultations. These trends suggest that older cancer patients may be denied valuable treatments that could potentially prolong their survival and improve the quality of their lives. On the other hand, it is well documented that all cancer treatments may more commonly have adverse outcomes in the elderly who have more comorbidities and reduced functional reserves. Surgical resection of localized cancers in octogenarians is associated with a perioperative mortality rate of 7% to 11% [11,12]. Complications related to surgery, such as operative leaks and infections, are not more common in older patients, but are more frequently fatal. Age- and disease-related sarcopenia and cachexia are prevalent in the elderly, and may lead to adverse outcomes with surgical complications. Cachexia, defined as weight loss of more than 5%, or of 2% to 5% when the body mass index is less than 20 kg/m^2, was present in 36% of patients with localized colorectal cancer and a mean age of 79.6 years old [13]. The prevalence of sarcopenia was 13% in the same series. Chemotherapy is also more toxic for elderly patients, and in many cases it is omitted, even when there is an oncologic indication for its administration [14]. Tools to predict high-grade adverse effects in older patients have been proposed, and play a role in improving the anticipation of adverse outcomes in individual patients, who may be then counseled against treatment, or be treated with modified doses or enhanced surveillance and support [9]. Therefore, a strategy with the specific patient in view, and which considers not only their age, but also their general status and individual wishes for treatment, would better serve this more challenging-to-treat patient age group.

In our cohort of stage I to III colorectal cancer patients over 80 years old, there were no significant differences in the distribution of genders, location of the tumor in the colon or grade of the tumor compared to a younger cohort. A trend toward a lower incidence of family history of cancers and a lower prevalence of incidentally and screening-diagnosed cancers in the older group was present. This is related to the fact that, although screening colonoscopies decrease the incidence of colorectal cancer diagnosis, guidelines advise for selective-only screening over the age of 75 [15–17]. A decreased incidence of screening-diagnosed cancer has also been reported in other cancers, such as breast cancer, in the elderly, as guidelines advise against routine screening [18]. The two age groups did not differ in their baseline CEA, rate of thrombocytosis or hypoalbuminemia, but older patients more frequently had decreased renal function. Although younger patients had significant higher rates of obesity, and the rate of diabetes did not differ between the groups, older patients had a higher frequency of hypertension, cardiovascular disease and dyslipidemia. Significant differences were observed in treatments, with the older patients less frequently receiving all types of cancer therapies, besides palliative radiation. In addition, the type of adjuvant chemotherapy differed between the groups, with the majority of older patients receiving fluoropyrimidine-based monotherapy, and three-fourths of the patients having a reduced dose of chemotherapy. As this was a retrospective analysis, the treatment decisions had been made by the treating physicians in a non-randomized manner. Therefore, it cannot be ascertained by the current analysis whether the process of treatment allocation in individual patients was based on age considerations alone, or whether it considered other factors, such as comorbidities and frailty. However, the process of multi-parametric decision making is routine in oncology. Moreover, a significant proportion of older patients in the study (28%) had indeed received combination chemotherapy, suggesting that additional patient factors, in addition to age, were taken into consideration in deciding the most appropriate treatment for the individual patient. Despite the treatment differences, and despite that, as expected, older patients had worse overall survival than younger patients, progression-free survival did not differ significantly between the two groups. Given the similar progression-free survival in the two groups, and the fact that baseline characteristics were well balanced (Tables 1 and 2), no multivariate analysis was performed.

The location of the cancer in the right or left colon is of biological and clinical importance, as right-sided cancers tend to more often be developing along the microsatellite instability pathway, and tend to have a better prognosis when localized. Some studies have reported a higher incidence of right-sided colon primaries in older patients, although this has not been observed by other investigators [14,19,20]. Given their better prognosis, stage II right-sided colon cancers with microsatellite instability may be managed without adjuvant treatment. Ongoing clinical studies are examining whether more advanced localized stages with microsatellite instability may be successfully treated with immunotherapy instead of chemotherapy, based on the success of these treatments in treating microsatellite-unstable metastatic disease [21]. In our series, a non-significant trend for a higher incidence of right-sided colon primaries in the older population was observed.

Although all cancer treatment modalities, including surgery, radiation and chemotherapy, were used less frequently in patients older than 80 years than in younger patients in our cohort, most patients received treatment appropriate for the stage of their cancer. For example, 83.7% of octogenarians and older patients had surgical resection of their colorectal cancer. The feasibility and acceptable outcomes of surgical resection of colorectal cancer in octogenarians and nonagenarians in contemporary practice have been documented, with post-operative 90-day survival rates of 98.1% and 98.1%, respectively, and post-operative 180-day survival rates of 93.1% and 88.9%, respectively [22].

Adjuvant chemotherapy is recommended for all stage III colorectal cancer patients that have an adequate performance status for receiving the treatment, and it was administered in 68.7% of octogenarians and older patients in our cohort. Monotherapy with capecitabine was favored in this population as a less toxic treatment, and dose adjustments were frequently performed. The overall rate of chemotherapy administration in our elderly cohort was higher than the rate reported in other series and databases which ranges from 3% to 25%, suggesting that, with appropriate dose and intensity adjustments, adjuvant therapy is feasible [14,23]. Adjuvant chemotherapy in patients over 80 years old with stage III colorectal cancer has been associated with improved survival. In a study on the United States National Cancer Database, patients over the age of 80 years old with stage III colorectal cancer who received adjuvant chemotherapy had a median overall survival of 61.7 months, while similar patients who did not receive adjuvant chemotherapy had a median overall survival of 35 months [24]. The progression-free survival outcomes observed in our older cohort suggest that less intense chemotherapy regimens may provide results that are similar to those obtained with combination adjuvant treatments employed in younger patients. Combination chemotherapy with a fluoropyrimidine and oxaliplatin is the standard of care in the adjuvant setting for stage III colorectal cancer, based on its superior efficacy compared to fluoropyrimidines alone [25]. However, the pivotal trials that established this standard excluded older patients over the age of 75 years old. Capecitabine monotherapy may be adequate as an adjuvant therapy for stage III colorectal cancer patients aged over 80 years old, and provides a survival benefit compared to no adjuvant treatment [26]. Geriatric tools to predict high-grade toxicity from chemotherapy in the elderly may provide further guidance for the advisability of adjuvant treatment in the elderly, and could serve as a safeguard against advising therapy in patients predicted to have an unacceptably high risk of toxicity [27]. A tool devised by the Cancer and Aging

Research Group (CARG) provides a validated scale for the prediction of chemotherapy toxicity in the elderly, and is endorsed by the American Society of Clinical Oncology (ASCO) [28]. The CARG tool assigns a low, intermediate or high risk for toxicity to geriatric patients aged above 70 years old, based on 11 parameters, which include an age above 72 years old, a diagnosis a gastrointestinal or genitourinary cancer, the dose and number of chemotherapy drugs, anemia, renal insufficiency, hearing loss, previous falls, an inability to take medications, mobility restrictions and social activity [28]. A simpler prediction tool based on just four parameters—Eastern Co-operative Oncology Group (ECOG) performance status, hypoalbuminemia, renal insufficiency and presence of a metastatic cancer—has been proposed and found to perform similarly to the CARG tool [29,30]. However, this tool has not been validated more broadly. The European Society of Medical Oncology, in collaboration with the International Society of Geriatric Oncology (SIOG), has advocated, in a position paper, for the use of geriatric assessments for the optimization of the management of geriatric cancer patients [31].

The current study has certain limitations. The cohort was studied retrospectively and was recruited from a single cancer center. Although the current study included over one hundred stage I to III colorectal cancer patients older than 80 years old, which is one of the highest numbers of patients studied in this population reported in the literature, the number of included patients was still comparatively small. The source records had incomplete data on patients' performance status and quality of life evaluations. Therefore, an analysis of these parameters could not be performed in the current study. Moreover, the role of comorbidities in the difference in OS between the two groups of patients was not assessed. No molecular data regarding mismatch repair status and other mutations were available in the current report. However, other studies have confirmed a higher prevalence of mismatch repair deficiency in colorectal cancer patients and a higher prevalence of cases with a high tumor mutation burden in this population [6,32,33]. Both molecular markers provide opportunities for treatment with checkpoint inhibitor immunotherapy in the metastatic setting, and this treatment could be expanded in the localized setting if ongoing trials confirm its benefit. Common cancer-associated alterations of colorectal cancer, including mutations in the tumor suppressors *APC*, *TP53* and in the oncogenes *KRAS* and *PIK3CA*, have shown no significant differences in prevalence between age groups [32–34].

In conclusion, the treatment of stage I to III colorectal cancer in octogenarians is a conundrum frequently faced by physicians treating cancer in daily practice. Older colorectal cancer patients differ from younger patients in their organ function reserves, notably their renal function, which limits their ability to receive more intensive treatments. Indeed, we have observed lower rates of chemotherapy use and a lower intensity of treatments in the older patients. Particularly, the presence of comorbidities affects the intensity of the chemotherapy used. A multidisciplinary approach should be influenced by the individual patient's general status and wishes, and should take advantage of all available therapies tailored to the specific patient. The optimization of treatment has the potential to provide beneficial outcomes of localized colorectal cancer in octogenarians and older patients that are similar to those obtained in younger patients.

Author Contributions: M.R.Y.: Data collection, data analysis, manuscript writing, manuscript review, manuscript approval. I.A.V.: Study conception, protocol writing, data analysis, supervision, manuscript writing, manuscript revision, manuscript approval. All authors have read and agreed to the published version of the manuscript.

Funding: This research was partially funded by the Mach-Gaensslen foundation.

Institutional Review Board Statement: The study was conducted in accordance with the Declaration of Helsinki, and approved by the Ethics Review Board of Sault Area Hospital, Sault Ste Marie, Canada (Research Ethics Board number 2021-05-01, date of approval: 1 May 2021).

Informed Consent Statement: This was a retrospective study, and the Ethics Review Board has waived the requirement for informed consent.

Data Availability Statement: All the data generated in this study are presented in the article, and no additional data are available.

Conflicts of Interest: The authors declare no conflicts of interest related to this study.

References

1. Bray, F.; Laversanne, M.; Sung, H.; Ferlay, J.; Siegel, R.L.; Soerjomataram, I.; Jemal, A. Global cancer statistics 2022: GLOBOCAN estimates of incidence and mortality worldwide for 36 cancers in 185 countries. *CA Cancer J. Clin.* **2024**, *74*, 229–263. [CrossRef] [PubMed]
2. Benson, A.B.; Venook, A.P.; Adam, M.; Chang, G.; Chen, Y.J.; Ciombor, K.K.; Cohen, S.A.; Cooper, H.S.; Deming, D.; Garrido-Laguna, I.; et al. Colon Cancer, Version 3.2024, NCCN Clinical Practice Guidelines in Oncology. *J. Natl. Compr. Canc Netw.* **2024**, *22*, e240029. [CrossRef] [PubMed]
3. Angelakas, A.; Christodoulou, T.; Kamposioras, K.; Barriuso, J.; Braun, M.; Hasan, J.; Marti, K.; Misra, V.; Mullamitha, S.; Saunders, M.; et al. Is early-onset colorectal cancer an evolving pandemic? Real-world data from a tertiary cancer center. *Oncologist* **2024**, *29*, e1680–e1691. [CrossRef] [PubMed]
4. Goldvaser, H.; Purim, O.; Kundel, Y.; Shepshelovich, D.; Shochat, T.; Shemesh-Bar, L.; Sulkes, A.; Brenner, B. Colorectal cancer in young patients: Is it a distinct clinical entity? *Int. J. Clin. Oncol.* **2016**, *21*, 684–695. [CrossRef] [PubMed]
5. Siegel, R.L.; Wagle, N.S.; Cercek, A.; Smith, R.A.; Jemal, A. Colorectal cancer statistics, 2023. *CA A Cancer J. Clin.* **2023**, *73*, 233–254. [CrossRef] [PubMed]
6. Voutsadakis, I.A. Presentation, Molecular Characteristics, Treatment, and Outcomes of Colorectal Cancer in Patients Older than 80 Years Old. *Medicina* **2023**, *59*, 1574. [CrossRef] [PubMed] [PubMed Central]
7. Kajiwara, Y.; Ueno, H. Essential updates 2022–2023: Surgical and adjuvant therapies for locally advanced colorectal cancer. *Ann. Gastroenterol. Surg.* **2024**, *8*, 977–986. [CrossRef] [PubMed] [PubMed Central]
8. Goldvaser, H.; Katz Shroitman, N.; Ben-Aharon, I.; Purim, O.; Kundel, Y.; Shepshelovich, D.; Shochat, T.; Sulkes, A.; Brenner, B. Octogenarian patients with colorectal cancer: Characterizing an emerging clinical entity. *World J. Gastroenterol.* **2017**, *23*, 1387–1396. [CrossRef] [PubMed] [PubMed Central]
9. Voutsadakis, I.A. Clinical tools for chemotherapy toxicity prediction and survival in geriatric cancer patients. *J. Chemother.* **2018**, *30*, 266–279. [CrossRef] [PubMed]
10. Habbous, S.; Alibhai, S.M.H.; Menjak, I.B.; Forster, K.; Holloway, C.M.B.; Darling, G. The effect of age on the opportunity to receive cancer treatment. *Cancer Epidemiol.* **2022**, *81*, 102271. [CrossRef] [PubMed]
11. Claassen, Y.H.M.; Bastiaannet, E.; van Eycken, E.; Van Damme, N.; Martling, A.; Johansson, R.; Iversen, L.H.; Ingeholm, P.; Lemmens, V.E.P.P.; Liefers, G.J.; et al. Time trends of short-term mortality for octogenarians undergoing a colorectal resection in North Europe. *Eur. J. Surg. Oncol.* **2019**, *45*, 1396–1402. [CrossRef] [PubMed]
12. Diers, J.; Baum, P.; Lehmann, K.; Uttinger, K.; Baumann, N.; Pietryga, S.; Hankir, M.; Matthes, N.; Lock, J.F.; Germer, C.T.; et al. Disproportionately high failure to rescue rates after resection for colorectal cancer in the geriatric patient population—A nationwide study. *Cancer Med.* **2022**, *11*, 4256–4264. [CrossRef] [PubMed] [PubMed Central]
13. Dolin, T.G.; Mikkelsen, M.K.; Jakobsen, H.L.; Vinther, A.; Zerahn, B.; Nielsen, D.L.; Johansen, J.S.; Lund, C.M.; Suetta, C. The prevalence of sarcopenia and cachexia in older patients with localized colorectal cancer. *J. Geriatr. Oncol.* **2023**, *14*, 101402. [CrossRef] [PubMed]
14. Kotake, K.; Asano, M.; Ozawa, H.; Kobayashi, H.; Sugihara, K. Tumour characteristics, treatment patterns and survival of patients aged 80 years or older with colorectal cancer. *Colorectal Dis.* **2015**, *17*, 205–215. [CrossRef] [PubMed]
15. Kahi, C.J.; Myers, L.J.; Slaven, J.E.; Haggstrom, D.; Pohl, H.; Robertson, D.J.; Imperiale, T.F. Lower endoscopy reduces colorectal cancer incidence in older individuals. *Gastroenterology* **2014**, *146*, 718–725.e3. [CrossRef] [PubMed]
16. Heidelbaugh, J.J. The Adult Well-Male Examination. *Am. Fam. Physician* **2018**, *98*, 729–737. [PubMed]
17. Ness, R.M.; Llor, X.; Abbass, M.A.; Bishu, S.; Chen, C.T.; Cooper, G.; Early, D.S.; Friedman, M.; Fudman, D.; Giardiello, F.M.; et al. NCCN Guidelines® Insights: Colorectal Cancer Screening, Version 1.2024. *J. Natl. Compr. Cancer Netw.* **2024**, *22*, 438–446. [CrossRef] [PubMed]
18. Bertolo, A.; Rosso, C.; Voutsadakis, I.A. Breast Cancer in Patients 80 Years-Old and Older. *Eur. J. Breast Health* **2020**, *16*, 208–212. [CrossRef] [PubMed] [PubMed Central]

19. Sell, N.M.; Qwaider, Y.Z.; Goldstone, R.N.; Stafford, C.E.; Cauley, C.E.; Francone, T.D.; Ricciardi, R.; Bordeianou, L.G.; Berger, D.L.; Kunitake, H. Octogenarians present with a less aggressive phenotype of colon adenocarcinoma. *Surgery* **2020**, *168*, 1138–1143. [CrossRef] [PubMed] [PubMed Central]
20. Lee, S.M.; Shin, J.S. Colorectal Cancer in Octogenarian and Nonagenarian Patients: Clinicopathological Features and Survivals. *Ann. Coloproctol.* **2020**, *36*, 323–329. [CrossRef] [PubMed] [PubMed Central]
21. André, T.; Shiu, K.K.; Kim, T.W.; Jensen, B.V.; Jensen, L.H.; Punt, C.; Smith, D.; Garcia-Carbonero, R.; Benavides, M.; Gibbs, P.; et al. Pembrolizumab in Microsatellite-Instability-High Advanced Colorectal Cancer. *N. Engl. J. Med.* **2020**, *383*, 2207–2218. [CrossRef] [PubMed]
22. Høydahl, Ø.; Edna, T.H.; Xanthoulis, A.; Lydersen, S.; Endreseth, B.H. Octogenarian patients with colon cancer—Postoperative morbidity and mortality are the major challenges. *BMC Cancer* **2022**, *22*, 302. [CrossRef] [PubMed] [PubMed Central]
23. Vermeer, N.C.A.; Claassen, Y.H.M.; Derks, M.G.M.; Iversen, L.H.; van Eycken, E.; Guren, M.G.; Mroczkowski, P.; Martling, A.; Johansson, R.; Vandendael, T.; et al. Treatment and Survival of Patients with Colon Cancer Aged 80 Years and Older: A EURECCA International Comparison. *Oncologist* **2018**, *23*, 982–990. [CrossRef] [PubMed] [PubMed Central]
24. Bergquist, J.R.; Thiels, C.A.; Spindler, B.A.; Shubert, C.R.; Hayman, A.V.; Kelley, S.R.; Larson, D.W.; Habermann, E.B.; Pemberton, J.H.; Mathis, K.L. Benefit of Postresection Adjuvant Chemotherapy for Stage III Colon Cancer in Octogenarians: Analysis of the National Cancer Database. *Dis. Colon. Rectum* **2016**, *59*, 1142–1149. [CrossRef] [PubMed]
25. André, T.; de Gramont, A.; Vernerey, D.; Chibaudel, B.; Bonnetain, F.; Tijeras-Raballand, A.; Scriva, A.; Hickish, T.; Tabernero, J.; Van Laethem, J.L.; et al. Adjuvant Fluorouracil, Leucovorin, and Oxaliplatin in Stage II to III Colon Cancer: Updated 10-Year Survival and Outcomes According to BRAF Mutation and Mismatch Repair Status of the MOSAIC Study. *J. Clin. Oncol.* **2015**, *33*, 4176–4187. [CrossRef] [PubMed]
26. Shibutani, M.; Maeda, K.; Kashiwagi, S.; Hirakawa, K.; Ohira, M. Effect of Adjuvant Chemotherapy on Survival of Elderly Patients With Stage III Colorectal Cancer. *Anticancer Res.* **2021**, *41*, 3615–3624. [CrossRef] [PubMed]
27. Mohile, S.G.; Dale, W.; Somerfield, M.R.; Schonberg, M.A.; Boyd, C.M.; Burhenn, P.S.; Canin, B.; Cohen, H.J.; Holmes, H.M.; Hopkins, J.O.; et al. Practical Assessment and Management of Vulnerabilities in Older Patients Receiving Chemotherapy: ASCO Guideline for Geriatric Oncology. *J. Clin. Oncol.* **2018**, *36*, 2326–2347. [CrossRef] [PubMed] [PubMed Central]
28. Hurria, A.; Togawa, K.; Mohile, S.G.; Owusu, C.; Klepin, H.D.; Gross, C.P.; Lichtman, S.M.; Gajra, A.; Bhatia, S.; Katheria, V.; et al. Predicting chemotherapy toxicity in older adults with cancer: A prospective multicenter study. *J. Clin. Oncol.* **2011**, *29*, 3457–3465. [CrossRef] [PubMed] [PubMed Central]
29. Reed, M.; Patrick, C.; Quevillon, T.; Walde, N.; Voutsadakis, I.A. Prediction of hospital admissions and grade 3-4 toxicities in cancer patients 70 years old and older receiving chemotherapy. *Eur. J. Cancer Care* **2019**, *28*, e13144. [CrossRef] [PubMed]
30. Lewis, A.; Reed, M.; Walde, N.; Voutsadakis, I.A. An evaluation of the Index4 tool for chemotherapy toxicity prediction in cancer patients older than 70 years old. *Sci. Rep.* **2023**, *13*, 1082. [CrossRef] [PubMed] [PubMed Central]
31. Loh, K.P.; Liposits, G.; Arora, S.P.; Neuendorff, N.R.; Gomes, F.; Krok-Schoen, J.L.; Amaral, T.; Mariamidze, E.; Biganzoli, L.; Brain, E.; et al. Adequate assessment yields appropriate care-the role of geriatric assessment and management in older adults with cancer: A position paper from the ESMO/SIOG Cancer in the Elderly Working Group. *ESMO Open* **2024**, *9*, 103657. [CrossRef] [PubMed] [PubMed Central]
32. Cancer Genome Atlas Network. Comprehensive molecular characterization of human colon and rectal cancer. *Nature* **2012**, *487*, 330–337. [CrossRef] [PubMed] [PubMed Central]
33. Giannakis, M.; Mu, X.J.; Shukla, S.A.; Qian, Z.R.; Cohen, O.; Nishihara, R.; Bahl, S.; Cao, Y.; Amin-Mansour, A.; Yamauchi, M.; et al. Genomic Correlates of Immune-Cell Infiltrates in Colorectal Carcinoma. *Cell Rep.* **2016**, *17*, 1206. [CrossRef] [PubMed] [PubMed Central]
34. Roelands, J.; Kuppen, P.J.K.; Ahmed, E.I.; Mall, R.; Masoodi, T.; Singh, P.; Monaco, G.; Raynaud, C.; de Miranda, N.F.C.C.; Ferraro, L.; et al. An integrated tumor, immune and microbiome atlas of colon cancer. *Nat. Med.* **2023**, *29*, 1273–1286. [CrossRef] [PubMed] [PubMed Central]

cancers

MDPI

Article

Advocate-BREAST80+: A Comprehensive Patient and Advocate-Led Study to Enhance Breast Cancer Care Delivery and Patient-Centered Research in Women Aged ≥80 Years

Ciara C. O'Sullivan [1,*], Robert A. Vierkant [2], Nicole L. Larson [2], Mary Lou Smith [3,4], Cynthia Chauhan [4], Fergus J. Couch [5], Janet E. Olson [2], Stacy D'Andre [1], Aminah Jatoi [1] and Kathryn J. Ruddy [1]

1 Department of Oncology, Mayo Clinic, Rochester, MN 55905, USA; dandre.stacy@mayo.edu (S.D.); jatoi.aminah@mayo.edu (A.J.); ruddy.kathryn@mayo.edu (K.J.R.)

2 Department of Quantitative Health Sciences, Mayo Clinic College of Medicine and Science, Mayo Clinic, Rochester, MN 55905, USA; vierkant.robert@mayo.edu (R.A.V.); larson.nicole2@mayo.edu (N.L.L.); olsonj@mayo.edu (J.E.O.)

3 Research Advocacy Network, Plano, TX 75093, USA; mlsmith@researchadvocacy.org

4 Patient Advocate, Mayo Clinic Breast Cancer Specialized Program of Research Excellence (SPORE), Mayo Clinic, Rochester, MN 55905, USA; cynthiachauhan@aol.com

5 Department of Experimental Pathology & Laboratory Medicine, Mayo Clinic, Rochester, MN 55905, USA; couch.fergus@mayo.edu

* Correspondence: osullivan.ciara@mayo.edu; Tel.: +1-507-293-0526

Simple Summary: The high-level aims of the Advocate-BREAST initiative are to study and improve the overall experience of patients with breast cancer (BC) through education, shared decision making, and patient-centered clinical trials. Advocate-BREAST80+ is a survey substudy that specifically focused on the unique needs and perspectives of BC patients aged ≥80 years. Although patients aged ≥80 years experienced less anxiety and symptom-related distress compared with younger patients, they were significantly less satisfied with information regarding short and long term side effects of BC therapies, as well as the management of same. Older patients were significantly less likely to have participated in a clinical trial or be open to considering this option in future. Future research should address unique educational needs and barriers to research participation in older BC patients. Focused interviews could assist with better comprehension of the lived experience of these patients, given the smaller number of BC patients ≥80 years in many available databases.

Abstract: Background: There are limited evidence-based data to guide treatment recommendations for breast cancer (BC) patients ≥80 years (P80+). Identifying and addressing unmet needs are critical. Aims: Advocate-BREAST80+ compared the needs of P80+ vs. patients < 80 years (P80−). Methods: In 12/2021, a REDCap survey was electronically circulated to 6918 persons enrolled in the Mayo Clinic Breast Disease Registry. The survey asked about concerns and satisfaction with multiple aspects of BC care. Results: Overall, 2437 participants responded (35% response rate); 202 (8.3%) were P80+. P80+ were less likely to undergo local regional and systemic therapies vs. P80− ($p < 0.01$). Notably, P80+ were significantly less satisfied with information about the short and long-term side effects of BC therapies and managing toxicities. P80+ were also less likely to have participated in a clinical trial ($p < 0.001$) or to want to do so in the future ($p = 0.0001$). Conclusions: Although P80+ experienced less anxiety and symptom-related distress compared with P80−, they were significantly less satisfied with information regarding the side effects of BC therapies and their management. P80+ were significantly less likely to have participated in a clinical trial or be open to considering this option. Future studies should address educational needs pertaining to side effects and barriers to research participation in P80+.

Keywords: advocacy; breast cancer; older patients

1. Introduction

In 2023, approximately 297,790 American women were diagnosed with invasive breast cancer (BC) [1], and ~12% were aged ≥80 years [2]. Despite important advances in BC care, there are limited evidence-based data to guide treatment recommendations in patients ≥80 years (P80+), which can lead to both under and over-treatment [3], as well as limited data on these patients' perspectives on cancer and cancer therapy. Unique challenges in this patient population include concerns regarding treatment-related toxicities, comorbidities and limited life expectancy, and underrepresentation in clinical trials [4]. Furthermore, although BC biology in older women is often indolent [5], older patients may experience worse BC-specific outcomes when controlling for disease subtype and stage [4,6]. Older women with BC may also differ from younger women in their educational needs, but there are limited data regarding these needs [7]. Online patient resources devoted to this population are limited [8]. Therefore, identifying and addressing gaps will be a critical step toward the optimization of care for older BC patients and should be a clinical and research priority [9].

The Advocate-BREAST project, "Advocates and Patients' Advice to Enhance Breast Cancer Care Delivery, Patient Experience and Patient Centered Research", is a collaboration between breast oncologists at Mayo Clinic in Rochester (MCR), Minnesota, USA and Mayo Clinic BC Specialized Program of Research Excellence (SPORE) advocates. Its high level aims are to study and improve the overall patient experience through education, shared decision-making, and patient-centered clinical trials. The primary objective is to identify areas of unmet need in BC care delivery and research with the goal of improving patient experience and driving further research. We initially conducted a patient experience survey in BC survivors enrolled in the Mayo Clinic Breast Disease Registry (MCBDR) [10]. This paper presents the results of Advocate-BREAST80+, a survey substudy that compares the perspectives of P80+ with BC patients < 80 years (P80−) after having experienced a diagnosis of BC.

2. Methods

2.1. Advocate-BREAST Project Approach and Committee Formation

The Advocate-BREAST project uses a five-step framework: Connecting, Comprehending, Analyzing, Implementing, and Reflecting (Figure 1). The overall goals are outlined in Figure 2. The Mayo Clinic project management team included two Breast Medical Oncologists [C.O.S. and K.J.R.], a Research Program Co-Ordinator [N.L.], a statistician [R.V.], and two senior Mayo Clinic SPORE BC advocates [M.L.S. and C.C.].

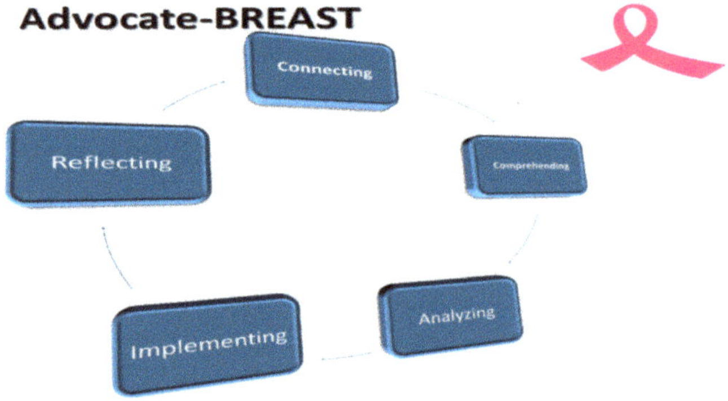

Figure 1. The Advocate-BREAST Project. Legend: The Advocate BREAST project involves 5 distinct steps as follows: 1. Connecting with advocates and patients to determine scope and focus of projects; 2. Comprehending the lived experience of EBC and MBC patients; 3. Developing, circulating surveys and analyzing results in partnership with patient advocates; 4. Implementing results to promote patient centered BC research and treatment; 5.Reflecting on process and considering ways to improve and repeat cycle.

1. Survey a population/populations of breast cancer patients to address satisfaction with aspects of Breast Cancer Care Delivery and Research (adjuvant vs. metastatic) **2022**
2. Analysis, presentation and publication of results **2022-2023**
3. Survey a population/populations of patient advocates to determine areas of unmet need in Breast Cancer Care Delivery and Research (adjuvant vs. metastatic) **2022**
4. Analysis, presentation and publication of results **2022-2023**
5. Identify ideas for pilot studies/projects and potentially clinical trials, prioritizing those which patient centered, and have the potential to make positive and tangible changes in a time sensitive manner **2022-2023**
6. Involve Research Advocacy Groups and Research Co-operative Groups **2023**
7. Determine and apply for funding sources (Grants, Other) **2024**
8. Conduct study/project/trial (s)(single center vs. multicenter) **2024 Onwards**

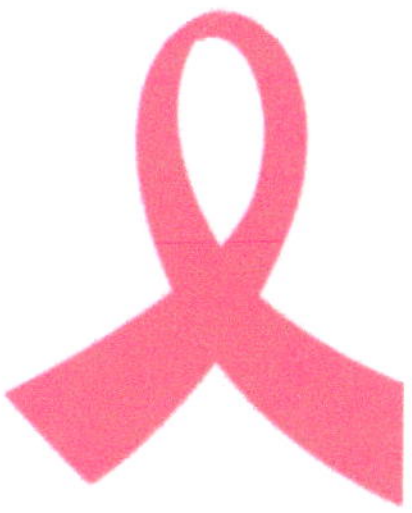

Figure 2. Goals of the Advocate BREAST Project.

2.2. Study Design and Recruitment

The Mayo Clinic Comprehensive Cancer Center (MCCC) is an NCI-designated comprehensive cancer center with three main campuses in Minnesota (MCR), Florida and Arizona. We conducted a retrospective cohort study of patients enrolled in the MCBDR, a prospective longitudinal cohort study that enrolls patients with stage 0–4 BC who were seen at least once at MCR within one year of diagnosis (2001–2021). Informed consent was obtained prior to registry enrollment. Patients were excluded if they had received an initial BC diagnosis more than one year prior, did not speak English, or did not live within the USA.

2.3. Data Collection and Processing

In MCBDR, demographic information, histopathological tumor characteristics and treatment-related factors are abstracted from the electronic medical record by trained nursing personnel. For this study, we accessed age, sex, date of BC diagnosis and disease stage. Patients were classified into three groups: ductal carcinoma in situ (DCIS; stage 0), invasive non-metastatic BC (stage 1–3), and metastatic breast cancer (MBC; stage 4) at time of survey completion. ZIP codes of residence were mapped to rural–urban commuting area (RUCA) codes, and rurality was defined as RUCA code 10 (i.e., >60 min road travel (one-way) to the closest edge of an urbanized area) [11]. The Mayo Clinic Institutional Review Board (IRB1815-04) reviewed and approved this study. Data were handled in a manner consistent with both US laws and the Declaration of Helsinki.

In addition to medical chart review, participants completed a survey developed by the study team (see below) addressing satisfaction with (i) multiple aspects of cancer care delivery and (ii) the education and/or support they receive(d) regarding practical, financial, emotional, societal and spiritual concerns linked to their diagnosis. Racial/ethnic, educational, rural/urban, and financial status data were used to inform the development of novel resources to address patient-reported gaps in care. Participants were also asked to rank potential QI projects in order of the likelihood the proposal could improve quality of life for patients and their families. Patients were also asked to comment on how care for BC patients might be improved, and their thoughts on what research topics should be prioritized. Feedback from P80+ was initially reviewed by the research program coordinator, who categorized the content. The Breast Medical Oncology team further reviewed the qualitative data and classified each theme as either major or minor based on the number of responses. Comments regarding suggestions for further research were noted separately. Responses were collected via anonymous local language questionnaires.

2.4. Survey

Our 23-page survey, containing 147 items, was developed to assess patient levels of concern and satisfaction with various aspects of their BC diagnosis and treatment. We used REDCap, a secure web application for developing and managing online surveys and databases that is specifically tailored to support online and offline data capture for research studies. A questionnaire was electronically sent to all MCBDR participants who were consented, alive, and had an e-mail address on file on 12/9/2021. Non-respondents were sent two reminder e-mails on 12/16 and 12/23/2021.

The questionnaire captured: 1. Demographic Information; 2. BC Treatment; 3. Concerns Regarding Side Effects of BC Treatment; 4. BC Clinical Care Concerns ([i] level of symptoms experienced during the first year after BC diagnosis and [ii] level of concern regarding health-related, practical, financial, emotional, societal and spiritual issues related to BC during that time); 5. Clinical Care BC Patient Experience ([i] overall satisfaction with BC care, [ii] satisfaction with information and support received from the care team as regards symptom management during first year after BC diagnosis, and [iii] satisfaction with information and support received from BC care team as regards practical, financial, emotional, societal and spiritual issues related to BC during the first year after diagnosis); 6. Ranking of Proposed QI Projects; 7. Integrative Medicine; 8. Medical Second Opinions; 9. Clinical Trial Participation; and 10. Thoughts/suggestions (patient comments) on [i] how care for BC patients could be improved and [ii] what research topics should be prioritized in BC.

Sections 3–5 of the questionnaire contained different numbers of items to be scored, each on a 10-point Likert scale. For Section 3 and some items in Section 4, respondents were asked to score their responses (0 = not at all concerned, 10 = highly concerned). Other items in Section 4 related to symptom severity, and were scored accordingly (0 = none, 10 = [symptom] as bad as I can imagine). For Section 5, respondents were asked to rate their overall satisfaction with their BC care (0 = very dissatisfied, 10 = extremely satisfied). For the satisfaction data, scores of 0–3 were rated as low satisfaction, scores of 4–6 were rated as moderate satisfaction, and scores of 7–10 were rated as high satisfaction. Section 6 of the questionnaire asked respondents to rate the likelihood that a proposed QI project would improve patient care (0 = none, vs. 10 = as much as I can imagine).

2.5. Statistical Analysis

Participants were dichotomized into two groups based on age at survey completion: those younger than 80 (hereafter referred to as P80−) and those 80 or older (P80+). Data were summarized using frequencies and percents for categorical variables and means, standard deviations (SDs), medians and interquartile ranges (IQRs) for continuous variables. We compared demographic and clinical characteristics across survey response status using chi-square tests of significance. Amongst those who returned surveys, associations of survey responses with dichotomized age were first univariately examined using two-sample t-tests for continuous variables and chi-square tests for categorical variables. All statistical tests were two-sided, and all analyses were carried out using the SAS System (SAS Institute, Inc., Cary, NC, USA).

3. Results

A total of 6918 MCBDR participants (6877 female) were sent surveys, and 2450 responses (response rate = 35.4%) were received. Thirteen males were excluded, resulting in a final study size of 2437. Overall, the mean age of participants was 64 (SD 11.8), and 202 (8.3%) were aged $\geq$80 years. The mean time from BC diagnosis at the time of the survey was 93.3 months (SD 70.2). Comparisons of the demographic and clinical characteristics of P80+ vs. P80− across survey response status are provided in Table 1. Survey responses are listed in Table 2.

Table 1. Demographic Information.

	Current Age			
	Under 80 (N = 2235)	**80 and Older (N = 202)**	**Total (N = 2437)**	***p*-Value**
	Demographic Characteristics			
Race, n (%)				0.0136 [1]
Non-White	65 (2.9%)	0 (0.0%)	65 (2.7%)	
White	2139 (97.1%)	201 (100.0%)	2340 (97.3%)	
Missing	31	1	32	
Ethnicity, n (%)				0.7161 [1]
Hispanic or Latino	27 (1.3%)	3 (1.6%)	30 (1.3%)	
Not Hispanic or Latino	2125 (98.7%)	189 (98.4%)	2314 (98.7%)	
Missing	83	10	93	
LGBTQIA, n (%)				0.0795 [1]
Yes	30 (1.4%)	0 (0.0%)	30 (1.3%)	
No	2166 (98.3%)	192 (99.0%)	2358 (98.4%)	
Unsure	7 (0.3%)	2 (1.0%)	9 (0.4%)	
Missing	32	8	40	
Marital status, n (%)				<0.0001 [1]
Married/living with someone	1811 (81.6%)	121 (61.1%)	1932 (79.9%)	
Separated/divorced	174 (7.8%)	9 (4.5%)	183 (7.6%)	
Widowed	126 (5.7%)	54 (27.3%)	180 (7.4%)	
Never been married	108 (4.9%)	14 (7.1%)	122 (5.0%)	
Missing	16	4	20	
Religion, n (%)				<0.0001 [1]
Catholic	630 (28.5%)	50 (25.1%)	680 (28.2%)	
Jewish/Ashkenazi Jewish	23 (1.0%)	2 (1.0%)	25 (1.0%)	
Protestant	830 (37.5%)	115 (57.8%)	945 (39.2%)	
Islam/Muslim	37 (1.7%)	7 (3.5%)	44 (1.8%)	
Other	392 (17.7%)	13 (6.5%)	405 (16.8%)	
None	302 (13.6%)	12 (6.0%)	314 (13.0%)	
Missing	21	3	24	
English is first language, n (%)				0.1874 [1]
Yes	2145 (97.5%)	196 (99.0%)	2341 (97.6%)	
No	55 (2.5%)	2 (1.0%)	57 (2.4%)	
Missing	35	4	39	
Residency based on Census tract, n (%)				0.0136 [1]
Non-Rural	2008 (90.2%)	171 (84.7%)	2179 (89.7%)	
Rural	219 (9.8%)	31 (15.3%)	250 (10.3%)	
Missing	8	0	8	
Patient has primary care provider at Mayo Clinic, n (%)				0.3645 [1]
No	1465 (65.5%)	126 (62.4%)	1591 (65.3%)	
Yes	770 (34.5%)	76 (37.6%)	846 (34.7%)	
Months since breast cancer diagnosis, n (%)				<0.0001 [1]
<12 months	181 (8.1%)	4 (2.0%)	185 (7.6%)	
12–23 months	183 (8.2%)	6 (3.0%)	189 (7.8%)	
24–35 months	222 (9.9%)	7 (3.5%)	229 (9.4%)	
36–59 months	397 (17.8%)	30 (14.9%)	427 (17.5%)	
60–119 months	530 (23.7%)	43 (21.3%)	573 (23.5%)	
120+ months	722 (32.3%)	112 (55.4%)	834 (34.2%)	

Table 1. *Cont.*

	Current Age			
	Under 80 (N = 2235)	80 and Older (N = 202)	Total (N = 2437)	*p*-Value
BC stage, n (%)				0.2571 [1]
Stage 0	361 (17.7%)	31 (15.7%)	392 (17.5%)	
Stage 1–3	1640 (80.4%)	165 (83.8%)	1805 (80.7%)	
Stage 4	40 (2.0%)	1 (0.5%)	41 (1.8%)	
Missing	194	5	199	
Primary Breast Cancer Treatment Location(s), n (%)				0.0531 [1]
Mayo Clinic Sites	1528 (68.8%)	152 (76.8%)	1680 (69.4%)	
Other (Non-Mayo Clinic)	135 (6.1%)	7 (3.5%)	142 (5.9%)	
Both (Mayo Clinic and Non-Mayo Clinic)	559 (25.2%)	39 (19.7%)	598 (24.7%)	
Missing	13	4	17	
Was surgery recommended, n (%)?				0.0062 [1]
Yes	2135 (96.9%)	181 (92.8%)	2316 (96.6%)	
No	58 (2.6%)	13 (6.7%)	71 (3.0%)	
Unsure	10 (0.5%)	1 (0.5%)	11 (0.5%)	
Missing	32	7	39	
If surgery was recommended, did you proceed with it, n (%)?				0.5643 [1]
Yes	2075 (98.6%)	175 (97.8%)	2250 (98.5%)	
No	28 (1.3%)	4 (2.2%)	32 (1.4%)	
Unsure	2 (0.1%)	0 (0.0%)	2 (0.1%)	
Missing	130	23	153	
Was chemotherapy recommended, n (%)?				<0.0001 [1]
Yes	950 (43.2%)	42 (21.8%)	992 (41.5%)	
No	1221 (55.6%)	142 (73.6%)	1363 (57.0%)	
Unsure	27 (1.2%)	9 (4.7%)	36 (1.5%)	
Missing	37	9	46	
If chemotherapy was recommended, did you proceed with it, n (%)?				0.1641 [1]
Yes	878 (93.4%)	36 (87.8%)	914 (93.2%)	
No	62 (6.6%)	5 (12.2%)	67 (6.8%)	
Missing	1295	161	1456	
Was radiotherapy recommended, n (%)?				0.0037 [1]
Yes	1463 (66.5%)	111 (58.4%)	1574 (65.9%)	
No	705 (32.0%)	71 (37.4%)	776 (32.5%)	
Unsure	32 (1.5%)	8 (4.2%)	40 (1.7%)	
Missing	35	12	47	
If radiotherapy was recommended, did you proceed with it, n (%)?				0.6635 [1]
Yes	1346 (93.9%)	102 (92.7%)	1448 (93.8%)	
No	82 (5.7%)	8 (7.3%)	90 (5.8%)	
Unsure	5 (0.3%)	0 (0.0%)	5 (0.3%)	
Missing	802	92	894	
Was endocrine (anti-estrogen) therapy recommended, n (%)?				<0.0001 [1]
Yes	1296 (59.2%)	68 (35.8%)	1364 (57.3%)	
No	708 (32.3%)	76 (40.0%)	784 (33.0%)	
Unsure	185 (8.5%)	46 (24.2%)	231 (9.7%)	
Missing	46	12	58	

Table 1. *Cont.*

	Current Age			
	Under 80 (N = 2235)	**80 and Older (N = 202)**	**Total (N = 2437)**	***p*-Value**
If endocrine therapy was recommended, did you proceed with it, n (%)?				0.0011 [1]
Yes	1154 (90.8%)	57 (85.1%)	1211 (90.5%)	
No	114 (9.0%)	8 (11.9%)	122 (9.1%)	
Unsure	3 (0.2%)	2 (3.0%)	5 (0.4%)	
Missing	964	135	1099	
Was targeted biologic therapy recommended, n (%)?				<0.0001 [1]
Yes	104 (4.8%)	5 (2.7%)	109 (4.6%)	
No	1707 (78.1%)	121 (65.1%)	1828 (77.1%)	
Unsure	374 (17.1%)	60 (32.3%)	434 (18.3%)	
Missing	50	16	66	
If targeted biologic therapy was recommended, did you proceed with it, n (%)?				0.0940 [1]
Yes	99 (96.1%)	4 (80.0%)	103 (95.4%)	
No	4 (3.9%)	1 (20.0%)	5 (4.6%)	
Missing	2132	197	2329	
Was immunotherapy recommended, n (%)?				<0.0001 [1]
Yes	100 (4.6%)	3 (1.6%)	103 (4.3%)	
No	1786 (81.3%)	138 (73.0%)	1924 (80.6%)	
Unsure	311 (14.2%)	48 (25.4%)	359 (15.0%)	
Missing	38	13	51	
If immunotherapy was recommended, did you proceed with it, n (%)?				0.0015 [1]
Yes	98 (98.0%)	2 (66.7%)	100 (97.1%)	
No	2 (2.0%)	1 (33.3%)	3 (2.9%)	
Missing	2135	199	2334	

[1] Chi-Square *p*-value.

Table 2. Survey Responses.

	Unweighted			Weighted		
	Under 80 (N = 2235)	80 and Older (N = 202)	*p*–Value	Under 80	80 and Older	*p*-Value
	Level of symptom experienced in first year after breast cancer diagnosis (10-point scale, 0 = none, 10 = as bad as I could imagine)					
Hair loss/thinning			<0.0001 [2]			0.0412 [4]
N	2180	191				
Mean (SD)	4.0 (4.23)	2.2 (3.41)		3.9 (3.21)	3.5 (9.37)	
Median (IQR)	2.0 (0.0, 9.0)	0.0 (0.0, 4.0)		2.0 (0.0–9.0)	2.0 (0.0–6.0)	
Hot flashes			<0.0001 [2]			<0.0001 [4]
N	2179	190				
Mean (SD)	3.8 (3.52)	1.5 (2.51)		3.8 (2.68)	1.6 (6.12)	
Median (IQR)	3.0 (0.0, 7.0)	0.0 (0.0, 2.0)		3.0 (0.0–7.0)	0.0 (0.0–2.0)	
Eyebrow/Eyelash thinning			<0.0001 [2]			<0.0001 [4]
N	2164	189				
Mean (SD)	3.6 (4.11)	1.6 (2.98)		3.5 (3.11)	2.2 (7.74)	
Median (IQR)	1.0 (0.0, 8.0)	0.0 (0.0, 2.0)		1.0 (0.0–8.0)	0.0 (0.0–4.0)	
Sexual dysfunction			<0.0001 [2]			<0.0001 [4]
N	2154	184				
Mean (SD)	3.2 (3.36)	0.9 (2.10)		3.2 (2.55)	1.0 (5.54)	
Median (IQR)	2.0 (0.0, 6.0)	0.0 (0.0, 0.0)		2.0 (0.0–6.0)	0.0 (0.0–0.0)	
Cognitive/memory issues (i.e., brain fog or chemo brain)			<0.0001 [2]			<0.0001 [4]
N	2180	192				
Mean (SD)	2.9 (3.25)	0.8 (1.73)		2.8 (2.47)	1.0 (4.46)	
Median (IQR)	2.0 (0.0, 6.0)	0.0 (0.0, 1.0)		1.0 (0.0–5.0)	0.0 (0.0–2.0)	
The numbness and/or tingling in your hands and/or feet			<0.0001 [2]			0.9199 [4]
N	2180	190				
Mean (SD)	2.1 (2.91)	1.2 (2.39)		2.0 (2.21)	2.0 (7.04)	
Median (IQR)	0.0 (0.0, 3.0)	0.0 (0.0, 1.0)		0.0 (0.0–3.0)	0.0 (0.0–3.0)	

Table 2. *Cont.*

	Unweighted			Weighted		
	Under 80 (N = 2235)	80 and Older (N = 202)	*p*–Value	Under 80	80 and Older	*p*-Value
The swelling in your arm or arms			0.0137 [2]			<0.0001 [4]
N	2176	191				
Mean (SD)	1.2 (2.24)	0.8 (1.84)		1.2 (1.71)	0.8 (4.28)	
Median (IQR)	0.0 (0.0, 1.0)	0.0 (0.0, 0.0)		0.0 (0.0–1.0)	0.0 (0.0–0.0)	
	Level of concern regarding issues within first year after breast cancer diagnosis (10-point scale, 0 = not at all concerned, 10 = highly concerned)					
Breast cancer recurrence or spread			<0.0001 [2]			<0.0001 [4]
N	2161	185				
Mean (SD)	4.9 (3.62)	2.7 (3.16)		4.8 (2.78)	3.3 (8.11)	
Median (IQR)	5.0 (1.0, 8.0)	2.0 (0.0, 5.0)		5.0 (1.0–8.0)	2.0 (0.0–5.0)	
Concerns as regards how loved ones will cope practically and emotionally if you pass away from breast cancer			<0.0001 [2]			<0.0001 [4]
N	2159	180				
Mean (SD)	4.7 (3.68)	2.7 (2.98)		4.6 (2.81)	3.6 (8.43)	
Median (IQR)	5.0 (1.0, 8.0)	2.0 (0.0, 5.0)		5.0 (1.0–8.0)	2.0 (0.0–6.0)	
Your diagnosis and prognosis			<0.0001 [2]			<0.0001 [4]
N	2158	181				
Mean (SD)	4.4 (3.39)	2.5 (3.02)		4.4 (2.58)	3.2 (8.21)	
Median (IQR)	4.0 (1.0, 8.0)	1.0 (0.0, 4.0)		4.0 (1.0–7.0)	2.0 (0.0–5.0)	
Fear of dying from breast cancer			<0.0001 [2]			<0.0001 [4]
N	2166	184				
Mean (SD)	4.0 (3.53)	2.0 (2.61)		4.0 (2.68)	2.5 (7.17)	
Median (IQR)	3.0 (1.0, 7.0)	1.0 (0.0, 3.0)		3.0 (1.0–7.0)	1.0 (0.0–5.0)	
Your weight and/or physical fitness level			<0.0001 [2]			<0.0001 [4]
N	2163	185				
Mean (SD)	3.9 (3.12)	1.9 (2.42)		3.9 (2.37)	2.4 (6.28)	
Median (IQR)	4.0 (1.0, 6.0)	1.0 (0.0, 4.0)		4.0 (1.0–6.0)	2.0 (0.0–4.0)	

Table 2. *Cont.*

	Unweighted			Weighted		
	Under 80 (N = 2235)	80 and Older (N = 202)	*p*-Value	Under 80	80 and Older	*p*-Value
Your emotional health			<0.0001 [2]			<0.0001 [4]
N	2149	182				
Mean (SD)	4.0 (3.19)	1.7 (2.42)		3.9 (2.43)	2.0 (6.17)	
Median (IQR)	4.0 (1.0, 7.0)	1.0 (0.0, 3.0)		3.0 (1.0–7.0)	1.0 (0.0–3.0)	
The emotional health of others (partner, children, other family members)			<0.0001 [2]			<0.0001 [4]
N	2161	185				
Mean (SD)	3.5 (3.17)	1.5 (2.26)		3.5 (2.42)	2.0 (6.32)	
Median (IQR)	3.0 (0.0, 6.0)	0.0 (0.0, 2.0)		3.0 (0.0–6.0)	1.0 (0.0–3.0)	
Your quality of life			<0.0001 [2]			<0.0001 [4]
N	2158	182				
Mean (SD)	3.5 (3.18)	1.9 (2.73)		3.4 (2.42)	2.3 (6.94)	
Median (IQR)	3.0 (0.0, 6.0)	0.0 (0.0, 3.0)		3.0 (0.0–6.0)	1.0 (0.0–4.0)	
Your bone health			0.0001 [2]			<0.0001 [4]
N	2163	183				
Mean (SD)	3.4 (3.22)	2.5 (2.90)		3.4 (2.44)	2.6 (6.66)	
Median (IQR)	3.0 (0.0, 6.0)	1.0 (0.0, 5.0)		3.0 (0.0–6.0)	2.0 (0.0–5.0)	
Your nutrition/diet			<0.0001 [2]			<0.0001 [4]
N	2159	183				
Mean (SD)	3.3 (3.07)	1.7 (2.42)		3.3 (2.33)	2.0 (5.96)	
Median (IQR)	3.0 (0.0, 5.0)	0.0 (0.0, 3.0)		3.0 (0.0–5.0)	1.0 (0.0–4.0)	
Your self-esteem/self-confidence			<0.0001 [2]			<0.0001 [4]
N	2157	185				
Mean (SD)	3.3 (3.17)	1.6 (2.43)		3.3 (2.42)	1.8 (6.32)	
Median (IQR)	2.0 (0.0, 6.0)	0.0 (0.0, 2.0)		2.0 (0.0–6.0)	0.0 (0.0–3.0)	
Changes in intimacy with your partner			<0.0001 [2]			<0.0001 [4]
N	2134	183				
Mean (SD)	3.4 (3.50)	0.8 (1.96)		3.3 (2.67)	1.0 (5.69)	
Median (IQR)	2.0 (0.0, 6.0)	0.0 (0.0, 0.0)		2.0 (0.0–6.0)	0.0 (0.0–0.0)	

Table 2. *Cont.*

	Unweighted			Weighted		
	Under 80 (N = 2235)	80 and Older (N = 202)	p–Value	Under 80	80 and Older	p-Value
Body image/attractiveness/sexuality			<0.0001 [2]			<0.0001 [4]
N	2156	184				
Mean (SD)	3.4 (3.37)	1.1 (2.10)		3.3 (2.57)	1.5 (5.82)	
Median (IQR)	2.0 (0.0, 6.0)	0.0 (0.0, 2.0)		2.0 (0.0–6.0)	0.0 (0.0–2.0)	
Existential Issues (anxiety and/or questions regarding the meaning of life and/or your purpose in life)			<0.0001 [2]			<0.0001 [4]
N	2155	183				
Mean (SD)	3.0 (3.25)	1.5 (2.33)		3.0 (2.48)	1.8 (6.17)	
Median (IQR)	2.0 (0.0, 5.0)	0.0 (0.0, 2.0)		2.0 (0.0–5.0)	0.0 (0.0–3.0)	
Pressure to keep positive about your breast cancer diagnosis			<0.0001 [2]			<0.0001 [4]
N	2157	183				
Mean (SD)	2.7 (3.18)	1.3 (2.35)		2.7 (2.42)	1.8 (6.82)	
Median (IQR)	1.0 (0.0, 5.0)	0.0 (0.0, 1.0)		1.0 (0.0–5.0)	0.0 (0.0–3.0)	
Your heart health			0.0005 [2]			0.0395 [4]
N	2161	186				
Mean (SD)	2.5 (3.00)	1.8 (2.62)		2.5 (2.28)	2.2 (7.20)	
Median (IQR)	1.0 (0.0, 5.0)	0.0 (0.0, 3.0)		1.0 (0.0–5.0)	0.0 (0.0–5.0)	
Genetic testing/counseling for family members			<0.0001 [2]			<0.0001 [4]
N	2143	182				
Mean (SD)	2.6 (3.27)	1.3 (2.49)		2.5 (2.48)	1.9 (6.47)	
Median (IQR)	1.0 (0.0, 5.0)	0.0 (0.0, 2.0)		1.0 (0.0–5.0)	0.0 (0.0–3.0)	
Advocating for yourself as it relates to your breast cancer diagnosis			<0.0001 [2]			<0.0001 [4]
N	2141	184				
Mean (SD)	2.6 (3.24)	1.1 (2.21)		2.6 (2.47)	1.5 (5.78)	
Median (IQR)	1.0 (0.0, 5.0)	0.0 (0.0, 1.0)		1.0 (0.0–5.0)	0.0 (0.0–2.0)	

Table 2. *Cont.*

	Unweighted			Weighted		
	Under 80 (N = 2235)	80 and Older (N = 202)	p–Value	Under 80	80 and Older	p-Value
Genetic testing/counseling for yourself			<0.0001 [2]			<0.0001 [4]
N	2143	181				
Mean (SD)	2.5 (3.18)	1.1 (2.40)		2.4 (2.41)	1.5 (6.51)	
Median (IQR)	1.0 (0.0, 5.0)	0.0 (0.0, 1.0)		1.0 (0.0–5.0)	0.0 (0.0–2.0)	
The impact of your cancer diagnosis on your home responsibilities			<0.0001 [2]			<0.0001 [4]
N	2158	181				
Mean (SD)	2.5 (2.98)	1.1 (2.06)		2.4 (2.26)	1.5 (6.18)	
Median (IQR)	1.0 (0.0, 5.0)	0.0 (0.0, 1.0)		1.0 (0.0–4.0)	0.0 (0.0–2.0)	
Changes in your relationships with friends and/or family members			<0.0001 [2]			<0.0001 [4]
N	2153	185				
Mean (SD)	2.3 (2.94)	0.7 (1.83)		2.2 (2.22)	1.2 (5.98)	
Median (IQR)	1.0 (0.0, 4.0)	0.0 (0.0, 0.0)		1.0 (0.0–4.0)	0.0 (0.0–1.0)	
Ease of access to/communication with your oncology care team			0.0229 [2]			0.0475 [4]
N	2154	182				
Mean (SD)	1.9 (2.95)	1.4 (2.71)		1.9 (2.25)	1.7 (6.78)	
Median (IQR)	0.0 (0.0, 3.0)	0.0 (0.0, 1.0)		0.0 (0.0–3.0)	0.0 (0.0–2.0)	
The impact of your cancer diagnosis on your employment status and your career			<0.0001 [2]			<0.0001 [4]
N	2153	183				
Mean (SD)	1.9 (3.04)	0.5 (1.99)		1.9 (2.29)	0.4 (3.78)	
Median (IQR)	0.0 (0.0, 3.0)	0.0 (0.0, 0.0)		0.0 (0.0–3.0)	0.0 (0.0–0.0)	
Pressure to keep family and friends updated as regards your breast cancer diagnosis and the plan for treatment			<0.0001 [2]			<0.0001 [4]
N	2150	182				
Mean (SD)	1.9 (2.57)	0.9 (2.09)		1.8 (1.96)	1.3 (6.22)	
Median (IQR)	1.0 (0.0, 3.0)	0.0 (0.0, 1.0)		1.0 (0.0–3.0)	0.0 (0.0–1.0)	

Table 2. *Cont.*

	Unweighted			Weighted		
	Under 80 (N = 2235)	**80 and Older (N = 202)**	***p*–Value**	**Under 80**	**80 and Older**	***p*-Value**
The need for privacy regarding your breast cancer diagnosis			<0.0001 [2]			<0.0001 [4]
N	2150	183				
Mean (SD)	1.8 (2.78)	1.0 (2.26)		1.8 (2.11)	1.1 (5.61)	
Median (IQR)	0.0 (0.0, 3.0)	0.0 (0.0, 0.0)		0.0 (0.0–3.0)	0.0 (0.0–1.0)	
The impact of your breast cancer diagnosis on dating and/or socializing			<0.0001 [2]			<0.0001 [4]
N	2146	184				
Mean (SD)	1.6 (2.72)	0.4 (1.51)		1.6 (2.07)	0.8 (4.26)	
Median (IQR)	0.0 (0.0, 2.0)	0.0 (0.0, 0.0)		0.0 (0.0–2.0)	0.0 (0.0–0.0)	
Your fertility			0.0012 [2]			<0.0001 [4]
N	2147	182				
Mean (SD)	0.5 (2.01)	0.0 (0.35)		0.5 (1.52)	0.0 (0.92)	
Median (IQR)	0.0 (0.0, 0.0)	0.0 (0.0, 0.0)		0.0 (0.0–0.0)	0.0 (0.0–0.0)	
Cultural and/or religious concerns related to your breast cancer diagnosis and treatment			0.9544 [2]			0.6661 [4]
N	2149	184				
Mean (SD)	0.4 (1.25)	0.4 (1.41)		0.4 (0.94)	0.4 (3.34)	
Median (IQR)	0.0 (0.0, 0.0)	0.0 (0.0, 0.0)		0.0 (0.0–0.0)	0.0 (0.0–0.0)	
Satisfaction of breast cancer patient experience (10-point scale, 0 = very dissatisfied, 10 = very satisfied)						
How satisfied have you been with your breast cancer care overall to date			0.1566 [2]			0.0015 [4]
N	2155	183				
Mean (SD)	8.9 (1.76)	9.1 (2.07)		8.9 (1.35)	9.1 (4.78)	
Median (IQR)	10.0 (8.0, 10.0)	10.0 (9.0, 10.0)		10 (8.0–10)	10 (9.0–10)	
How satisfied were/are you overall with the information and support you receive(d) from your cancer care teams			0.6385 [2]			0.9826 [4]
N	2159	183				
Mean (SD)	8.9 (1.83)	8.8 (2.46)		8.9 (1.41)	8.9 (5.91)	
Median (IQR)	10.0 (8.0, 10.0)	10.0 (9.0, 10.0)		10 (8.0–10)	10 (9.0–10)	

Table 2. *Cont.*

	Unweighted			Weighted		
	Under 80 (N = 2235)	**80 and Older (N = 202)**	***p*–Value**	**Under 80**	**80 and Older**	***p*-Value**
	Satisfaction of breast cancer information and support received from cancer care team for symptoms (10-point scale, 0 = very dissatisfied, 10 = very satisfied)					
The short-term side effects of breast cancer surgery			0.0140 [2]			0.5266 [4]
N	1844	119				
Mean (SD)	7.8 (2.77)	7.2 (3.41)		7.8 (2.12)	7.7 (8.27)	
Median (IQR)	9.0 (7.0, 10.0)	9.0 (5.0, 10.0)		9.0 (7.0–10)	9.0 (6.0–10)	
The short-term side effects of radiotherapy			<0.0001 [2]			<0.0001 [4]
N	1318	82				
Mean (SD)	7.7 (2.99)	6.3 (3.89)		7.6 (2.31)	6.8 (9.97)	
Median (IQR)	9.0 (7.0, 10.0)	8.0 (2.0, 10.0)		9.0 (6.0–10)	8.0 (5.0–10)	
The long-term side effects of breast cancer surgery			0.0730 [2]			0.7805 [4]
N	1825	118				
Mean (SD)	7.3 (2.97)	6.8 (3.63)		7.3 (2.28)	7.3 (8.81)	
Median (IQR)	8.0 (5.0, 10.0)	8.5 (4.0, 10.0)		8.0 (5.0–10)	9.0 (5.0–10)	
The side effects of endocrine therapy (i.e., hormone blocking treatment)			0.1811 [2]			0.0638 [4]
N	1256	64				
Mean (SD)	7.0 (3.09)	6.4 (3.75)		6.9 (2.35)	7.3 (8.61)	
Median (IQR)	8.0 (5.0, 10.0)	8.0 (4.0, 10.0)		8.0 (5.0–10)	9.0 (5.0–10)	
The short-term side effects of chemotherapy			<0.0001 [2]			<0.0001 [4]
N	942	49				
Mean (SD)	7.1 (3.30)	4.2 (3.99)		7.0 (2.51)	5.5 (10.5)	
Median (IQR)	8.0 (5.0, 10.0)	4.0 (0.0, 8.0)		8.0 (5.0–10)	6.0 (2.0–8.0)	
The long-term side effects of radiotherapy			0.0277 [2]			<0.0001 [4]
N	1287	76				
Mean (SD)	7.0 (3.24)	6.1 (3.87)		6.9 (2.47)	6.0 (9.99)	
Median (IQR)	8.0 (5.0, 10.0)	8.0 (2.5, 10.0)		8.0 (5.0–10)	8.0 (4.0–9.0)	

Table 2. *Cont.*

	Unweighted			Weighted		
	Under 80 (N = 2235)	80 and Older (N = 202)	*p*–Value	Under 80	80 and Older	*p*-Value
Hot flashes			<0.0001 [2]			<0.0001 [4]
N	1347	63				
Mean (SD)	7.0 (3.05)	4.8 (4.22)		7.0 (2.32)	4.5 (9.22)	
Median (IQR)	8.0 (5.0, 10.0)	5.0 (0.0, 10.0)		8.0 (5.0–10)	4.0 (0.0–10)	
The swelling in your arm or arms			<0.0001 [2]			<0.0001 [4]
N	933	67				
Mean (SD)	6.7 (3.64)	4.6 (4.24)		6.6 (2.78)	4.4 (11.1)	
Median (IQR)	8.0 (4.0, 10.0)	5.0 (0.0, 9.0)		8.0 (4.0–10)	4.0 (0.0–9.0)	
Hair loss/thinning			0.0030 [2]			0.0066 [4]
N	1214	77				
Mean (SD)	6.5 (3.40)	5.4 (3.74)		6.5 (2.58)	6.0 (9.64)	
Median (IQR)	8.0 (4.0, 10.0)	5.0 (2.0, 9.0)		8.0 (4.0–10)	7.0 (3.0–9.0)	
The numbness and/or tingling in your hands and/or feet			<0.0001 [2]			0.0062 [4]
N	1064	70				
Mean (SD)	6.5 (3.39)	4.3 (3.84)		6.4 (2.58)	5.8 (10.2)	
Median (IQR)	8.0 (4.0, 9.0)	4.0 (0.0, 8.0)		8.0 (4.0–9.0)	7.0 (3.0–10)	
Eyebrow/Eyelash thinning			0.0070 [2]			0.1417 [4]
N	1107	71				
Mean (SD)	6.3 (3.48)	5.1 (3.84)		6.2 (2.64)	5.9 (10.2)	
Median (IQR)	7.0 (4.0, 10.0)	5.0 (1.0, 9.0)		7.0 (4.0–10)	7.0 (3.0–9.0)	
The long-term side effects of chemotherapy			0.0021 [2]			0.4551 [4]
N	932	50				
Mean (SD)	6.2 (3.46)	4.6 (4.03)		6.1 (2.61)	6.0 (10.5)	
Median (IQR)	7.0 (3.0, 9.0)	5.0 (0.0, 8.0)		7.0 (3.0–9.0)	8.0 (3.0–8.0)	
Sexual dysfunction			<0.0001 [2]			<0.0001 [4]
N	1125	51				
Mean (SD)	5.8 (3.34)	3.0 (3.69)		5.8 (2.53)	2.7 (7.28)	
Median (IQR)	6.0 (3.0, 9.0)	2.0 (0.0, 5.0)		6.0 (3.0–9.0)	2.0 (0.0–3.0)	

Table 2. *Cont.*

	Unweighted			Weighted		
	Under 80 (N = 2235)	80 and Older (N = 202)	*p*–Value	Under 80	80 and Older	*p*-Value
The potential side effects of targeted biologic therapies			0.0008 [2]			0.0110 [4]
N	342	22				
Mean (SD)	4.9 (4.23)	1.8 (3.43)		4.8 (3.20)	3.7 (11.1)	
Median (IQR)	5.0 (0.0, 9.0)	0.0 (0.0, 2.0)		5.0 (0.0–9.0)	5.0 (0.0–5.0)	
The side effects of immunotherapy			0.0320 [2]			0.0293 [4]
N	343	26				
Mean (SD)	4.4 (4.07)	2.6 (3.91)		4.3 (3.08)	3.3 (9.81)	
Median (IQR)	4.0 (0.0, 9.0)	0.0 (0.0, 5.0)		4.0 (0.0–8.0)	0.0 (0.0–7.0)	
Satisfaction of breast cancer information and support received from cancer care team for concerns (10-point scale, 0 = very dissatisfied, 10 = very satisfied)						
Availability of information related to your cancer diagnosis (e.g., scan results, medical notes)			0.7445 [2]			0.0793 [4]
N	1878	133				
Mean (SD)	8.8 (2.09)	8.9 (2.34)		8.8 (1.61)	9.0 (5.74)	
Median (IQR)	10.0 (8.0, 10.0)	10.0 (9.0, 10.0)		10 (8.0–10)	10 (9.0–10)	
Ease of access to/communication with your cancer care team			0.8561 [2]			0.3358 [4]
N	1903	142				
Mean (SD)	8.8 (2.06)	8.7 (2.36)		8.8 (1.59)	8.7 (5.74)	
Median (IQR)	10.0 (8.0, 10.0)	10.0 (8.0, 10.0)		10 (8.0–10)	10 (9.0–10)	
The amount of information available to you about your breast cancer diagnosis and your treatment plan			0.9373 [2]			0.5537 [4]
N	1884	139				
Mean (SD)	8.7 (2.17)	8.7 (2.46)		8.7 (1.66)	8.6 (5.73)	
Median (IQR)	10.0 (8.0, 10.0)	10.0 (8.0, 10.0)		10 (8.0–10)	10 (8.0–10)	
Your diagnosis and prognosis			0.2169 [2]			0.5283 [4]
N	1843	123				
Mean (SD)	8.1 (2.41)	7.9 (3.02)		8.1 (1.84)	8.2 (6.91)	
Median (IQR)	9.0 (8.0, 10.0)	9.0 (7.0, 10.0)		9.0 (8.0–10)	9.0 (8.0–10)	

Table 2. *Cont.*

	Unweighted			Weighted		
	Under 80 (N = 2235)	80 and Older (N = 202)	*p*–Value	Under 80	80 and Older	*p*-Value
Advocating for yourself as it relates to your breast cancer diagnosis			0.6014 [2]			0.7448 [4]
N	1502	95				
Mean (SD)	7.9 (2.70)	8.1 (2.84)		7.9 (2.05)	8.0 (6.65)	
Median (IQR)	9.0 (7.0, 10.0)	10.0 (7.0, 10.0)		9.0 (7.0–10)	9.0 (8.0–10)	
Genetic testing/counseling for yourself			0.0239 [2]			<0.0001 [4]
N	1334	54				
Mean (SD)	7.9 (2.93)	6.9 (3.41)		7.8 (2.25)	7.0 (7.99)	
Median (IQR)	9.0 (7.0, 10.0)	8.0 (5.0, 10.0)		9.0 (7.0–10)	7.0 (5.0–10)	
Breast cancer recurrence or spread			0.0889 [2]			0.7230 [4]
N	1686	111				
Mean (SD)	7.6 (2.64)	7.1 (3.36)		7.6 (2.01)	7.5 (8.16)	
Median (IQR)	8.0 (6.0, 10.0)	8.0 (5.0, 10.0)		8.0 (6.0–10)	9.0 (6.0–10)	
The need for privacy regarding your breast cancer diagnosis			0.1535 [2]			<0.0001 [4]
N	1127	62				
Mean (SD)	7.5 (3.11)	6.9 (3.73)		7.5 (2.38)	6.1 (10.1)	
Median (IQR)	9.0 (5.0, 10.0)	8.0 (5.0, 10.0)		9.0 (5.0–10)	7.0 (2.0–10)	
Your quality of life			0.9638 [2]			0.5924 [4]
N	1583	94				
Mean (SD)	7.4 (2.74)	7.4 (3.41)		7.4 (2.10)	7.5 (7.90)	
Median (IQR)	8.0 (5.0, 10.0)	9.0 (7.0, 10.0)		8.0 (6.0–10)	8.0 (7.0–10)	
Your bone health			0.8132 [2]			0.0122 [4]
N	1522	104				
Mean (SD)	7.3 (2.87)	7.2 (3.05)		7.3 (2.19)	7.7 (7.07)	
Median (IQR)	8.0 (5.0, 10.0)	8.0 (5.0, 10.0)		8.0 (5.0–10)	8.0 (5.0–10)	
Your emotional health			0.0583 [2]			0.0023 [4]
N	1620	89				
Mean (SD)	7.2 (2.81)	6.7 (3.46)		7.2 (2.14)	6.8 (7.86)	
Median (IQR)	8.0 (5.0, 10.0)	8.0 (5.0, 10.0)		8.0 (5.0–10)	8.0 (5.0–10)	

Table 2. *Cont.*

	Unweighted			Weighted		
	Under 80 (N = 2235)	80 and Older (N = 202)	p–Value	Under 80	80 and Older	p-Value
Ability to perform home responsibilities			0.3528 [2]			0.6902 [4]
N	1276	79				
Mean (SD)	7.2 (2.98)	6.9 (3.67)		7.2 (2.27)	7.3 (7.69)	
Median (IQR)	8.0 (5.0, 10.0)	9.0 (4.0, 10.0)		8.0 (5.0–10)	8.0 (6.0–10)	
Your self-esteem/self-confidence			0.1390 [2]			0.0012 [4]
N	1469	97				
Mean (SD)	7.1 (2.91)	7.5 (3.15)		7.1 (2.22)	7.6 (7.27)	
Median (IQR)	8.0 (5.0, 10.0)	9.0 (6.0, 10.0)		8.0 (5.0–10)	8.0 (7.0–10)	
Your weight and/or physical fitness level			0.0790 [2]			0.0242 [4]
N	1487	84				
Mean (SD)	7.1 (2.81)	6.5 (3.24)		7.1 (2.15)	6.8 (7.17)	
Median (IQR)	8.0 (5.0, 10.0)	8.0 (5.0, 9.0)		8.0 (5.0–10)	8.0 (5.0–9.0)	
Nutrition/diet			0.3873 [2]			0.2325 [4]
N	1499	84				
Mean (SD)	7.1 (2.89)	6.8 (3.35)		7.1 (2.19)	6.9 (7.85)	
Median (IQR)	8.0 (5.0, 10.0)	8.0 (5.0, 10.0)		8.0 (5.0–10)	8.0 (5.0–9.0)	
Fear of dying from breast cancer			0.4561 [2]			0.8885 [4]
N	1444	94				
Mean (SD)	7.0 (2.93)	6.8 (3.29)		7.0 (2.24)	7.0 (7.72)	
Median (IQR)	8.0 (5.0, 10.0)	8.0 (5.0, 10.0)		8.0 (5.0–10)	9.0 (5.0–9.0)	
Genetic testing/counseling for family members			0.2136 [2]			0.0271 [4]
N	1072	52				
Mean (SD)	7.0 (3.34)	6.4 (3.52)		7.0 (2.55)	6.5 (9.12)	
Median (IQR)	8.0 (5.0, 10.0)	7.0 (4.5, 10.0)		8.0 (5.0–10)	7.0 (5.0–10)	
Amount of information available to you about diet, nutrition and supplements			0.2805 [2]			0.2207 [4]
N	1675	102				
Mean (SD)	6.9 (3.09)	7.3 (3.11)		7.0 (2.34)	7.1 (7.35)	
Median (IQR)	8.0 (5.0, 10.0)	8.0 (5.0, 10.0)		8.0 (5.0–10)	8.0 (5.0–10)	

Table 2. *Cont.*

	Unweighted			Weighted		
	Under 80 (N = 2235)	**80 and Older (N = 202)**	***p*–Value**	**Under 80**	**80 and Older**	***p*-Value**
Your heart health			0.7540 [2]			0.0305 [4]
N	1355	91				
Mean (SD)	6.9 (2.98)	6.8 (3.16)		7.0 (2.26)	7.3 (7.06)	
Median (IQR)	8.0 (5.0, 10.0)	8.0 (5.0, 10.0)		8.0 (5.0–10)	8.0 (5.0–10)	
Amount of information available to you and your next of kin about advanced care directives, palliative medicine, hospice			0.4259 [2]			0.8057 [4]
N	969	70				
Mean (SD)	6.9 (3.34)	7.2 (3.57)		6.9 (2.55)	6.8 (8.38)	
Median (IQR)	8.0 (5.0, 10.0)	9.0 (5.0, 10.0)		8.0 (5.0–10)	7.0 (5.0–10)	
Pressure to keep family and friends updated as regards your breast cancer diagnosis and the plan for treatment			0.2879 [2]			0.0286 [4]
N	1086	69				
Mean (SD)	6.9 (3.10)	7.3 (3.57)		6.9 (2.37)	7.3 (8.67)	
Median (IQR)	8.0 (5.0, 10.0)	9.0 (5.0, 10.0)		8.0 (5.0–10)	9.0 (6.0–10)	
Pressure to keep positive about your breast cancer diagnosis			0.6017 [2]			0.8120 [4]
N	1182	74				
Mean (SD)	6.7 (3.14)	6.9 (3.61)		6.7 (2.39)	6.8 (8.75)	
Median (IQR)	8.0 (5.0, 10.0)	8.5 (5.0, 10.0)		8.0 (5.0–10)	8.0 (5.0–10)	
The emotional health of others (partner, children, other family members)			0.2264 [2]			0.8171 [4]
N	1389	78				
Mean (SD)	6.7 (3.05)	6.3 (3.42)		6.7 (2.32)	6.8 (8.06)	
Median (IQR)	8.0 (5.0, 10.0)	7.0 (4.0, 9.0)		8.0 (5.0–10)	8.0 (5.0–9.0)	
Cultural and/or religious concerns related to your breast cancer diagnosis and treatment			0.8936 [2]			0.0895 [4]
N	585	39				
Mean (SD)	6.5 (3.92)	6.4 (4.27)		6.5 (2.99)	7.0 (9.43)	
Median (IQR)	8.0 (3.0, 10.0)	9.0 (0.0, 10.0)		8.0 (3.0–10)	9.0 (6.0–10)	

Table 2. *Cont.*

	Unweighted			Weighted		
	Under 80 (N = 2235)	80 and Older (N = 202)	*p*–Value	Under 80	80 and Older	*p*-Value
Amount of information available to you about alternative medicine/complementary and integrative medicine			0.8773 [2]			0.0001 [4]
N	1488	80				
Mean (SD)	6.5 (3.35)	6.5 (3.64)		6.5 (2.55)	5.8 (9.58)	
Median (IQR)	7.0 (4.0, 10.0)	8.0 (4.0, 10.0)		7.0 (4.0–10)	6.0 (4.0–10)	
Body image/attractiveness/sexuality			0.3225 [2]			0.0132 [4]
N	1293	68				
Mean (SD)	6.4 (3.13)	6.0 (3.52)		6.4 (2.38)	5.9 (8.63)	
Median (IQR)	7.0 (5.0, 9.0)	6.0 (3.5, 9.0)		7.0 (4.0–9.0)	6.0 (4.0–9.0)	
Existential Issues (anxiety and/or questions regarding the meaning of life and/or your purpose in life)			0.5402 [2]			0.6197 [4]
N	1079	71				
Mean (SD)	6.3 (3.21)	6.1 (3.82)		6.3 (2.45)	6.4 (8.96)	
Median (IQR)	7.0 (4.0, 9.0)	7.0 (3.0, 10.0)		7.0 (4.0–9.0)	7.0 (4.0–10)	
Changes in your relationships with friends and/or family members			0.7054 [2]			0.2676 [4]
N	1057	63				
Mean (SD)	6.3 (3.28)	6.4 (3.90)		6.3 (2.50)	6.5 (9.33)	
Median (IQR)	7.0 (4.0, 9.0)	8.0 (3.0, 10.0)		7.0 (4.0–9.0)	8.0 (3.0–10)	
The impact of your cancer diagnosis on your employment status and your career			0.0565 [2]			<0.0001 [4]
N	904	23				
Mean (SD)	6.3 (3.53)	4.9 (4.63)		6.3 (2.69)	4.4 (9.22)	
Median (IQR)	7.0 (4.0, 10.0)	5.0 (0.0, 10.0)		7.0 (4.0–10)	2.0 (0.0–9.0)	
Cognitive/memory issues (i.e., brain fog or chemo brain)			0.3290 [2]			0.3409 [4]
N	1167	61				
Mean (SD)	6.3 (3.06)	5.9 (3.36)		6.3 (2.32)	6.1 (7.82)	
Median (IQR)	7.0 (4.0, 9.0)	6.0 (4.0, 9.0)		7.0 (4.0–9.0)	7.0 (4.0–8.0)	

Table 2. *Cont.*

	Unweighted			Weighted		
	Under 80 (N = 2235)	**80 and Older (N = 202)**	***p*–Value**	**Under 80**	**80 and Older**	***p*-Value**
Concerns as regards how loved ones will cope practically and emotionally if you pass away from breast cancer			0.5934 [2]			0.0022 [4]
N	1170	76				
Mean (SD)	6.3 (3.15)	6.1 (3.19)		6.2 (2.40)	6.8 (8.14)	
Median (IQR)	7.0 (4.0, 9.0)	6.0 (4.0, 9.0)		7.0 (4.0–9.0)	8.0 (5.0–10)	
Changes in intimacy with your partner			0.5182 [2]			0.0314 [4]
N	1164	51				
Mean (SD)	6.0 (3.20)	5.7 (3.83)		6.0 (2.43)	5.6 (9.16)	
Median (IQR)	6.0 (4.0, 9.0)	5.0 (2.0, 10.0)		6.0 (4.0–9.0)	5.0 (2.0–9.0)	
The impact of your breast cancer diagnosis on dating and/or socializing			0.2502 [2]			0.2292 [4]
N	756	29				
Mean (SD)	5.8 (3.58)	5.0 (4.61)		5.9 (2.73)	5.5 (11.3)	
Median (IQR)	6.0 (3.0, 9.0)	5.0 (0.0, 10.0)		6.0 (3.0–9.0)	5.0 (2.0–10)	
Your fertility			0.0019 [2]			<0.0001 [4]
N	367	11				
Mean (SD)	5.0 (4.26)	0.9 (3.02)		4.9 (3.23)	0.6 (4.84)	
Median (IQR)	5.0 (0.0, 10.0)	0.0 (0.0, 0.0)		5.0 (0.0–10)	0.0 (0.0–0.0)	
Quality of life How much do you think the following research ideas have to improve quality of life for patients with breast cancer and their families (10-point scale, 0 = none, 10 = as much as I can imagine)						
Lifetime Access to Online Patient Educational Resources			0.2588 [2]			0.3132 [4]
N	1883	136				
Mean (SD)	8.4 (2.34)	8.2 (2.75)		8.4 (1.79)	8.5 (6.03)	
Median (IQR)	10.0 (8.0, 10.0)	10.0 (7.0, 10.0)		10 (8.0–10)	10 (8.0–10)	
A Breast Cancer Wellness Program for EBC and MBC patients			0.0926 [2]			<0.0001 [4]
N	1879	137				
Mean (SD)	8.4 (2.31)	8.0 (2.75)		8.4 (1.77)	7.9 (6.51)	
Median (IQR)	9.0 (8.0, 10.0)	10.0 (7.0, 10.0)		9.0 (8.0–10)	9.0 (6.0–10)	

Table 2. *Cont.*

	Unweighted			Weighted		
	Under 80 (N = 2235)	80 and Older (N = 202)	p–Value	Under 80	80 and Older	p-Value
A study focusing on educational, practical, emotional and holistic support for patients with MBC			0.5105 [2]			0.0004 [4]
N	1865	137				
Mean (SD)	8.4 (2.27)	8.2 (2.61)		8.4 (1.74)	7.9 (6.94)	
Median (IQR)	9.0 (8.0, 10.0)	10.0 (7.0, 10.0)		9.0 (8.0–10)	10 (6.0–10)	
A study in patients with MBC to make the transition from oncology treatment to palliative/hospice care as smooth as possible			0.7291 [2]			0.0581 [4]
N	1850	134				
Mean (SD)	8.3 (2.38)	8.3 (2.74)		8.3 (1.81)	8.5 (6.38)	
Median (IQR)	9.0 (8.0, 10.0)	10.0 (8.0, 10.0)		9.0 (8.0–10)	10 (8.0–10)	
A study to train oncology providers about the specific/different needs of EBC vs. MBC patients			0.3198 [2]			0.0754 [4]
N	1872	135				
Mean (SD)	8.1 (2.43)	8.3 (2.66)		8.1 (1.86)	8.3 (5.89)	
Median (IQR)	9.0 (7.0, 10.0)	10.0 (8.0, 10.0)		9.0 (7.0–10)	10 (8.0–10)	
Virtual Second Opinion Breast Cancer Clinic			0.9879 [2]			0.5364 [4]
N	1879	135				
Mean (SD)	8.1 (2.56)	8.1 (2.86)		8.1 (1.96)	8.0 (7.04)	
Median (IQR)	9.0 (7.0, 10.0)	10.0 (7.0, 10.0)		9.0 (7.0–10)	9.0 (8.0–10)	
A study focusing on educational, practical, emotional and holistic support for patients with EBC			0.8702 [2]			0.0116 [4]
N	1881	138				
Mean (SD)	8.1 (2.44)	8.1 (2.80)		8.1 (1.86)	7.8 (7.96)	
Median (IQR)	9.0 (7.0, 10.0)	10.0 (7.0, 10.0)		9.0 (7.0–10)	10 (6.0–10)	
A study focusing on educational, practical, emotional and holistic support for caregivers/family members of patients with MBC			0.8983 [2]			0.0018 [4]
N	1871	137				
Mean (SD)	7.9 (2.49)	7.9 (2.86)		7.9 (1.90)	7.5 (7.64)	
Median (IQR)	9.0 (7.0, 10.0)	10.0 (6.0, 10.0)		9.0 (7.0–10)	9.0 (5.0–10)	

Table 2. *Cont.*

	Unweighted			Weighted		
	Under 80 (N = 2235)	80 and Older (N = 202)	p–Value	Under 80	80 and Older	p-Value
A Complementary and Integrative Medicine Workshop promoting emotional wellbeing and addressing spiritual suffering			0.6165 [2]			0.0025 [4]
N	1873	136				
Mean (SD)	7.5 (2.78)	7.4 (2.96)		7.5 (2.11)	7.1 (6.99)	
Median (IQR)	8.0 (6.0, 10.0)	8.0 (5.0, 10.0)		8.0 (6.0–10)	8.0 (5.0–10)	
A study focusing on educational, practical, emotional and holistic support for caregivers/family members of patients with EBC			0.6659 [2]			0.0002 [4]
N	1873	137				
Mean (SD)	7.3 (2.73)	7.4 (3.10)		7.3 (2.08)	6.8 (8.52)	
Median (IQR)	8.0 (5.0, 10.0)	9.0 (5.0, 10.0)		8.0 (5.0–10)	8.0 (5.0–10)	
A couples workshop to address relationship stresses and intimacy issues in patients with EBC vs. MBC			0.4301 [2]			<0.0001 [4]
N	1869	133				
Mean (SD)	6.8 (3.06)	6.6 (3.60)		6.8 (2.33)	5.9 (8.85)	
Median (IQR)	8.0 (5.0, 10.0)	8.0 (5.0, 10.0)		8.0 (5.0–10)	7.0 (3.0–9.0)	
Reconnect oncology providers with a past patient			0.8533 [2]			0.4414 [4]
N	1869	133				
Mean (SD)	6.3 (3.21)	6.3 (3.55)		6.3 (2.44)	6.4 (8.59)	
Median (IQR)	7.0 (4.0, 9.0)	7.0 (4.0, 10.0)		7.0 (4.0–9.0)	6.0 (4.0–10)	
Integrative medicine						
Have you ever seen an integrative medicine or complementary medicine provider for breast cancer symptoms or treatments, n (%)			0.0003 [1]			<0.0001 [3]
Yes	400 (20.9%)	11 (7.6%)		20.3% (19.4%–21.3%)	7.6% (7.2%–8.1%)	
No	1415 (73.9%)	122 (84.1%)		74.5% (73.3%–75.6%)	83.0% (82.1%–83.9%)	
Unsure	101 (5.3%)	12 (8.3%)		5.2% (4.9%–5.5%)	9.4% (8.8%–9.9%)	
Missing	319	57				

Table 2. *Cont.*

	Unweighted			Weighted		
	Under 80 (N = 2235)	80 and Older (N = 202)	p–Value	Under 80	80 and Older	p-Value
If so, did you ever take vitamins, minerals, herbal supplements or intravenous medications recommended by that provider, n (%)			0.0056 [1]			0.1463 [3]
Yes	174 (43.7%)	4 (36.4%)		43.1% (39.9%–46.4%)	47.3% (41.3%–53.3%)	
No	215 (54.0%)	5 (45.5%)		54.5% (51.2%–57.7%)	45.9% (39.9%–51.9%)	
Unsure	9 (2.3%)	2 (18.2%)		2.4% (2.1%–2.7%)	6.8% (5.3%–8.3%)	
Missing	1837	191				
If so, did your Oncology team know that you were taking these treatments, n (%)			0.0884 [1]			<0.0001 [3]
Yes	151 (87.3%)	2 (50.0%)		87.4% (85.1%–89.6%)	24.0% (17.7%–30.4%)	
No	9 (5.2%)	1 (25.0%)		4.8% (3.9%–5.8%)	70.4% (63.1%–77.7%)	
Unsure	13 (7.5%)	1 (25.0%)		7.8% (6.4%–9.3%)	5.5% (3.7%–7.4%)	
Missing	2062	198				
Saw integrative medicine or complementary medicine provider to strengthen immune system, n (%)			0.3369 [1]			0.0885 [3]
No	273 (68.3%)	6 (54.5%)		68.4% (65.5%–71.2%)	79.2% (75.2%–83.2%)	
Yes	127 (31.8%)	5 (45.5%)		31.6% (28.8%–34.5%)	20.8% (16.8%–24.8%)	
Missing	1835	191				
Saw integrative medicine or complementary medicine provider to support conventional medicine, n (%)			0.3688 [1]			0.0642 [3]
No	237 (59.3%)	8 (72.7%)		59.0% (55.8%–62.2%)	46.2% (40.2%–52.2%)	
Yes	163 (40.8%)	3 (27.3%)		41.0% (37.8%–44.2%)	53.8% (47.8%–59.8%)	
Missing	1835	191				
Saw integrative medicine or complementary medicine provider to combat side effects of cancer and traditional cancer treatments, n (%)			0.0267 [1]			<0.0001 [3]
No	158 (39.5%)	8 (72.7%)		40.1% (37.0%–43.3%)	74.6% (70.0%–79.1%)	
Yes	242 (60.5%)	3 (27.3%)		59.9% (56.7%–63.0%)	25.4% (20.9%–30.0%)	
Missing	1835	191				

Table 2. *Cont.*

	Unweighted			Weighted		
	Under 80 (N = 2235)	80 and Older (N = 202)	*p*–Value	Under 80	80 and Older	*p*-Value
Saw integrative medicine or complementary medicine provider because lack of confidence in traditional/ Western medicine, n (%)			0.4029 [1]			0.6881 [3]
No	384 (96.0%)	10 (90.9%)		95.6% (95.1%–96.2%)	96.7% (96.0%–97.5%)	
Yes	16 (4.0%)	1 (9.1%)		4.4% (3.8%–4.9%)	3.3% (2.5%–4.0%)	
Missing	1835	191				
Saw integrative medicine or complementary medicine provider because of other reason, n (%)			0.2631 [1]			0.0072 [3]
No	359 (89.8%)	11 (100.0%)		89.9% (88.8%–91.1%)	100% (100%–100%)	
Yes	41 (10.3%)	0 (0.0%)		10.1% (8.9%–11.2%)	0.0% (0.0%–0.0%)	
Missing	1835	191				
How satisfied were you with the care you received an integrative medicine or complementary medicine provider, n (%)			0.0002 [1]			<0.0001 [3]
Very satisfied	201 (50.9%)	4 (40.0%)		50.6% (47.3%–53.9%)	31.2% (26.0%–36.5%)	
Satisfied	135 (34.2%)	4 (40.0%)		34.2% (31.3%–37.2%)	61.4% (55.7%–67.2%)	
Neither satisfied or dissatisfied	48 (12.2%)	0 (0.0%)		12.5% (11.0%–13.9%)	0.0% (0.0%–0.0%)	
Dissatisfied	10 (2.5%)	1 (10.0%)		2.5% (2.2%–2.8%)	3.7% (2.8%–4.5%)	
Very dissatisfied	1 (0.3%)	1 (10.0%)		0.3% (0.2%–0.3%)	3.7% (2.8%–4.5%)	
Missing	1840	192				
Medical Second Opinion						
Have you ever received a second opinion regarding your breast cancer diagnosis and treatment plan, n (%)			<0.0001 [1]			<0.0001 [3]
Yes	792 (41.5%)	29 (20.0%)		40.9% (39.5%–42.3%)	21.7% (20.6%–22.9%)	
No	1102 (57.8%)	114 (78.6%)		58.4% (57.0%–59.9%)	77.5% (76.4%–78.7%)	
Unsure	14 (0.7%)	2 (1.4%)		0.7 % (0.7 %–0.7 %)	0.7 % (0.7 %–0.8 %)	
Missing	327	57				

Table 2. *Cont.*

	Unweighted			Weighted		
	Under 80 (N = 2235)	**80 and Older (N = 202)**	***p*–Value**	**Under 80**	**80 and Older**	***p*-Value**
If so, did you find it beneficial, n (%)			0.0596 [1]			<0.0001 [3]
Yes	752 (95.9%)	25 (92.6%)		95.9% (95.6%–96.3%)	83.7% (81.6%–85.8%)	
No	21 (2.7%)	0 (0.0%)		2.7 % (2.4 %–2.9 %)	0.0 % (0.0 %–0.0 %)	
Unsure	10 (1.3%)	2 (7.4%)		1.3 % (1.2 %–1.4 %)	16.3% (14.2%–18.4%)	
Not applicable	1 (0.1%)	0 (0.0%)		0.1 % (0.1 %–0.1 %)	0.0 % (0.0 %–0.0 %)	
Missing	1451	175				
Have patient advocates ever assisted you with decision making and the logistics of breast cancer treatment, n (%)			0.0029 [1]			<0.0001 [3]
Yes	371 (19.4%)	28 (19.4%)		19.3% (18.4%–20.2%)	25.7% (24.4%–26.9%)	
No	1371 (71.7%)	91 (63.2%)		71.8% (70.6%–73.0%)	57.2% (55.6%–58.8%)	
Unsure	169 (8.8%)	25 (17.4%)		8.9 % (8.4 %–9.4 %)	17.1% (16.2%–18.1%)	
Missing	324	58				
Clinical Trials						
Since being diagnosed with breast cancer, have you participated in a clinical trial, n (%)			<0.0001 [1]			<0.0001 [3]
Yes	907 (47.2%)	60 (40.5%)		46.2% (44.7%–47.7%)	47.3% (45.6%–48.9%)	
No	822 (42.8%)	54 (36.5%)		43.2% (41.7%–44.6%)	29.4% (28.1%–30.8%)	
Unsure	192 (10.0%)	34 (23.0%)		10.6% (10.1%–11.2%)	23.3% (22.1%–24.5%)	
Missing	314	54				
If you have not participated in a clinical trial for breast cancer patients, would you be open to doing so in the future, n (%)			0.0001 [1]			<0.0001 [3]
Yes	612 (62.0%)	35 (40.7%)		61.6% (59.7%–63.6%)	45.5% (43.3%–47.8%)	
No	84 (8.5%)	16 (18.6%)		8.5 % (7.9 %–9.2 %)	10.2% (9.4 %–11.1%)	
Unsure	291 (29.5%)	35 (40.7%)		29.8% (28.1%–31.5%)	44.2% (42.0%–46.5%)	
Missing	1248	116				

[1] Chi-Square *p*-value; [2] Two sample *t*-test; [3] Propensity score-weighted chi-square *p*-value; [4] Propensity score-weighted *t*-tests.

Advocate-BREAST80+ Substudy Results

- Demographic Information

Compared with responding P80−, responding P80+ were more likely to be white (p = 0.0136), widowed (<0.0001), living in a rural location (0.0136), and initially diagnosed with BC $\geq$ 24 months prior to completing the survey (<0.0001). For P80+, the mean time from BC diagnosis at the time of survey completion was 128.5 months (SD 74.4) compared with 90.1 months (SD 68.9) for P80− ($p \leq 0.001$). The BC stage distribution for patients (Stage 0–4) was similar in P80+ compared to P80− (p = 0.2571). Based on these results, the following variables were used to calculate propensity scores for subsequent weighted analyses: race, marital status, religion, time since BC diagnosis, primary BC treatment location, and recommendation status for surgery, chemotherapy, radiotherapy, endocrine therapy, biologic therapy, and immunotherapy.

- Treatment Recommendations

Overall, P80+ were less likely to report that they had been advised to undergo local regional and systemic therapies than P80−. Specifically, surgery was recommended less frequently for P80+ compared with P80− (p = 0.0062, Table 1). However, when surgery was recommended, P80+ were as likely to proceed with the same as P80− (p = 0.5643). Adjuvant radiation therapy was also less likely to be recommended for P80+ compared with P80− (p = 0.0037); however, there was no difference between the groups regarding the likelihood of proceeding with radiation therapy if advised (p = 0.6635).

Regarding systemic therapies, P80+ were less likely to be advised to pursue chemotherapy, immunotherapy, targeted biologic therapy or endocrine therapy compared with P80− ($p \leq 0.0001$ for each of these treatments). Furthermore, although P80+ were less likely to proceed with recommended endocrine therapy (p = 0.0011), targeted biologic therapy (p = 0.0940), and immunotherapy (p = 0.0015), they were as likely as P80− to proceed with chemotherapy if recommended (p = 0.1641).

- Symptom Severity

Overall, the most severe symptom experienced by patients in their first year following BC diagnosis was hair loss/thinning, followed by hot flashes, eyebrow/eyelash thinning, sexual dysfunction, cognitive/memory issues, neuropathy and lymphedema. Compared with P80−, P80+ were significantly less impacted by hot flashes, eyebrow/eyelash thinning, sexual dysfunction, cognitive/memory issues and lymphedema ($p < 0.0001$ each).

- Level of Concern Regarding Issues within the First Year after Breast Cancer Diagnosis

The main concerns patients of all ages recalled in the first year following their BC diagnosis were (i) fear of BC recurrence/spread, (ii) concerns about loved ones coping, (iii) diagnosis and prognosis, (iv) fear of dying of BC, (v) weight/physical fitness, and vi) their emotional health. P80+ were significantly less impacted than P80− regarding these issues ($p < 0.0001$ for each item), although they were still identified as top concerns overall.

- Overall Satisfaction with BC Patient Experience

Patients reported a high level of overall satisfaction with BC care received (>90%). Specifically, P80+ reported higher overall satisfaction with BC care than P80− (p = 0.0015). P80+ reported similar satisfaction overall with the information and support received from their cancer care teams compared to P80− (0.9826).

- Satisfaction with BC Information and Support Received Regarding Symptoms/Side Effects of Treatment

In the first year after BC diagnosis, patients of all ages were least satisfied with the information provided regarding (i) the side effects of immunotherapy, (ii) the side effects of targeted biologic therapies, (iii) sexual dysfunction, (iv) the long-term side effects of chemotherapy, and (v) eyebrow/eyelash thinning.

When compared with P80−, P80+ were significantly less satisfied with information they received regarding (i) the potential side effects of immunotherapy ($p = 0.0320$), targeted biologic therapies ($p = 0.008$), sexual dysfunction ($p < 0.0001$), peripheral neuropathy ($p < 0.0001$), hair loss/thinning ($p = 0.0030$), lymphedema ($p < 0.0001$), hot flashes ($p < 0.0001$), the short and long-term side effects of radiotherapy ($p < 0.0001$ and 0.0277, respectively) and the short term side effects of chemotherapy ($p < 0.001$).

- Satisfaction with BC Support Received Regarding Concerns

In the first year after BC diagnosis, patients of all ages reported high satisfaction overall with support provided (~90%). Specifically, there were no significant differences between P80+ and P80− regarding satisfaction with the availability of information pertaining to their BC diagnosis, access to their care team, and the amount of information available regarding their treatment plan. However, P80+ reported lower satisfaction with information provided regarding genetic testing (self) ($p = 0.0239$).

- Ranking of Quality Improvement (QI) projects

Compared to P80−, P80+ similarly prioritized proposed QI interventions focusing on (i) the provision of lifetime access to online educational resources ($p = 0.2588$). QI interventions focused on (i) wellness for early breast cancer (EBC) and metastatic breast cancer (MBC) patients and (ii) educational, practical, emotional and holistic support for patients with MBC were also considered high priority but did not differ across age.

- Integrative Medicine

P80+ were less likely to have visited an integrative medicine provider for BC treatment than P80− ($p = 0.0003$). P80+ who met with integrative medicine were as likely to have taken supplements or vitamins recommended as P80− ($p = 0.0056$). Despite lower care satisfaction reported overall compared with P80− ($p = 0.0002$), 80% of P80+ were satisfied/very satisfied with care received from integrative medicine. However, data from this section should be cautiously interpreted given the small number of P80+ who responded to these questions.

- Medical Second Opinions and Clinical Trial Participation

P80+ were less likely to have received a second opinion ($p < 0.0001$). P80+ were also more likely to have received assistance from a patient advocate regarding BC-related logistics and treatment decisions ($p = 0.0029$).

Regarding clinical trials, 40.5% of P80+ reported prior study participation vs. 47.2% of P80− ($p < 0.001$), and P80+ were less open to participating in a trial in the future ($p = 0.0001$) compared with P80− (18.6% responded "No" and 40.7% responded unsure).

- Qualitative Data: Suggestions to Improve BC Care and Prioritization for BC Research

Overall, 77 of 202 P80+ answered the open-ended survey questions (Table 3).

The major themes identified were (1) BC Education, (2) Side Effects of BC Treatment, and (3) Emotional Support During and After BC Diagnosis. Regarding BC education, suggestions included avoiding multiple printed resources unrelated to the patient's diagnosis and treatment plan, instead providing tailored information based on patient preferences (more vs. less information). Patients also advised that clinicians use less medical terminology and provide thorough information regarding all treatment options. Regarding managing the side effects of BC treatment, suggestions included more detailed information regarding the short and long-term sequelae of local and systemic therapy. Regarding emotional support, patients noted the importance of ongoing access to BC and community support groups. The need for provider education and ongoing efforts to optimize emotional support for BC patients was also highlighted. Other themes included (4) Care Concerns/Provider Sensitivity (need to consider patient frailty, vulnerability and increased susceptibility to discomfort during medical procedures), (5) Survivorship/Long Term Sequelae of BC treatment (advice about surveillance, prosthesis selection, etc.), (6) Diversity, Ethnicity and Inclusion (questions regarding the applicability of BC data for ethnic minorities), (7) BC Care Access (faster surgery and test results), (8) Dense Breast Tissue

Screening (insurance coverage), (9) Diet and Exercise (nutrition consultations) and (10) Sexual Dysfunction. Regarding thoughts on what areas of research should be championed, respondents prioritized focusing on efforts to determine the causes of BC, as well as to prevent and cure the same.

Table 3. Qualitative Data from Survey Respondents Aged 80+ Years.

Category	Feedback/Comment(s)	Patients' Age at Survey Completion
Breast Cancer Education	"Don't overwhelm patient with printed materials. Much is duplication and much does not relate to patient and patient's condition"	81
	"I think this depends on the individual patients. Some do not want to have so much information that they just feel confused about making a decision. They just want a more directed approach. Then there are others who have the opposite views and need to get all the info that is available"	83
	"I would have liked to have more information regarding the impact of genetic testing on such issues as insurance factors for my daughters. I would have liked to participate in genetic testing if insurance issues had not been a factor"	83
	"Develop a breast cancer app that includes info on the individual that would be immediately available to be shown to a new provider. Connect it to online resources and new information the patient can access over time"	80
	"Better non-medical terms information about the pros and cons of chemotherapy before or after surgery, and the choices between breast removal and lumpectomies. From what I hear from current patients, the providers are telling patients what they should do instead of giving them complete explanations of choices and the pros and cons"	84
Side-Effects of Breast Cancer Treatment	"Would have liked to have known the effects of radiation on breast prior to having radiation. . .. Would have liked to have had discussion of lymphedema prior to surgery again just to prepare me before I got it in my breast not arm"	80
	"I would suggest much more detailed information concerning side affects of radiation. The information provided does not share the possibility of the burning of the skin-simply states slight sunburn. . ."	81
	"inform them more about possibility of lymphademia (sic). I have it.	84
	". . .I should have been told the difficulty of reconstruction and also been told that because of previous radiation treatments for breast cancer that the skin and tissues were damaged and that there was a chance the implant would not hold. I went through the treatments only to have the implant fall and needed to be removed"	80
	"I am not sure if the pills I took for the five years following surgery were estrogen inhibitors or not, but they did affect my skeleton. That is the only aspect of treatment that truly upset me, since I had a very strong skeleton for my age and developed osteopenia because of the medicine. . .."	80
Survivorship/Long Term Sequelae of Breast Cancer Treatment	"Focus on post surgical mastectomy and what is available as a prosthesis and where items can be purchased"	86
	"I don't like to think of my self as a "breast cancer patient." I had breast cancer, and I may have it again, but it doesn't define me"	80
	"The first year check up was far more painful than I thought it would be"	83
Emotional Support During and After Diagnosis	"Connect breast cancer survivors with groups/activities in the community"	80
	"Patients need an ongoing source of physical and emotional assistance which they can rely on from the beginning to the end of their journey of healing"	82

Table 3. *Cont.*

Category	Feedback/Comment(s)	Patients' Age at Survey Completion
Emotional Support During and After Diagnosis	"Access to network of support persons. I live in [redacted] where people in health care had no suggestions. I was new to the community and did not know what to do. I needed to find someone who experienced my situation"	83
	"Discussing it with family. My family does not want to discuss it at all. It's like if they don't talk about it, it does not exist"	80
	"Continue open discussions and followups like this"	86
	"Training for the nurse practitioner to enable her/him to emotionally support and care for the patient, even as the years post op extend toward five"	80
	"Use of volunteers and survivors for group or individuals"	81
Care Concerns and Provider Sensitivity	"View each patient individually and try to treat at the level they are comfortable"	83
	"What I am most " upset" about is the doctor who informed me I had cancer!!"	81
	"My experience with Radiology . . ..I complained of the positioning which was causing my neck to hurt. I was told there was nothing they could do. Eventually, they did listen and apologized and adjustments were made. . ."	81
	"The oncologist . . .was not interested in the pain I was receiving from radiation.	88
	"Cooperation among hospitals/providers is important"	86
	"I was concerned that they seemed to be delaying getting treatment started and I was anxious about that delay. . ..I was confused by all the diagnostic testing"	84
	"I think the emotional impact is probably related to age. If I were younger, I think I would have a much different perspective. That said, it bothers me a little to hear references to my age and longevity aspects"	80
Diversity, Ethnicity and Inclusion	"What is the percentage of Hispanic women patients over the age of 79 that gets care at the Breast Clinic?"	81
	"As a Hispanic woman. . .. I have seen a difference in the care I have received. It is a subtle change either due to my age or other factors such as less staff or staff that is less attentive for whatever reason"	81
Access to Breast Cancer Care	"Early surgical treatment should be available after diagnosis is made"	83
	"Faster mammogram reports"	82
Screening for Patients With Dense Breast Tissue	"I have dense breast tissue so I think women with this should have both the mammogram and MBI. For first years after surgery and treatment had both mammogram and MBI. Now these last few years alternate. I have mammogram one year and then the MBI the next."	86
	"Better insurance coverage for patients with dense breasts and further options for evaluation and treatment"	84
Diet and Exercise	"Have diet and exercise be a very important part of care"	82
	"I believe help from a dietitian to strongly suggest food planning that would be more beneficial to the recovery of the patient"	82
Sexual Dysfunction	"Help with sexual dysfunction"	82

Table 3. *Cont.*

Category	Feedback/Comment(s)	Patients' Age at Survey Completion
Research Advocacy	"Focus on a cure and preventing Breast Cancer"	81
	"I believe in continued research"	82
	"Just participating in a clinical trial and getting the results is very satisfying"	81
	"How do genetics affect breast cancer in the families of cancer pts?"	82
	"Hopefully, research will develop a vaccine to help prevent breast cancer. And research will help discover the causes of breast cancer"	81

4. Discussion

We present the results of a large patient experience survey completed by ~2500 BC patients, of whom >200 were P80+; a comparison of both groups shows that P80+ appear to be a distinct population with regard to demographics, treatment-related symptoms, and unmet educational needs. Differences in engagement with integrative medicine and clinical trial participation, as well as the likelihood of pursuing a medical second opinion, were also noted between both groups. Based on our findings, ways to improve BC care in P80+ include: (i) refining patient education materials and (ii) identifying and reducing unique barriers to research participation. On review of the qualitative data, the need for ongoing emotional support during and after BC treatment was also found to be a priority for this population.

A strength of this substudy is the number of P80+ who responded to the survey, as well as the qualitative data provided from P80+; the latter helped identify relevant themes in this understudied population. Other strengths include the high survey response rate (35%) and the inclusion of rural-dwelling BC patients (15.3% of respondents were P80+), as these patients are often underrepresented in BC care delivery research. Notably, our definition of rurality was strict (RUCA code of 10) and did not include small towns (RUCA codes 7–9 inclusive). Regarding study limitations, most survey respondents had stage 0–3 BC (n = 196; 97%); therefore, concerns germane to P80+ with MBC are not well evaluated. Furthermore, as most survey respondents were married/widowed and Caucasian Christians living in the Midwest of the US, our conclusions may not be generalizable. Therefore, a future study should enroll a more ethnically, racially, and geographically diverse cohort of P80+. Although our survey response rate of 35% was higher than observed in some studies, the substantial number of non-responders could also have contributed to response bias. The higher rate of clinical trial participation reported in our study could also have been a function of response bias, as people who participate in clinical trials are likely more willing to complete a survey. In addition, 155 (76.7%) of the P80+ survey respondents were diagnosed 5–10 years ago, which may have led to recall bias when reporting BC-related symptom severity and concerns. Nevertheless, the inclusion of these patients is important to capture the unique perspectives of P80+ survivors.

P80+ were less likely than younger patients to report that they had been advised to pursue all types of BC therapy. However, when they recalled that this had been recommended, these older patients were as likely as P80− to report that they did indeed receive surgery, radiation therapy and/or chemotherapy. Conversely, if they reported that they had been recommended to receive endocrine therapy or immunotherapy, P80+ were less likely than P80− to report that they had indeed received that treatment. The reasons for therapy decline in older patients may include the duration of therapy, perceived unclear benefit of therapy, concerns regarding the potential for therapies to exacerbate preexisting medical conditions and/or cause new problems, financial concerns, and communication barriers (e.g., hearing or visual impairments that make it difficult to understand the benefits of a given cancer treatment) [12,13]. While the avoidance of potentially toxic therapies is often appropriate in P80+ as risks may outweigh benefits, some older BC patients do benefit from adjuvant chemotherapy [14,15]. The ADVANCE (ADjuVANt Chemotherapy in the Elderly) trial assessed the feasibility of two (neo)adjuvant chemotherapy regimens in parallel-enrolling cohorts of older persons (≥70 years) with human epidermal growth factor receptor 2 (HER2)-negative BC [16]. Although neither regimen met target feasibility goals, trials such as ADVANCE inform the development of tolerable, evidence-based regimens for older BC patients who need chemotherapy. Better age-specific data and personalized decision tools are needed to assist with provider and patient decision-making [17–19], as well as the greater integration of existing tools into oncology clinical practice [20–22].

From an educational perspective, the level of satisfaction regarding information and support provided to address BC therapy side effects was lower in P80+ than in P80−. Specifically, P80+ were significantly less satisfied with information regarding the potential side effects of immunotherapy, targeted biologic therapies, the short and long-term side effects of radiotherapy, and the short and long-term side effects of chemotherapy. As these topics encompass much of what is discussed at the initial BC consultation(s), the provision of improved educational resources tailored to older patients (e.g., larger print materials and PC use if internet access is available) with additional concessions (e.g., longer visit times and nurse navigator assistance) may improve comprehension and retention of information. Furthermore, a short interval follow-up visit with a care team representative may aid patient decision-making and decrease overwhelming feelings. Even though P80+ were less likely to request a second opinion, those that obtained the same reported a similar level of satisfaction to P80−. A second consultation with an oncology provider provides additional education and may reinforce initial recommendations and improve comprehension [23,24]. A "refresher" visit with a care team representative shortly after the initial consultation to provide a reminder regarding accessing suitable educational materials/resources could be helpful. As P80+ in our substudy also reported less satisfaction with information/education regarding sexual dysfunction, peripheral neuropathy, hair loss/thinning, lymphedema, and several other topics compared with P80−, an institutional pilot study focusing on the delivery of age-appropriate, concise education for P80+ could be implemented. An initial approach could be to focus on one side effect, with patient satisfaction levels assessed thereafter. Given our aging population, strategies focusing on catering to the educational needs of elderly BC patients will increasingly need to be prioritized [25,26].

With regard to the main concerns experienced during the first year after a BC diagnosis, although P80+ reported less anxiety and symptom-related distress compared with P80−, their primary concerns were similar (i.e., emotional distress and anxiety related to the BC diagnosis). Despite the lower levels of emotional distress experienced overall, ongoing access to psychosocial support (in person or virtual) was valued. The importance of "wellness" was stressed, with physical fitness reported as a leading concern. Although P80+ were less inclined to visit an integrative medicine provider, the majority who did were satisfied with their experience; however, these results are based on a relatively small sample size. Given the many benefits of integrative medicine regarding holistic health and pain and symptom management (including for cancer patients) [26,27], efforts to educate older patients and foster connections with licensed professionals should be encouraged.

With regard to clinical trial participation, 60 (40.5%) P80+ reported that they had already participated in a trial (a higher proportion than the general population), but these older patients were significantly less open to doing so in the future compared with P80− (16 [18.6%] stated no and 35 [40.7%] were unsure). Unfortunately, the percentage of P80+ who have participated in/are open to participating in clinical trials is considerably lower in underserved and/or ethnically diverse patients [28,29]. Initiatives to prioritize the inclusion of older persons in research are urgently needed.

P80+ and P80− were well-aligned in recommending the implementation of the following QI initiatives: (i) the provision of lifetime access to online concise patient educational resources; (ii) educational, practical, emotional and holistic support programs for MBC patients; and (iii) BC Wellness Programs for EBC and MBC patients. This implies that, irrespective of age, patients with BC prioritize concise educational resources, continuity of care, ongoing psychological support, and holistic care.

5. Conclusions

Efforts to refine care and to address unique challenges in older patients must be a clinical and research priority. Strategies focusing on tailoring educational materials to BC patients diagnosed in their 80s and 90s should be prioritized, as should initiatives that aim to increase clinical trial accrual and promote psychological well-being for P80+. In the future, focused interviews with P80+ could inform interventions to enhance continuity of care, communication, holistic care, and long-term psychosocial support.

Author Contributions: Conception or design of the work: C.C.O., R.A.V., K.J.R., M.L.S. and C.C.; data collection: C.C.O., R.A.V. and N.L.L.; data analysis and interpretation: C.C.O., R.A.V., N.L.L., K.J.R., J.E.O., M.L.S. and C.C.; drafting the article: C.C.O., R.A.V., N.L.L., K.J.R. and J.E.O.; critical revision of the article: C.C.O., R.A.V., N.L.L., M.L.S., C.C., F.J.C., J.E.O., S.D., A.J. and K.J.R.; final approval of the version to be published: C.C.O., R.A.V., N.L.L., M.L.S., C.C., F.J.C., J.E.O., S.D., A.J. and K.J.R. All authors have read and agreed to the published version of the manuscript.

Funding: This work was supported by a Mayo Clinic Population Sciences Grant (P30 CA015083).

Institutional Review Board Statement: This research was conducted in accordance with the Declaration of Helsinki, and the study protocol was reviewed by the Mayo Clinic Institutional Review Board (IRB 1815-04).

Informed Consent Statement: Informed consent was obtained from all participants prior to enrollment to the registry.

Data Availability Statement: The datasets for this study are available from the corresponding author upon request.

Acknowledgments: This work was supported by a Mayo Clinic Comprehensive Cancer Center pilot grant (P30 CA015083).

Conflicts of Interest: Ciara C. O'Sullivan—Dr. O'Sullivan has received research funding through Mayo Clinic from Lilly, Seagen Inc., Bavarian Nordic, Minnemarita Therapeutics, nFerence, AstraZeneca and Biovica. Mary Lou Smith—Serves on consulting/advisory boards with Bayer, Eisai, Novartis, Pfizer, and Rising Tide; received institutional grant funding from Genentech, Foundation Medicine, Novartis, Seagen, Eli Lilly, Exact Sciences, Daiichi, ECOG-ACRIN Medical Research Foundation, Pfizer, Prelude DX, International Association for Study of Lung Cancer, Conquer Cancer Foundation, and Cholangiocarcinoma Foundation; serves as Co-Chair of Cancer Research Advocate Committee and Member of Breast Core Committee, ECOG ACRIN Research Group; was a member of the following: Breast Cancer Treatment Guidelines Committee, National Comprehensive Cancer Network (NCCN); External Advisory Board, University of Wisconsin Comprehensive Cancer Center; Board of Directors, National Accreditation Program for Breast Centers; Board of Directors, Gateway for Cancer Research; NCI BOLD Task Force; Mayo Clinic Breast SPORE; Steering Committee, ASCO TAPUR Study; Stakeholder Advisory Board, COMET study; Advisory Board, PRO-TECT study; Advisory Committee, NCI-NCORP; Breast Cancer Guidelines Advisory Group, American Society of Clinical Oncology (ASCO); EVOLV Study; NCI Tolerability Consortium; and Women's Advisory Board, TMIST study. Janet E. Olson—Research support: Grail, Inc. Research grant: Exact Sciences, Exact-001.

References

1. Siegel, R.L.; Miller, K.D.; Wagle, N.S.; Jemal, A. Cancer statistics, 2023. *CA Cancer J. Clin.* **2023**, *73*, 17–48. [CrossRef] [PubMed]
2. Bertolo, A.; Rosso, C.; Voutsadakis, I.A. Breast Cancer in Patients 80 Years-Old and Older. *Eur. J. Breast Health* **2020**, *16*, 208–212. [CrossRef] [PubMed]
3. Shachar, S.S.; Hurria, A.; Muss, H.B. Breast Cancer in Women Older Than 80 Years. *J. Oncol. Pract.* **2016**, *12*, 123–132. [CrossRef] [PubMed]
4. Freedman, R.A.; Keating, N.L.; Lin, N.U.; Winer, E.P.; Vaz-Luis, I.; Lii, J.; Exman, P.; Barry, W.T. Breast cancer-specific survival by age: Worse outcomes for the oldest patients. *Cancer* **2018**, *124*, 2184–2191. [CrossRef] [PubMed]

5. Van Herck, Y.; Feyaerts, A.; Alibhai, S.; Papamichael, D.; Decoster, L.; Lambrechts, Y.; Pinchuk, M.; Bechter, O.; Herrera-Caceres, J.; Bibeau, F.; et al. Is cancer biology different in older patients? *Lancet Healthy Longev.* **2021**, *2*, e663–e677. [CrossRef] [PubMed]
6. Fleurier, C.; De Wit, A.; Pilloy, J.; Boivin, L.; Jourdan, M.L.; Arbion, F.; Body, G.; Ouldamer, L. Outcome of patients with breast cancer in the oldest old (≥80 years). *Eur. J. Obstet. Gynecol. Reprod. Biol.* **2020**, *244*, 66–70. [CrossRef] [PubMed]
7. Wong, J.J.; D'Alimonte, L.; Angus, J.; Paszat, L.; Soren, B.; Szumacher, E. What do older patients with early breast cancer want to know while undergoing adjuvant radiotherapy? *J. Cancer Educ.* **2011**, *26*, 254–261. [CrossRef] [PubMed]
8. Baskin, A.S.; Wang, T.; Mott, N.M.; Hawley, S.T.; Jagsi, R.; Dossett, L.A. Gaps in Online Breast Cancer Treatment Information for Older Women. *Ann. Surg. Oncol.* **2021**, *28*, 950–957. [CrossRef] [PubMed]
9. Bagegni, N.A.; Peterson, L.L. Age-related disparities in older women with breast cancer. *Adv. Cancer Res.* **2020**, *146*, 23–56. [CrossRef]
10. O'Sullivan, C.C.; Larson, N.; Vierkant, R.A.; Smith, M.L.; Chauhan, C.; Couch, F.J.; Olson, J.; Ruddy, K.J. Advocate-BREAST: Advocates and Patients' Advice to Enhance Breast Cancer Care Delivery, Patient Experience and Patient Centered Research by 2025. *Cancer Res.* **2023**, *83* (Suppl. S5), P6-05-41. [CrossRef]
11. (Dataset) USDA Economic Research Service. Rural-Urban Commuting Area Codes. 2022; Economic Research Service, Department of Agriculture. Available online: https://data.nal.usda.gov/dataset/rural-urban-commuting-area-codes (accessed on 5 December 2022).
12. White, M.J.; Kolbow, M.; Prathibha, S.; Praska, C.; Ankeny, J.S.; LaRocca, C.J.; Jensen, E.H.; Tuttle, T.M.; Hui, J.Y.C.; Marmor, S. Chemotherapy refusal and subsequent survival in healthy older women with high genomic risk estrogen receptor-positive breast cancer. *Breast Cancer Res. Treat.* **2023**, *198*, 309–319. [CrossRef]
13. Gopal, N.; Kozikowski, A.; Barginear, M.F.; Fishbein, J.; Pekmezaris, R.; Wolf-Klein, G. Reasons for Chemotherapy Refusal or Acceptance in Older Adults With Cancer. *South. Med. J.* **2017**, *110*, 47–53. [CrossRef] [PubMed]
14. Morita, M.; Shimomura, A.; Tokuda, E.; Horimoto, Y.; Kawamura, Y.; Ishizuka, Y.; Sekine, K.; Obayashi, S.; Kojima, Y.; Uemura, Y.; et al. Is adjuvant chemotherapy necessary in older patients with breast cancer? *Breast Cancer* **2022**, *29*, 498–506. [CrossRef] [PubMed]
15. Roy, S.; Lakritz, S.; Schreiber, A.R.; Molina, E.; Kabos, P.; Wood, M.; Elias, A.; Kondapalli, L.; Bradley, C.J.; Diamond, J.R. Clinical outcomes of adjuvant taxane plus anthracycline versus taxane-based chemotherapy regimens in older adults with node-positive, triple-negative breast cancer: A SEER-Medicare study. *Eur. J. Cancer* **2023**, *185*, 69–82. [CrossRef] [PubMed]
16. Freedman, R.A.; Li, T.; Sedrak, M.S.; Hopkins, J.O.; Tayob, N.; Faggen, M.G.; Sinclair, N.F.; Chen, W.Y.; Parsons, H.A.; Mayer, E.L.; et al. 'ADVANCE' (a pilot trial) ADjuVANt chemotherapy in the elderly: Developing and evaluating lower-toxicity chemotherapy options for older patients with breast cancer. *J. Geriatr. Oncol.* **2023**, *14*, 101377. [CrossRef] [PubMed]
17. Reid-Agboola, C.; Klukowska, A.; Malcolm, F.L.; Harrison, C.; Parks, R.M.; Cheung, K.L. Comprehensive Geriatric Assessment for Older Women with Early-Stage (Non-Metastatic) Breast Cancer-An Updated Systematic Review of the Literature. *Curr. Oncol.* **2023**, *30*, 8294–8309. [CrossRef] [PubMed]
18. Klepin, H.; Mohile, S.; Hurria, A. Geriatric assessment in older patients with breast cancer. *J. Natl. Compr. Cancer Netw.* **2009**, *7*, 226–236. [CrossRef]
19. Okonji, D.O.; Sinha, R.; Phillips, I.; Fatz, D.; Ring, A. Comprehensive geriatric assessment in 326 older women with early breast cancer. *Br. J. Cancer* **2017**, *117*, 925–931. [CrossRef]
20. Mohile, S.G.; Dale, W.; Somerfield, M.R.; Schonberg, M.A.; Boyd, C.M.; Burhenn, P.S.; Canin, B.; Cohen, H.J.; Holmes, H.M.; Hopkins, J.O.; et al. Practical Assessment and Management of Vulnerabilities in Older Patients Receiving Chemotherapy: ASCO Guideline for Geriatric Oncology. *J. Clin. Oncol.* **2018**, *36*, 2326–2347. [CrossRef]
21. Webster, S.; Lawn, S.; Chan, R.; Koczwara, B. The role of comorbidity assessment in guiding treatment decision-making for women with early breast cancer: A systematic literature review. *Support. Care Cancer* **2020**, *28*, 1041–1050. [CrossRef] [PubMed]
22. Li, D.; Sun, C.L.; Kim, H.; Soto-Perez-de-Celis, E.; Chung, V.; Koczywas, M.; Fakih, M.; Chao, J.; Cabrera Chien, L.; Charles, K.; et al. Geriatric Assessment-Driven Intervention (GAIN) on Chemotherapy-Related Toxic Effects in Older Adults With Cancer: A Randomized Clinical Trial. *JAMA Oncol.* **2021**, *7*, e214158. [CrossRef]
23. Tattersall, M.H.; Dear, R.F.; Jansen, J.; Shepherd, H.L.; Devine, R.J.; Horvath, L.G.; Boyer, M.L. Second opinions in oncology: The experiences of patients attending the Sydney Cancer Centre. *Med. J. Aust.* **2009**, *191*, 209–212. [CrossRef] [PubMed]
24. Hillen, M.A.; Medendorp, N.M.; Daams, J.G.; Smets, E.M.A. Patient-Driven Second Opinions in Oncology: A Systematic Review. *Oncol.* **2017**, *22*, 1197–1211. [CrossRef] [PubMed]
25. Tjong, M.C.; Menjak, I.; Trudeau, M.; Mehta, R.; Wright, F.; Leahey, A.; Ellis, J.; Gallagher, D.; Gibson, L.; Bristow, B.; et al. The Perceptions and Expectations of Older Women in the Establishment of the Senior Women's Breast Cancer Clinic (SWBCC): A Needs Assessment Study. *J. Cancer Educ.* **2017**, *32*, 850–857. [CrossRef] [PubMed]
26. Champarnaud, M.; Villars, H.; Girard, P.; Brechemier, D.; Balardy, L.; Nourhashémi, F. Effectiveness of Therapeutic Patient Education Interventions for Older Adults with Cancer: A Systematic Review. *J. Nutr. Health Aging* **2020**, *24*, 772–782. [CrossRef] [PubMed]
27. Mao, J.J.; Ismaila, N.; Bao, T.; Barton, D.; Ben-Arye, E.; Garland, E.L.; Greenlee, H.; Leblanc, T.; Lee, R.T.; Lopez, A.M.; et al. Integrative Medicine for Pain Management in Oncology: Society for Integrative Oncology-ASCO Guideline. *J. Clin. Oncol.* **2022**, *40*, 3998–4024. [CrossRef] [PubMed]

28. Green, A.K.; Tabatabai, S.M.; Aghajanian, C.; Landgren, O.; Riely, G.J.; Sabbatini, P.; Bach, P.B.; Begg, C.B.; Lipitz-Snyderman, A.; Mailankody, S. Clinical Trial Participation Among Older Adult Medicare Fee-for-Service Beneficiaries With Cancer. *JAMA Oncol.* **2022**, *8*, 1786–1792. [CrossRef]
29. Bumanlag, I.M.; Jaoude, J.A.; Rooney, M.K.; Taniguchi, C.M.; Ludmir, E.B. Exclusion of Older Adults from Cancer Clinical Trials: Review of the Literature and Future Recommendations. *Semin. Radiat. Oncol.* **2022**, *32*, 125–134. [CrossRef]

cancers

MDPI

Article

Pre-Frailty and Frailty in Hospitalized Older Adults: A Comparison Study in People with and without a History of Cancer in an Acute Medical Unit

Chad Yixian Han [1,*], Raymond Javan Chan [1,2], Huah Shin Ng [3,4], Yogesh Sharma [3,5], Alison Yaxley [1], Claire Baldwin [1] and Michelle Miller [1]

1 Caring Futures Institute, College of Nursing and Health Sciences, Flinders University, Adelaide, SA 5042, Australia; raymond.chan@flinders.edu.au (R.J.C.); alison.yaxley@flinders.edu.au (A.Y.); claire.baldwin@flinders.edu.au (C.B.); michelle.miller@flinders.edu.au (M.M.)
2 Faculty of Health, Queensland University of Technology, Brisbane, QLD 4000, Australia
3 College of Medicine and Public Health, Flinders University, Adelaide, SA 5042, Australia; huahshin.ng@flinders.edu.au (H.S.N.); yogesh.sharma@sa.gov.au (Y.S.)
4 SA Pharmacy, SA Health, Adelaide, SA 5001, Australia
5 Department of Acute and General Medicine, Flinders Medical Centre, Adelaide, SA 5042, Australia
* Correspondence: chad.han@flinders.edu.au

Simple Summary: A prospective observational study was conducted in a cohort of 329 hospitalized older adults ≥65 years admitted to the acute medical unit (AMU) of a tertiary hospital. Statistical models compared older adults with and without a history of cancer to determine characteristics associated with pre-frailty/frailty and length of hospital stay (LOS). About one-fifth of the cohort had a history of cancer. The prevalence of pre-frailty/frailty among older adults with a history of cancer was 58%. In patients with a history of cancer, pre-frailty/frailty was associated with eight and nine times more likelihood of experiencing polypharmacy and malnutrition, respectively. The risk of having a longer LOS was 24% higher in older adults with a history of cancer than those without. Further investigations are warranted for improvement to systematic assessments to identify those at risk and provide interventions to meet the complex needs of this vulnerable population.

Abstract: A prospective observational study was conducted in a cohort of older adults ≥65 years (n = 329), admitted to the acute medical unit (AMU) of a tertiary hospital, to describe and compare characteristics including frailty status and clinical outcomes. Multivariable models compared older adults with and without a history of cancer to determine characteristics associated with frailty and pre-frailty. An adjusted Poisson regression model was used to compare the length of hospital stay (LOS) between the two groups. About one-fifth (22%) of the cohort had a history of cancer. The most common cancer types were prostate (n = 20), breast (n = 13), lung (n = 8) and gastrointestinal (n = 8). There was no difference in the prevalence of pre-frailty/frailty among patients with or without a history of cancer (58% vs. 57%, $p > 0.05$). Pre-frailty/frailty was associated with polypharmacy (OR 8.26, 95% CI: 1.74 to 39.2) and malnutrition (OR 8.91, 95% CI: 2.15 to 36.9) in patients with a history of cancer. Adjusted analysis revealed that the risk of having a longer LOS was 24% higher in older adults with a history of cancer than those without (IRR 1.24, 95% CI 1.10 to 1.41, $p < 0.001$). Clinicians in the AMU should be aware that older adults with a history of cancer have a higher risk of a longer LOS compared to those without.

Keywords: older adults; frailty; pre-frailty; cancer; hospitalized; acute medical unit

1. Introduction

Frailty and pre-frailty can significantly impact older adults who are admitted to hospital, influencing their treatment outcomes, quality of life, healthcare utilization and mortality rates [1,2]. This is of particular importance for those with a history of cancer. Older adults make up a significant percentage of people with cancer and cancer deaths [3]. The prevalence of pre-frailty and frailty vary across settings, i.e., community (ambulatory and population-based), nursing home and hospital; with the highest prevalence of pre-frailty reported in hospital settings [4]. The incidence of frailty is particularly high among older adults with cancer, considering that the disease itself and its treatments are stressors that significantly tax their physiologic reserve [5]. Previous research has demonstrated that older adults with cancer who are frail have decreased chemotherapy tolerance, increased risk of postoperative complications and disease progression, and mortality [6].

The Fried frailty criteria phenotype model and the Rockwood frailty deficit-accumulation model are two generally recognized models/theories underpinning instruments used to identify frailty and pre-frailty in older adults [7]. There are many instruments developed to identify frailty and pre-frailty, and the Edmonton Frail Scale (EFS) is one of the most commonly used pre-frailty and frailty assessment tools for hospitalized older adults [8,9].

Although many frailty-specific screening and assessment tools have been developed, with a subset of them also validated for the oncology population, there continues to be a lack of knowledge and their implementation amongst oncological healthcare professionals worldwide [10,11]. At present, there is no consensus on the optimum frailty screening or assessment tool for the geriatric oncology population [12]. In fact, frailty and pre-frailty can also be detected using non-frailty-specific assessment tools used in oncology populations (e.g., the scored patient-generated subjective global assessment (PG-SGA)), which is primarily a nutritional assessment tool [13]. While there is significant variability in how studies categorize frailty and pre-frailty within the older adult oncology population, addressing these conditions remains a priority in geriatric oncology research [12,14].

Studies examining frailty and pre-frailty in older adults with a history of cancer have been limited to outpatient settings [15]. Limited studies have determined the prevalence and outcomes of frailty depending on a history of cancer in acutely hospitalized older adults.

This study had two aims. First, to expand the limited knowledge of characteristics related to frailty and cancer by describing and comparing the frailty status and patient characteristics between older adults with a history of cancer and those without who are admitted to the acute medical unit (AMU) of a tertiary hospital. Second, to better understand the impact of a history of cancer on clinical outcomes during hospital stay by comparing hospital length of stay (LOS) and inpatient mortality between these two groups. We hypothesize that there will be a difference in frailty statuses between older adults with and without a history of cancer and that those with a history of cancer will have a poorer clinical outcome compared to those without.

2. Materials and Methods

2.1. Study Design and Setting

A prospective observational study was conducted in a cohort of hospitalized older adults ≥65 years (n = 329), admitted to the AMU, Flinders Medical Centre, Adelaide, South Australia. The AMU is a 30-bed medical unit that accepts patients who are referred directly from the emergency department for medical admission. This includes short-stay medical patients who require admission for ≤48 h and are discharged directly from the AMU. Patients may also be referred to long-stay medical wards from the AMU if they are deemed, by their attending physician, that they need further care after 48 h. The AMU also admits patients for the geriatric services of the hospital, including older patients who require input from the Older Persons Assessment Liaison team and nursing home patients who are seen by the Residential Care Outreach Service team.

2.2. Recruitment and Ethics

All eligible patients ≥65 years, admitted between February and September 2020 to the AMU, were approached for participation in this study within 48 h of their hospital admission. As many of the assessments were only available in English and had components that required patients to self-assess, patients who were unable to speak English, or those with cognitive impairment (Mini-Mental State Examination (MMSE) score $\leq$ 24), [16] and were unable to provide valid consent, were excluded. Patients who were under palliative care/severely or critically ill were deemed by the treating clinical team as unsafe to participate in this research study and were also excluded. This study was approved by the Southern Adelaide Clinical Human Research Ethics Committee (HREC reference number: HREC/19/SAC/240), within which the work was undertaken and conforms to the provisions of the Declaration of Helsinki in 1995 (as revised in Edinburgh 2000). Written informed consent was obtained from each participant. Participants were recruited by research staff not involved in their usual care. This study was reported in accordance with the Strengthening the Reporting of Observational Studies in Epidemiology (STROBE) guidelines [17].

2.3. Measures

2.3.1. Frailty Status

The EFS was used to assess frailty status. The EFS assesses nine domains contributing to frailty–cognition, general health status, functional independence, social support, medication use, nutrition, mood, continence and functional performance [9]. The EFS score ranges from 0 to 17 points with higher scores indicative of a greater severity of frailty [6]. The total score categorizes the patient into one of the following five categories: not frail; pre-frail; mildly frail; moderately frail; and severely frail. For this study, we simplified the frailty categories by dividing the EFS score into three categories—robust (0–5), pre-frail (6–7) and frail ($\geq$8)—as the degree of frailty was not a primary focus.

2.3.2. History of Cancer

Information on the history of or existing cancer(s), type and current status(es) of cancer was collected from electronic medical records and patient case files at the time of recruitment.

2.3.3. Other Patient Factors and Clinical Outcomes

The following patient factors of all participants were collected from electronic medical records and case files: age, sex, weight (kg), height (m), day of admission, comorbidities, number of medications, vitamin D supplementation, living status (living alone or with partner/friend), income and education level. The body mass index (BMI), kg/height (m^2), was calculated from weight and height. The Mini-Mental State Examination (MMSE) was used to ascertain cognition [18]. A research dietitian conducted nutritional assessments on all participants using the PG-SGA and scored PG-SGA [19]. The Charlson Comorbidity Index (CCI) was used to assess the burden of comorbidities [20]. The clinical outcomes of interest for this study, hospital LOS and in-patient mortality, were also recorded.

2.4. Statistical Analysis

All statistical analyses were performed with SAS software version 9.3, IBM SPSS Statistics version 28.0 (IBM Corp, Armonk, NY, USA) and STATA version 18.0, and two-sided p-values < 0.05 were considered statistically significant. The sample size for this study was determined using a sample size calculator with the "CI for one proportion" method, based on a previously reported frailty prevalence of 0.7, and with an alpha level of 0.05. The sample size calculator from the Australian Bureau of Statistics was utilized, considering the population of older adults in South Australia in 2019 and prevalence data from two earlier studies [21–23]. Normality tests, one-way ANOVA, t-test and Chi-square tests of independence using a range of demographic and clinical variables compared "older adults with history of cancer" and "older adults without cancer". Additional Kruskal–Wallis H tests were conducted for CCI. We used multivariable models for older adults with a history of cancer and those without to identify the characteristics associated with frailty and pre-frailty, with robust individuals serving as the reference group. The results were reported as odds ratio (OR) with 95% confidence interval (CI). Additionally, we employed multivariable Poisson regression, adjusting for various patient characteristics (age, sex, BMI, CCI, number of medications, use of vitamin D, living situation, education and income level and malnutrition status) to compare hospital LOS between older adults with and without a history of cancer, and the findings reported as an incidence rate ratio (IRR) with 95% CI.

3. Results

Figure 1 illustrates the flow of patient recruitment wherein 329 consecutive older adult patients were included in the study. Normality tests revealed a normal distribution for all measures except for CCI and LOS.

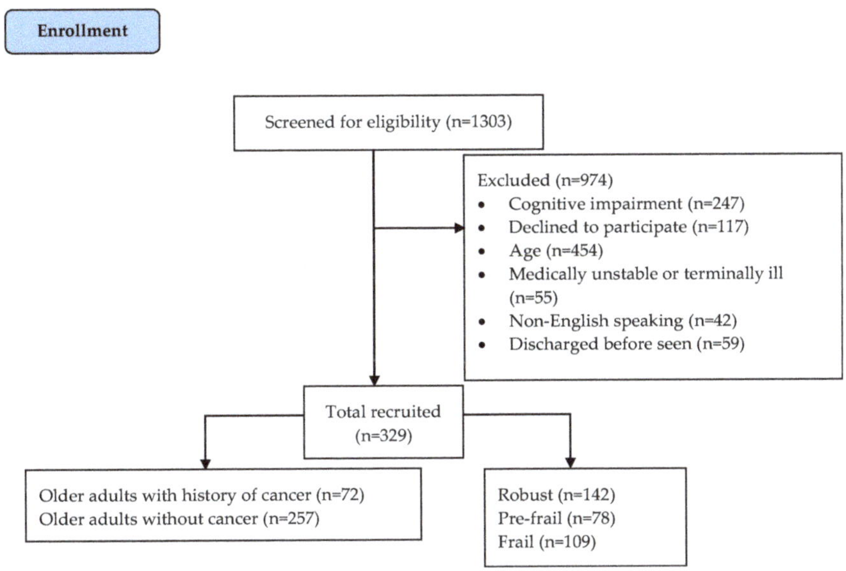

Figure 1. Flowchart of consecutive patient recruitment for present analyses.

3.1. Patient Characteristics

Characteristics of the study cohort organized by a history of cancer are presented in Table 1. Overall, 22% of hospitalized older adults (n = 72) had a history of cancer. The cancer types were prostate (n = 20), breast (n = 13), lung (n = 8), gastrointestinal (n = 8), skin (n = 6), colorectal (n = 5), head and neck (n = 2), liver (n = 3), ovarian (n = 2) and others (n = 4). Eight participants had cancers that were metastatic. There was no significant difference in the prevalence of pre-frailty/frailty among patients with or without a history of cancer (58% vs. 56%, respectively, $p > 0.05$). Older adults with a history of cancer were significantly more likely to be male, with a higher comorbidity burden, and poorer nutritional status when compared to those without a history of cancer ($p < 0.05$ for all).

Table 1. Characteristics of cohort by history of cancer (n = 329).

	History of Cancer (n = 72)	Without Cancer (n = 257)	p-Value [a]
Age [b]	79.7 ± 6.5	78.9 ± 8.6	0.483
Age (years) [c]			
65–79	37 (51%)	137 (53%)	0.773
≥80	35 (49%)	120 (47%)	

Table 1. *Cont.*

	History of Cancer (n = 72)	Without Cancer (n = 257)	p-Value [a]
BMI [b]	26.4 ± 5.4	27.1 ± 6.5	0.396
BMI [c]			
Under/healthy weight	31 (43%)	105 (41%)	0.738
Overweight/obese	41 (57%)	153 (59%)	
Sex [c]			
Male	46 (64%)	105 (41%)	<0.001
Female	26 (36%)	152 (59%)	
CCI score [b]	4.9 ± 2.0	4.3 ± 1.3	0.003
CCI score [c]			
0–3	19 (26%)	77 (30%)	0.556
≥4	53 (74%)	180 (70%)	
No. of medications [b]	6.8 ± 3.7	6.1 ± 3.6	0.155
No. of medications [c]			
0–4	24 (33%)	90 (35%)	0.790
≥5	48 (67%)	167 (65%)	
On vitamin D [c]			
Yes	20 (28%)	89 (35%)	0.275
No	52 (73%)	168 (65%)	
Living alone [c]			
Yes	24 (33%)	117 (46%)	0.065
No	48 (68%)	140 (54%)	
Education level [c]			
Tertiary	31 (43%)	114 (44%)	0.844
Up to secondary	41 (57%)	143 (56%)	
Income level [c]			
≤20 k	36 (50%)	105 (41%)	0.166
>20 k	36 (50%)	152 (59%)	
PG-SGA [c]			
Well nourished	34 (47%)	175 (68%)	0.001
Malnourished	38 (53%)	82 (32%)	
EFS category [c]			
Robust	30 (42%)	112 (44%)	0.772
Pre-frail/Frail	42 (58%)	145 (56%)	

BMI: Body Mass Index; CCI: Charlson comorbidity index; PG-SGA: Patient-generated Subjective Global Assessment; EFS: Edmonton Frail Scale; [a] p-values obtained by one-way ANOVA or t-tests for continuous variables and Chi-square tests for categorical variables; [b] values reflect the mean (standard deviation) for continuous variables; [c] values expressed as absolute numbers (percentage) for categorical variables; percentage may not add up due to rounding.

3.2. Characteristics and Clinical Outcomes Associated with Frailty and Pre-Frailty

According to the multivariate model (Table 2) that included all participants with a history of cancer, pre-frailty/frailty demonstrated significant associations with both polypharmacy (OR 8.26, 95% CI: 1.74 to 39.2) and malnutrition (OR 8.91, 95% CI: 2.15 to 36.9). Conversely, among older adults without a history of cancer, pre-frailty/frailty was associated with a higher CCI (OR 2.64, 95% CI: 1.13 to 6.20) and a lower education level (OR 2.64, 95% CI: 1.13 to 6.20), in addition to polypharmacy (OR 2.98, 95% CI: 1.57 to 5.66) and malnutrition (OR 9.03, 95% CI: 4.25 to 19.2). In older adults with a history of cancer, while the median (IQR) hospital LOS was longer compared to those without cancer, the result was not statistically significant (3 (2, 6) versus 2 (2, 4) days, $p = 0.085$). Unadjusted analysis indicated that the risk of experiencing a prolonged LOS was 41% higher in older adults with a history of cancer than in those without (incidence risk ratio (IRR) 1.41, 95% CI 1.26 to 1.58, $p < 0.001$). Following adjusted analysis which accounted for factors such as age, gender, BMI, living status, Charlson index, vitamin D supplementation, SGA status, income level, prior admissions and EFS score, the LOS remained significantly longer in older adults with a history of cancer than in those without (IRR 1.24, 95% CI 1.10 to 1.41, $p < 0.001$). In-patient mortality was not analyzed due to the occurrence of only one death during hospitalization.

Table 2. Multivariate models examining the characteristics associated with pre-frailty/frailty status (versus robust) in older adults with a history of cancer and those without cancer.

Characteristics	History of Cancer OR (95% CI)	Without Cancer OR (95% CI)
Age		
65–79	Reference	Reference
≥80	0.88 (0.18–4.39)	1.60 (0.77–3.36)
Sex		
Male	Reference	Reference
Female	1.51 (0.35–6.55)	1.04 (0.55–1.95)
BMI		
Underweight/healthy weight	Reference	Reference
Overweight/obese	3.03 (0.76–12.03)	1.84 (0.98–3.44)
CCI score		
0–3	Reference	Reference
≥4	0.91 (0.14–5.90)	2.64 (1.13–6.20) *
No. of medications		
0–4	Reference	Reference
≥5	8.26 (1.74–39.16) *	2.98 (1.57–5.66) *
On vitamin D		
Yes	Reference	Reference
No	0.68 (0.14–3.38)	1.36 (0.72–2.57)
Living alone		
No	Reference	Reference
Yes	1.76 (0.39–7.96)	1.09 (0.59–2.01)
Education level		
Tertiary	Reference	Reference
Up to secondary	1.78 (0.47–6.73)	2.14 (1.17–3.91) *
Income level		
>20 k	Reference	Reference
≤20 k	0.29 (0.07–1.17)	1.18 (0.64–2.18)
PG-SGA		
Well nourished	Reference	Reference
Malnourished/malnutrition	8.91 (2.15–36.89) *	9.03 (4.25–19.20) *

OR: odds ratio; CI: confidence interval; BMI: Body Mass Index; CCI: Charlson comorbidity index; PG-SGA: Patient-generated Subjective Global Assessment. * $p < 0.05$.

4. Discussion

Our study found more than one-fifth of hospitalized older adults in the AMU had a history of cancer. The prevalence of pre-frailty and frailty amongst them were comparable to those without a history of cancer. Regardless of cancer history, pre-frailty/frailty was independently associated with polypharmacy and malnutrition. However, the risk of having a prolonged LOS was 24% higher in older adults with a history of cancer than those without, prompting further investigations for systematic assessment and timely interventions for older adults with a history of cancer admitted to the AMU.

The results of this study concur with a recent review of 20 studies evaluating frailty and pre-frailty in older cancer patients (inpatient, hospital outpatient and community settings), which revealed that frailty/pre-frailty affected more than half of patients (median prevalence of 68%; range of 12% to 89%) [15]. Although frailty is prevalent across hospital wards, its distribution varies, contingent upon factors such as ward type, whether medical or surgical, which may account for the diversity in prevalence rates. Findings from this study support routine screening and assessment of frailty and pre-frailty in older adults admitted to the AMU, including those with a history of cancer, to inform decisions on treatment and intervention.

Findings from the present study also highlight polypharmacy and malnutrition as two important factors associated with pre-frailty/frailty in older inpatients, regardless of their cancer history, aligning with previous research in acute care and community settings [24,25]. These results have implications for clinical practice, especially in the AMU. Pre-frail and frail older adults often have several co-existing chronic conditions that require pharmacological management, leading to multiple medications being prescribed. Given the significance of polypharmacy in this group of patients, the establishment of a medication reconciliation service at the AMU could foster better communication between pharmacists and physicians. This initiative has the potential not only to deprescribe unnecessary medications but also to mitigate medication errors and ultimately reduce hospital LOS [26].

Likewise, malnutrition is still often missed in hospital settings due to suboptimal nutrition screening practices in hospitalized older adults, including those with cancers [27]. To alleviate malnutrition, strategies to prevent and treat frailty and pre-frailty can consider services to implement dietary change [28]. Referrals for such nutritional interventions should also be coupled with exercise to improve frailty and frailty-related indicators in hospitalized older adults [29,30]. While it is important to treat malnutrition during hospitalization, efforts should also target prevention and early intervention at the primary care level through multidisciplinary teams involving exercise health professionals and dietitians [31,32]. Whilst acknowledging the increasing burden of geriatric and oncological care on general practitioners in primary care settings, a recent novel study provided preliminary evidence that dietitians could potentially act as first contact practitioners for older adults at risk of malnutrition (and frailty) as part of the practice multidisciplinary team [33].

Further to their association with frailty and pre-frailty, polypharmacy and malnutrition can be interrelated. A recent review demonstrated a significant association between polypharmacy (defined as the use of five or more medications) and malnutrition [34]. The use of drugs is associated with a number of side effects, some of which can impact nutritional intake such as nausea, decreased appetite and decreased saliva production [35]. While malnutrition may not be a direct causal factor for more medication, patients who are malnourished have a higher risk of adverse events which may require additional medications as part of its management. For example, post-operative infections may require antibiotic treatment, or individuals undergoing cancer therapy may experience more pronounced side effects, leading to the need for additional medications [36].

The median LOS found in this study from the AMU corresponds with and adds to reports from other studies: a cohort study of hospitalization in cancer patients (i.e., cancer types: breast, prostate, lung, gastrointestinal and colorectal) with LOS of the median (IQR) of 3 (2–7) days, and another retrospective study of in-hospital LOS after surgical oncological procedures with LOS of median (IQR) of 4 (2–7) days [37,38]. Furthermore, similar to another study, a comparison between cancer and non-cancer diagnoses has shown that hospital LOS was longer for patients with cancer [39].

There could be several reasons for older adults with a history of cancer have a longer hospital LOS compared to their non-cancer counterparts. Older adults with active cancers deal with acute side effects of treatment or cancer itself, while those that survive have to cope with long-term and/or late effects of treatments—physical and psychological issues, e.g., lymphoedema, osteoporosis, pain, fatigue, altered sleep and cognition [40,41]. Consequently, admission to an acute care setting can sometimes exacerbate these symptoms and could trigger a cascade of additional investigations that may not be directly related to the presenting problem. In addition, cancer care often involves input from a multidisciplinary team of specialists including oncologists, nurses and allied health professionals, and delays in organizing care among these different specialties may extend the hospital stay [42]. It is worth highlighting that, in this cohort, 11% of the older adults with a history of cancer were living with metastatic cancers. Future research could prioritize enhancing access to specialist advice and triage services within the community settings. By doing so, we can proactively address the intricate needs of older adults with a history of cancer, intervening before these needs escalate to emergency department visits or inpatient hospitalizations [43].

Several strategies have been proposed to bridge existing health services across settings for older adults with cancer so these services can better meet their complex needs. Montroni and colleagues proposed a six-step multidimensional, multiphase pathway to optimize the care of older adults with cancer undergoing surgery that included co-management in the long term, as recovery continues after hospital discharge, e.g., linking operative service with prehabilitation and transitional care management [44]. Another strategy, which is probably more achievable within the community, is the integration of comprehensive geriatric assessment into community oncology practices, which has been associated with improved patient-centered communication, reduced hospital LOS and treatment toxicity in older adults with cancer [45,46].

While a longer LOS may seem burdensome, it can serve as an opportunity for beneficial interventions, especially in older adults with complex health needs. Unplanned hospitalization can be an opportunity in disguise to allow for conducting geriatric and frailty assessments, which can help identify gaps in care and pinpoint areas for improvement. These assessments may help healthcare professionals tailor treatment plans and make referrals to appropriate services, ultimately improving outcomes for older patients [47].

This study has several strengths. Frailty and pre-frailty were measured with a validated assessment tool in older adults with and without cancer that incorporates the multidimensional domains (cognition, general health status, functional independence and performance, social support, medication use, nutrition, mood, continence) included in a comprehensive geriatric assessment [48–50]. The consecutive sampling also reduced bias in the selection of participants during the data collection period. However, this study is not without limitations. A sensitivity analysis replacing frailty defined by EFS with another frailty assessment tool could not be conducted, as frailty was not concurrently measured with another validated tool. Future studies can consider measuring frailty with different tools to assess the relationship between frailty status and LOS and other outcome measures. Participants in this study may not represent older adults who were unable to speak in English, with mild to severe cognitive impairments, or those directly admitted to general wards from the emergency department. Therefore, the generalizability of the results to other populations or settings may be limited. Lastly, inpatient mortality could not be examined due to the lack of incidences reported within this study period.

5. Conclusions

The prevalence of frailty/pre-frailty did not differ between older adults with a history of cancer and those without in the AMU. Factors associated with frailty/pre-frailty, regardless of history of cancer, are not different from those reported in other settings; polypharmacy and malnutrition are two important factors in both older adults with and without a history of cancer. Acutely hospitalized older adults with a history of cancer had a higher risk of a longer LOS compared to those without cancer. This prompts further investigations not only into systematic assessment to identify those at risk but also into trialing new models of care or evolving existing health services to provide early interventions that extend to the community to meet the complex needs of this vulnerable population.

Author Contributions: Conceptualization, C.Y.H., R.J.C., A.Y., Y.S., C.B. and M.M.; methodology, C.Y.H., H.S.N., A.Y., Y.S., C.B. and M.M.; formal analysis, C.Y.H., H.S.N. and Y.S.; resources, C.Y.H. and M.M.; writing—original draft preparation, C.Y.H.; writing—review and editing, R.J.C., H.S.N., A.Y., Y.S., C.B. and M.M.; supervision, A.Y., Y.S., C.B. and M.M.; project administration, C.Y.H. Funding, C.Y.H. and M.M. All authors have read and agreed to the published version of the manuscript.

Funding: This study is partially supported by Flinders University's College of Nursing and Health Sciences Research Student Maintenance and the Australian Government Research Training Program Scholarship. In addition, in-kind support for the staff working on this project has been provided by the Flinders Medical Centre, Southern Adelaide Local Health Network. The funder had no role in the design and conduct of the study; the collection, management, analysis and interpretation of the data; preparation, review, or approval of the manuscript; and the decision to submit the manuscript for publication.

Institutional Review Board Statement: This study was approved by the Southern Adelaide Clinical Human Research Ethics Committee (HREC reference number: HREC/19/SAC/240) on 4 December 2019, within which the work was undertaken and conforms to the provisions of the Declaration of Helsinki in 1995 (as revised in Edinburgh 2000).

Informed Consent Statement: A written informed consent was obtained from each participant regarding the use of their data for the purposes of this research study.

Data Availability Statement: The raw data supporting the conclusions of this article will be made available by the authors upon request.

Acknowledgments: All authors would like to thank the respective heads of departments and nurse managers at the Flinders Medical Centre for facilitating this study, and all the participants who have taken time from their schedules to contribute to improving healthcare services.

Conflicts of Interest: The authors declare no conflicts of interest.

References

1. Cunha, A.I.L.; Veronese, N.; de Melo Borges, S.; Ricci, N.A. Frailty as a predictor of adverse outcomes in hospitalized older adults: A systematic review and meta-analysis. *Ageing Res. Rev.* **2019**, *56*, 100960. [CrossRef] [PubMed]
2. Boucher, E.L.; Gan, J.M.; Rothwell, P.M.; Shepperd, S.; Pendlebury, S.T. Prevalence and outcomes of frailty in unplanned hospital admissions: A systematic review and meta-analysis of hospital-wide and general (internal) medicine cohorts. *eClinicalMedicine* **2023**, *59*, 101947. [CrossRef]
3. Siegel, R.L.; Miller, K.D.; Fuchs, H.E.; Jemal, A. Cancer statistics, 2022. *CA Cancer J. Clin.* **2022**, *72*, 524–541. [CrossRef] [PubMed]
4. Veronese, N.; Custodero, C.; Cella, A.; Demurtas, J.; Zora, S.; Maggi, S.; Barbagallo, M.; Sabba, C.; Ferrucci, L.; Pilotto, A. Prevalence of multidimensional frailty and pre-frailty in older people in different settings: A systematic review and meta-analysis. *Ageing Res. Rev.* **2021**, *72*, 101498. [CrossRef] [PubMed]
5. Mohile, S.G.; Xian, Y.; Dale, W.; Fisher, S.G.; Rodin, M.; Morrow, G.R.; Neugut, A.; Hall, W. Association of a cancer diagnosis with vulnerability and frailty in older Medicare beneficiaries. *J. Natl. Cancer Inst.* **2009**, *101*, 1206–1215. [CrossRef] [PubMed]
6. Ethun, C.G.; Bilen, M.A.; Jani, A.B.; Maithel, S.K.; Ogan, K.; Master, V.A. Frailty and cancer: Implications for oncology surgery, medical oncology, and radiation oncology. *CA Cancer J. Clin.* **2017**, *67*, 362–377. [CrossRef] [PubMed]
7. Goede, V. Frailty and cancer: Current perspectives on assessment and monitoring. *Clin. Interv. Aging* **2023**, *18*, 505–521. [CrossRef] [PubMed]
8. Apóstolo, J.; Cooke, R.; Bobrowicz-Campos, E.; Santana, S.; Marcucci, M.; Cano, A.; Vollenbroek-Hutten, M.; Germini, F.; Holland, C. Predicting risk and outcomes for frail older adults: An umbrella review of frailty screening tools. *JBI Evid. Synth.* **2017**, *15*, 1154–1208. [CrossRef] [PubMed]
9. Rolfson, D.B.; Majumdar, S.R.; Tsuyuki, R.T.; Tahir, A.; Rockwood, K. Validity and reliability of the edmonton frail scale. *Age Ageing* **2006**, *35*, 526–529. [CrossRef] [PubMed]
10. Banna, G.L.; Cantale, O.; Haydock, M.M.; Battisti, N.M.L.; Bambury, K.; Musolino, N.; O'Carroll, E.; Maltese, G.; Garetto, L.; Addeo, A.; et al. International survey on frailty assessment in patients with cancer. *Oncologist* **2022**, *27*, e796–e803. [CrossRef] [PubMed]
11. Huisingh-Scheetz, M.; Walston, J. How should older adults with cancer be evaluated for frailty? *J. Geriatr. Oncol.* **2017**, *8*, 8–15. [CrossRef] [PubMed]
12. Fletcher, J.A.; Logan, B.; Reid, N.; Gordon, E.H.; Ladwa, R.; Hubbard, R.E. How frail is frail in oncology studies? A scoping review. *BMC Cancer* **2023**, *23*, 498. [CrossRef] [PubMed]
13. Han, C.Y.; Sharma, Y.; Yaxley, A.; Baldwin, C.; Miller, M. Use of the patient-generated subjective global assessment to identify pre-frailty and frailty in hospitalized older adults. *J. Nutr. Health Aging* **2021**, *25*, 1229–1234. [CrossRef] [PubMed]
14. Extermann, M.; Brain, E.; Canin, B.; Cherian, M.N.; Cheung, K.L.; de Glas, N.; Devi, B.; Hamaker, M.; Kanesvaran, R.; Karnakis, T.; et al. Priorities for the global advancement of care for older adults with cancer: An update of the international society of geriatric oncology priorities initiative. *Lancet Oncol.* **2021**, *22*, e29–e36. [CrossRef] [PubMed]
15. Handforth, C.; Clegg, A.; Young, C.; Simpkins, S.; Seymour, M.T.; Selby, P.J.; Young, J. The prevalence and outcomes of frailty in older cancer patients: A systematic review. *Ann. Oncol.* **2015**, *26*, 1091–1101. [CrossRef] [PubMed]

16. Independent Hospital Pricing Authority. Standardised Mini-Mental State Examination. 2019. Available online: https://www.ihpa.gov.au/what-we-do/standardised-mini-mental-state-examination-smmse (accessed on 25 September 2019).
17. Von Elm, E.; Altman, D.G.; Egger, M.; Pocock, S.J.; Gøtzsche, P.C.; Vandenbroucke, J.P. The strengthening the reporting of observational studies in epidemiology (strobe) statement: Guidelines for reporting observational studies. *Bull. World Health Organ.* **2007**, *85*, 867–872. [CrossRef] [PubMed]
18. Pangman, V.C.; Sloan, J.; Guse, L. An examination of psychometric properties of the mini-mental state examination and the standardized mini-mental state examination: Implications for clinical practice. *Appl. Nurs Res.* **2000**, *13*, 209–213. [CrossRef] [PubMed]
19. Ottery, F.D.; Isenring, E.; Kasenic, S.; DeBolt, S.P.; Sealy, M.; Jager-Wittenaar, H. *Patient-Generated Subjective Global Assessment*; Hanzehogeschool Groningen: Groningen, The Netherlands, 2015.
20. Charlson, M.E.; Pompei, P.; Ales, K.L.; MacKenzie, C.R. A new method of classifying prognostic comorbidity in longitudinal studies: Development and validation. *J. Chronic Dis.* **1987**, *40*, 373–383. [CrossRef] [PubMed]
21. Australia Bureau of Statistics. Sample Size Calculator. 2019. Available online: https://www.abs.gov.au/websitedbs/D3310114.nsf/home/Sample+Size+Calculator (accessed on 25 September 2019).
22. Joosten, E.; Demuynck, M.; Detroyer, E.; Milisen, K. Prevalence of frailty and its ability to predict in hospital delirium, falls, and 6-month mortality in hospitalized older patients. *BMC Geriatr.* **2014**, *14*, 1. [CrossRef] [PubMed]
23. Andela, R.M.; Dijkstra, A.; Slaets, J.P.; Sanderman, R. Prevalence of frailty on clinical wards: Description and implications. *Int. J. Nurs. Pract.* **2010**, *16*, 14–19. [CrossRef]
24. Hammami, S.; Zarrouk, A.; Piron, C.; Almas, I.; Sakly, N.; Latteur, V. Prevalence and factors associated with frailty in hospitalized older patients. *BMC Geriatr.* **2020**, *20*, 144. [CrossRef] [PubMed]
25. Liu, J.; Zhu, Y.; Tan, J.K.; Ismail, A.H.; Ibrahim, R.; Hassan, N.H. Factors associated with frailty in older adults in community and nursing home settings: A systematic review with a meta-analysis. *J. Clin. Med.* **2024**, *13*, 2382. [CrossRef]
26. Park, B.; Baek, A.; Kim, Y.; Suh, Y.; Lee, J.; Lee, E.; Lee, J.Y.; Lee, E.; Lee, J.; Park, H.S.; et al. Clinical and economic impact of medication reconciliation by designated ward pharmacists in a hospitalist-managed acute medical unit. *Res. Social Adm. Pharm.* **2022**, *18*, 2683–2690. [CrossRef] [PubMed]
27. Sharma, Y.; Thompson, C.; Shahi, R.; Hakendorf, P.; Miller, M. Malnutrition in acutely unwell hospitalized elderly—"The skeletons are still rattling in the hospital closet". *J. Nutr. Health Aging* **2017**, *21*, 1210–1215. [CrossRef] [PubMed]
28. Ni Lochlainn, M.; Cox, N.J.; Wilson, T.; Hayhoe, R.P.; Ramsay, S.E.; Granic, A.; Isanejad, M.; Roberts, H.C.; Wilson, D.; Welch, C.; et al. Nutrition and frailty: Opportunities for prevention and treatment. *Nutrients* **2021**, *13*, 2349. [CrossRef] [PubMed]
29. Han, C.Y.; Miller, M.; Yaxley, A.; Baldwin, C.; Woodman, R.; Sharma, Y. Effectiveness of combined exercise and nutrition interventions in prefrail or frail older hospitalised patients: A systematic review and meta-analysis. *BMJ Open* **2020**, *10*, e040146. [CrossRef] [PubMed]
30. Han, C.Y.; Sharma, Y.; Yaxley, A.; Baldwin, C.; Woodman, R.; Miller, M. Individualized hospital to home, exercise-nutrition self-managed intervention for pre-frail and frail hospitalized older adults: The independence randomized controlled pilot trial. *Clin. Interv. Aging* **2023**, *18*, 809–825. [CrossRef] [PubMed]
31. Joseph, R.; Hart, N.H.; Bradford, N.; Agbejule, O.A.; Koczwara, B.; Chan, A.; Wallen, M.P.; Chan, R.J. Diet and exercise advice and referrals for cancer survivors: An integrative review of medical and nursing perspectives. *Support Care Cancer* **2022**, *30*, 8429–8439. [CrossRef] [PubMed]
32. Joseph, R.; Hart, N.H.; Bradford, N.; Wallen, M.P.; Han, C.Y.; Pinkham, E.P.; Hanley, B.; Lock, G.; Wyld, D.; Wishart, L.; et al. Essential elements of optimal dietary and exercise referral practices for cancer survivors: Expert consensus for medical and nursing health professionals. *Support Care Cancer* **2023**, *31*, 46. [CrossRef] [PubMed]
33. Hickson, M.; Child, J.; Collinson, A. Impact of a dietitian in general practice: Care of the frail and malnourished. *J. Hum. Nutr. Diet.* **2022**, *35*, 145–153. [CrossRef] [PubMed]
34. Kok, W.; Haverkort, E.; Algra, Y.; Mollema, J.; Hollaar, V.R.Y.; Naumann, E.; de van der Schueren, M.A.E.; Jerković-Ćosić, K. The association between polypharmacy and malnutrition (risk) in older people: A systematic review. *Clin. Nutr. ESPEN* **2022**, *49*, 163–171. [CrossRef] [PubMed]
35. Omlin, A.; Blum, D.; Wierecky, J.; Haile, S.R.; Ottery, F.D.; Strasser, F. Nutrition impact symptoms in advanced cancer patients: Frequency and specific interventions, a case–control study. *J. Cachexia Sarcopenia Muscle* **2013**, *4*, 55–61. [CrossRef] [PubMed]
36. Riad, A.; Knight, S.R.; Ghosh, D.; Kingsley, P.A.; Lapitan, M.C.; Parreno-Sacdalan, M.D.; Sundar, S.; Qureshi, A.U.; Valparaiso, A.P.; Pius, R.; et al. Impact of malnutrition on early outcomes after cancer surgery: An international, multicentre, prospective cohort study. *Lancet Glob. Health* **2023**, *11*, e341–e349. [CrossRef] [PubMed]
37. Feliciana Silva, F.; Macedo da Silva Bonfante, G.; Reis, I.A.; André da Rocha, H.; Pereira Lana, A.; Leal Cherchiglia, M. Hospitalizations and length of stay of cancer patients: A cohort study in the brazilian public health system. *PLoS ONE* **2020**, *15*, e0233293. [CrossRef] [PubMed]
38. Nazzani, S.; Preisser, F.; Mazzone, E.; Tian, Z.; Mistretta, F.A.; Shariat, S.F.; Saad, F.; Graefen, M.; Tilki, D.; Montanari, E.; et al. In-hospital length of stay after major surgical oncological procedures. *Eur. J. Surg. Oncol.* **2018**, *44*, 969–974. [CrossRef] [PubMed]
39. Numico, G.; Zanelli, C.; Ippoliti, R.; Rossi, M.; Traverso, E.; Antonuzzo, A.; Bellini, R. The hospital care of patients with cancer: A retrospective analysis of the characteristics of their hospital stay in comparison with other medical conditions. *Eur. J. Cancer* **2020**, *139*, 99–106. [CrossRef] [PubMed]

40. Fitch, M.I.; Nicoll, I.; Lockwood, G.; Strohschein, F.J.; Newton, L. Main challenges in survivorship transitions: Perspectives of older adults with cancer. *J. Geriatr. Oncol.* **2021**, *12*, 632–640. [CrossRef]
41. Emery, J.; Butow, P.; Lai-Kwon, J.; Nekhlyudov, L.; Rynderman, M.; Jefford, M. Management of common clinical problems experienced by survivors of cancer. *Lancet* **2022**, *399*, 1537–1550. [CrossRef] [PubMed]
42. Presley, C.J.; Krok-Schoen, J.L.; Wall, S.A.; Noonan, A.M.; Jones, D.C.; Folefac, E.; Williams, N.; Overcash, J.; Rosko, A.E. Implementing a multidisciplinary approach for older adults with cancer: Geriatric oncology in practice. *BMC Geriatr.* **2020**, *20*, 231. [CrossRef] [PubMed]
43. Chen, H.; Johnson, M.; Boland, E.; Seymour, J.; Macleod, U. Emergency admissions and subsequent inpatient care through an emergency oncology service at a tertiary cancer centre: Service users' experiences and views. *Support Care Cancer* **2019**, *27*, 451–460. [CrossRef] [PubMed]
44. Montroni, I.; Saur, N.M.; Shahrokni, A.; Suwanabol, P.A.; Chesney, T.R. Surgical considerations for older adults with cancer: A multidimensional, multiphase pathway to improve care. *J. Clin. Oncol.* **2021**, *39*, 2090. [CrossRef] [PubMed]
45. Mohile, S.G.; Epstein, R.M.; Hurria, A.; Heckler, C.E.; Canin, B.; Culakova, E.; Duberstein, P.; Gilmore, N.; Xu, H.; Plumb, S. Communication with older patients with cancer using geriatric assessment: A cluster-randomized clinical trial from the national cancer institute community oncology research program. *JAMA Oncol.* **2020**, *6*, 196–204. [CrossRef] [PubMed]
46. Zuccarino, S.; Monacelli, F.; Antognoli, R.; Nencioni, A.; Monzani, F.; Ferrè, F.; Seghieri, C.; Antonelli Incalzi, R. Exploring cost-effectiveness of the comprehensive geriatric assessment in geriatric oncology: A narrative review. *Cancers* **2022**, *14*, 3235. [CrossRef] [PubMed]
47. Mariano, C.; Williams, G.; Deal, A.; Alston, S.; Bryant, A.L.; Jolly, T.; Muss, H.B. Geriatric assessment of older adults with cancer during unplanned hospitalizations: An opportunity in disguise. *Oncologist* **2015**, *20*, 767–772. [CrossRef] [PubMed]
48. Parker, S.G.; McCue, P.; Phelps, K.; McCleod, A.; Arora, S.; Nockels, K.; Kennedy, S.; Roberts, H.; Conroy, S. What is comprehensive geriatric assessment (cga)? An umbrella review. *Age Ageing* **2018**, *47*, 149–155. [CrossRef] [PubMed]
49. Meyers, B.M.; Al-Shamsi, H.O.; Rask, S.; Yelamanchili, R.; Phillips, C.M.; Papaioannou, A.; Pond, G.R.; Jeyabalan, N.; Zbuk, K.M.; Dhesy-Thind, S.K. Utility of the edmonton frail scale in identifying frail elderly patients during treatment of colorectal cancer. *J. Gastrointest. Oncol.* **2017**, *8*, 32. [CrossRef] [PubMed]
50. Røyset, I.M.; Eriksen, G.F.; Benth, J.Š.; Saltvedt, I.; Grønberg, B.H.; Rostoft, S.; Kirkevold, Ø.; Rolfson, D.; Slaaen, M. Edmonton frail scale predicts mortality in older patients with cancer undergoing radiotherapy—A prospective observational study. *PLoS ONE* **2023**, *18*, e0283507. [CrossRef] [PubMed]

cancers

MDPI

Article

Exploring the Language Used to Describe Older Patients at Multidisciplinary Cancer Conferences

Valerie S. Kim [1,2,†], Anthony Carrozzi [1,†], Efthymios Papadopoulos [3], Isabel Tejero [4], Thirisangi Thiruparanathan [5], Nathan Perlis [6], Andrew J. Hope [7,8], Raymond W. Jang [9] and Shabbir M. H. Alibhai [2,10,11,*]

1 Temerty Faculty of Medicine, University of Toronto, Toronto, ON M5S 1A8, Canada; valerie.kim@mail.utoronto.ca (V.S.K.); anthony.carrozzi@mail.utoronto.ca (A.C.)
2 Department of Medicine, University Health Network, Toronto, ON M5G 2C4, Canada
3 School of Kinesiology, Louisiana State University, Baton Rouge, LA 70802, USA; epap@lsu.edu
4 Department of Geriatrics, Hospital del Mar, 08003 Barcelona, Spain; itejero@psmar.cat
5 Department of Nursing, University Health Network, Toronto, ON M5G 2C4, Canada; thirisangi.thiruparanathan@mail.utoronto.ca
6 Division of Urology, Department of Surgical Oncology, University Health Network, Toronto, ON M5G 2C4, Canada; nathan.perlis@uhn.ca
7 Department of Radiation Oncology, University of Toronto, Toronto, ON M5T 1P5, Canada; andrew.hope@uhn.ca
8 Radiation Medicine Program, Princess Margaret Cancer Centre, Toronto, ON M5G 2M9, Canada
9 Division of Medical Oncology and Hematology, Princess Margaret Cancer Centre, Toronto, ON M5G 2M9, Canada; raymond.jang@uhn.ca
10 Department of Medicine, University of Toronto, Toronto, ON M5G 2C4, Canada
11 Institute of Health Policy, Management, and Evaluation, University of Toronto, Toronto, ON M5T 3M6, Canada
* Correspondence: shabbir.alibhai@uhn.ca
† These authors contributed equally to this work.

Simple Summary: Older adults with cancer are often the subject of much discussion at multidisciplinary cancer conferences (MCCs), yet little is known about the language used to describe frailty and other geriatric considerations at these meetings. Our objective was to explore how MCC presentations depict older patients. We found that MCCs frequently referred to comorbidity burden and projected treatment tolerance on the basis of subjective evaluations, rather than comprehensive geriatric assessments. We also noted that mentions of surrogate measures for frailty, such as chronological age and performance status, varied between tumour sites, presenter specialties, and presenter training levels. Overall, our results suggest that MCCs predominantly rely on age-based descriptions and, thus, engender risk of age-biased decision making. This work may guide future efforts aimed at standardizing the language at MCCs to include more objective terms and validated tools for considering different geriatric domains when discussing older adults with cancer.

Abstract: Older adults with cancer often present with distinct complexities that complicate their care, yet the language used to discuss their management at multidisciplinary cancer conferences (MCCs) remains poorly understood. A mixed methods study was conducted at a tertiary cancer centre in Toronto, Canada, where MCCs spanning five tumour sites were attended over six months. For presentations pertaining to a patient aged 75 or older, a standardized data collection form was used to record their demographic, cancer-related, and non-cancer-related information, as well as the presenter's specialty and training level. Descriptive statistics and thematic analysis were employed to explore MCC depictions of older patients (n = 75). Frailty status was explicitly mentioned in 20.0% of presentations, but discussions more frequently referenced comorbidity burden (50.7%), age (33.3%), and projected treatment tolerance (30.7%) as surrogate measures. None of the presentations included mentions of formal geriatric assessment (GA) or validated frailty tools; instead, presenters tended to feature select GA domains and subjective descriptions of appearance ("looks to be fit") or overall health ("relatively healthy"). In general, MCCs appeared to rely on age-focused language that may perpetuate ageism. Further work is needed to investigate how frailty and geriatric considerations can be objectively incorporated into discussions in geriatric oncology.

Keywords: multidisciplinary cancer conferences; tumour boards; geriatric oncology; geriatric assessment; frailty; communicate; language

1. Introduction

Older adults comprise a growing majority of patients with cancer, yet they remain disproportionately underrepresented in research trials and evidence-based guidelines [1,2]. As a result, clinical decision making for this demographic can be complicated and nuanced, particularly given the heterogeneity in their medical comorbidities, cognitive abilities, and functional levels [3–5].

Against this backdrop, older adults are often the subject of much discussion at multidisciplinary cancer conferences (MCCs) or "tumour boards", where health professionals with complementary areas of expertise convene to deliberate cases, review guidelines, and coordinate treatment plans [6]. According to a recent umbrella review, this forum can facilitate guideline-concordant diagnosis and treatment [7]. By fostering communication between cancer care team members and promoting discourse on best practices, MCCs represent key opportunities for collaborative decision making and high-quality care [6,7].

At these meetings, a high-level summary about each patient is presented and discussed in a time-sensitive manner [6,7]. The details shared and the language used can carry significant connotations and implications for treatment decisions: depictions of patients as "elderly" or "old", for instance, can influence clinicians' perceptions and subsequently their recommendations [6,8]. In fact, patients who are described as older may be less likely to be referred for adjuvant chemotherapy [9]. According to a recent literature-based perspective piece, age-biased decision making and stereotyping appear to pervade conversations related to diagnostic and therapeutic recommendations for older adults with cancer [10–12]. In one report, a reliance on disease-centred, rather than patient-centred, terminology when caring for this demographic emerged as one of the five common patterns of stigmatizing language [12]. The prevalence of such trends in the discussion of older adults and their care raises concerns about potential ageism [12].

In our clinical experience, most MCCs without the presence of a geriatrician or a geriatric oncologist tend to focus on oncologic factors with little mention of geriatric considerations [13]. For instance, mentions of activities of daily living (ADLs) remain lacking at these meetings, despite the relevance of this detail, not only to patients' suitability for treatment, but also to their decision-making priorities [13]. While their comorbidities are generally reported in comprehensive lists using precise medical terminology, non-cancer-related characteristics are poorly described with vague phrases (for instance, "pretty fit") [8,13]. In fact, the existing literature reveals that MCCs often allude to patients' fitness as an indicator of their general physical state or their eligibility for a specific intervention, yet consensus on the definition of "fit" remains unclear among the different clinicians and specialties [8]. Although clinical guidelines have recommended the use of the geriatric assessment (GA) in evaluating frailty, it is not commonly implemented, and it remains unclear whether GA domains are even being discussed at MCCs, both for patients in general and for the select few who have undergone a formal GA [2,13].

To date, little research has explored how MCCs depict older patients with attention to their frailty levels and geriatric considerations [8,13–19]. This has left a major gap in our understanding of the impact of language on cancer care. For these reasons, our study aimed to explore how MCCs presented older patients, their frailty considerations, and their GA domains.

2. Materials and Methods

2.1. Objectives

The study's primary objective was to explore whether and how frailty status and GA domains are discussed in relation to treatment decision making for older adults with cancer at MCCs. We sought to examine the depiction of frailty, in the form of explicit descriptions of patients as "frail" or "fit", mentions of chronological age as a proxy for frailty status, and references to other synonyms for frailty or fitness. We additionally sought to assess the incorporation of the GA, specifically with the inclusion of two or more GA domains, into MCC discussions.

As an exploratory objective, we also set out to compare case presentations by MCC site, by presenter specialty, and by presenter training level. The latter was included to potentially inform educational initiatives that may arise from our findings.

2.2. Study Design and Setting

For this mixed methods study, we attended weekly virtual general gastrointestinal, genitourinary, head and neck, thoracic, and upper gastrointestinal MCCs at the Princess Margaret Cancer Centre in Toronto, Canada. These five MCC streams were selected after reviewing the number of annual referrals and identifying the tumour sites with the highest proportion of new patients aged 75 or older. This cutoff was selected based on the consensus among geriatric oncology experts and among study investigators that all patients aged 75 or older should undergo a GA [20].

At each MCC, a presiding chairperson oversees presentations, ensuring that relevant disciplines (e.g., radiology, pathology, medical/radiation/surgical oncology) are in attendance. Cases are presented by the physician (either the attending or a senior trainee, such as a resident or fellow) who submitted the case to MCC: they share pertinent clinical context and the reason for presentation. As relevant, imaging and pathology are reviewed by the respective disciplines. Subsequently, all attendees are invited to weigh in and offer input on the diagnostic or therapeutic question at hand. The chairperson facilitates these discussions and ultimately summarizes recommendations for each case.

For all sites, a general summary about the project was circulated a week in advance to MCC chairs and attendees, who were provided with the opportunity to opt out should they wish to be excluded from our data collection and analysis.

Approval from the Research Ethics Board of University Health Network was obtained prior to study commencement. The requirement for informed patient consent was waived.

2.3. Data Collection

A data collection form (Appendix A) was developed and refined through iterative revisions to ensure comprehensive, standardized capture of data across the research team. As nonparticipating observers, alternating members of the team (V.S.K., medical student; A.C., medical student; E.P., postdoctoral researcher in exercise oncology; I.T., geriatric oncology fellow; and T.T., graduate nursing student) attended MCCs and electronically recorded our variables of interest for presentations pertaining to patients aged 75 or older. We organized these variables into two groups. The first group consisted of frailty-related variables: in the absence of a universally shared definition for frailty at these meetings, these variables included explicit terminology or assessment to describe patients as "frail" or "fit", as well as synonyms for frailty status, including activity, mobility, appearance, overall health, treatment tolerance, independence, and performance status. The second group consisted of GA-related variables encompassing the following domains: functional status, physical performance, falls, comorbidities, medications, cognition, mood, social support, and nutritional status.

The data collection form included a checklist, where the research team could indicate whether a variable was mentioned, as well as an area for free text, where frailty and GA-related descriptions could be recorded verbatim. Definitions and examples for each variable are provided in Table 1.

Table 1. Definitions and examples of frailty-related and GA-related variables.

	Variables	Definition	Examples
Frailty-Related	Frailty status	Description of patients as "frail", "vulnerable", or "fit"	"Quite frail". "Pretty fit".
	Age	Reiteration of age to suggest or emphasize frailty/fitness status	"Fine for age". "He's 86, but an okay 86".
	Activity level	Description of patients as "active" or "inactive"	"Pretty healthy, very active".
	Appearance	Description of patients' appearance	"Looks younger than 80". "Does not look like a candidate for anything".
	Independence	Description of patients as "independent" or "dependent" on others, without elaboration on specific ADLs or IADLs	"Fully independent".
	Mobility	Description of patients' ability to ambulate or move	"Very vigorous, moves well".
	Overall health	Description of patients' general health or well-being	"Otherwise quite healthy".
	Performance status	Mention of patients' performance status per ECOG	"ECOG 1". "Performance status poor, very symptomatic".
	Treatment tolerance	Prediction of a patient's ability to tolerate treatment	"No way fit for [chemotherapy]".
GA-Related	Comorbidities	Mention of patients' comorbidities (complete or incomplete) or comorbidity burden	"Many comorbidities, not a surgical candidate".
	Medications	Mention of patients' medication list (complete or incomplete)	"On apixaban".
	Cognition	Mention of the presence/absence of any cognitive impairment	"Baseline dementia".
	Falls	Mention of patients' falls or fall risk	"Had a fall and [subsequent] hip fracture with surgical repair".
	Functional status	Description of patients' ability to perform activities necessary for or desirable in daily life	"Fully independent, drives here for clinic appointments".
	Mood	Mention of patients' mood	"[Patient] has generalized low mood".
	Physical performance	Mention of objective measures of patients' physical function (for example, gait speed, grip strength)	N/A
	Nutrition	Mention of patients' appetite or nutritional status	"Struggling with malnutrition".
	Social support	Mention of a social support network, including mention of caregivers or loved ones involved in the patient's life	"Difficult social situation, [patient] lives alone, [with] family in [another country]".

Note: "ADL" = activities of daily living, "IADL" = instrumental activities of daily living, "ECOG" = Eastern Cooperative Oncology Group, "GA" = geriatric assessment, "N/A" = not available.

2.4. Data Analysis

Once completed, data collection forms were analyzed using convergent parallel mixed methods. While the overall cohort included representation from five tumour sites, the site-, specialty-, and training level-specific analyses excluded the head and neck presentations given the small sample size (n = 4). For the remaining four tumour sites, we anonymized their identities, as we were primarily interested in potential differences between the sites, rather than specific details about the individual sites themselves. We then enumerated the MCC presentations that included mentions of frailty- and GA-related variables. We were specifically interested in the proportion of discussions that explicitly described patients as frail or fit, that used chronological age as a proxy for frailty status, that alluded to frailty with nonage synonyms (for instance, overall health, performance status, projected treatment tolerance), and that included mentions of two or more GA domains. For these outcomes of interest, we stratified our observations by MCC site, presenter specialty, and presenter training level and used chi-square tests (with the Fisher's and Fisher-Freeman–Halton exact tests where applicable) to identify statistically significant differences. We also conducted a thematic analysis of terms and phrases shared during MCC discussions. One researcher (V.S.K.) reviewed all field notes to identify recurring themes in the representation of frailty descriptions and GA domains; synonyms for frailty and mentions of geriatric considerations were reviewed and consensually agreed upon by the core research team.

3. Results

3.1. Presentations in Overall Cohort

From January to June 2022, we attended 42 MCCs. A total of 75 case presentations pertained to patients aged 75 or older and included representation from the general gastrointestinal (n = 15), genitourinary (n = 18), head and neck (n = 4), thoracic (n = 19), and upper gastrointestinal (n = 19) sites. The mean age of included patients was 80.9 years (range 75–97 years), the majority (61.3%) were male, and more than half (55.5%) had a new diagnosis of cancer. With only a small proportion of cases (5.3%) centred around diagnostic uncertainty, the predominant reason (86.7%) for presentation was to deliberate options for treatment, which included chemotherapy (46.7%), radiotherapy (53.3%), surgery (49.3%), immunotherapy (5.3%), and best supportive care (8.0%). A small proportion of these discussions made mention of patient preferences (20.0%). Additional baseline demographic and clinical characteristics are reported in Table 2.

Table 2. Demographic and clinical characteristics of older patients discussed at MCCs (n = 75).

Mean patient age, years (range)		80.9 (75–97)
Patient sex, n (%)	Male	46 (61.3)
	Female	29 (38.7)
Presenter specialty, n	Medical oncology	22
	Radiation oncology	11
	Surgical oncology	45
Presenter level, n	Trainee	31
	Staff	38
	Both	2
Case presentations by site, n (%)	General gastrointestinal	4 (5.3)
	Genitourinary	19(25.3)
	Head and neck	19 (25.3)
	Thoracic	15 (20.0)
	Upper gastrointestinal	18 (24.0)
Presentation question, n (%)	Diagnostic	4 (5.3)
	Therapeutic	65 (86.7)
	Both	6 (8.0)
Cancer diagnosis, n (%)	Symptomatic	40 (53.3)
	Incidental	3 (4.0)
	Detection via surveillance	17 (22.7)
	Unclear or unspecified	15 (20.0)
Cancer treatment history, n (%)	New diagnosis	36 (48.0)
	Prior treatment	37 (49.3)
	Unclear or unspecified	2 (2.7)
Proposed treatment intent, n (%)	Curative	1 (1.3)
	Palliative	12 (16.0)
	Both	6 (8.0)
	Unclear or unspecified	56 (74.7)
Patient preferences, n (%)	Mentioned	15 (20.0)
Proposed treatment modalities, n (%)	Chemotherapy	35 (46.7)
	Radiotherapy	40 (53.3)
	Surgery	37 (49.3)
	Immunotherapy	4 (5.3)
	Best supportive care	6 (8.0)

3.2. Descriptions of Frailty in Overall Cohort

Across the five tumour sites comprising our overall cohort, 20.0% of the 75 case presentations explicitly identified individuals as "frail" or "fit". None, however, mentioned a validated assessment tool to explain how frailty status was determined. More frequently, discussions referred to patients' age (33.3%), projected treatment tolerance (30.7%), and overall health (21.3%) to hint at suspected frailty (Table 3, Figure 1).

Table 3. Presentation of frailty-related descriptors and GA domains in overall cohort (n = 75).

Frailty-related descriptors	Frailty status, n (%)	15 (20.0)
	Age, n (%)	24 (32.0)
	Activity level, n (%)	2 (2.7)
	Appearance, n (%)	8 (10.6)
	Appearance, n (%)	4 (5.3)
	Independence, n (%)	4 (5.3)
	Mobility, n (%)	16 (21.3)
	Overall health, n (%)	12 (16.0)
	Performance status, n (%)	15 (20.0)
	Treatment tolerance, n (%)	23 (30.7)
GA domains	Comorbidities, n (%)	39 (52.0)
	Medications, n (%)	16 (21.3)
	Cognition, n (%)	4 (5.3)
	Falls, n (%)	1 (1.3)
	Functional status, n (%)	5 (6.7)
	Mood, n (%)	1 (1.3)
	Physical performance, n (%)	0 (0)
	Nutrition, n (%)	3 (4.0)
	Social support, n (%)	7 (9.3)

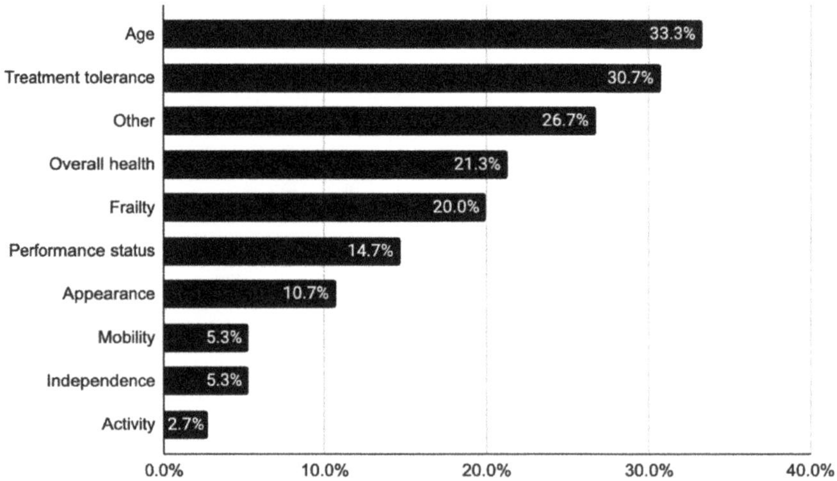

Figure 1. Descriptions of and synonyms for frailty across all case presentations (n = 75).

While age was consistently included as part of identifying data, it was often reiterated to suggest either fitness or frailty. For instance, one presenter described their patient as "an okay 86 [year-old]", while another pointed out that their patient was "very fit . . . for her age". Conversely, MCC discussions restated age to portray a patient as frail. In one instance, a patient was noted to be "87 [years-old], so elderly and frail".

Age was also highlighted to suggest poor treatment tolerance. A potential regimen was described as "a lot for an 82-year-old", while some presenters directly stated that "chemotherapy [was] obviously not at play given his age" or that "at that age, we wouldn't be doing [surgery]". Other frailty-related descriptions tended to be vague, such as "not the most robust", or "pretty healthy, very active", and "looks good, moves well". In most cases, little elaboration, if any, was provided to justify frailty assignments with objective measures of physical performance or functional independence, for instance.

3.3. Mentions of GA Domains in Overall Cohort

Across the 75 MCC discussions, 22 case presentations (31.0%) made reference to at least two GA domains. The most frequently mentioned GA domain was comorbidity status, which was included in more than half (52.0%) of the case presentations, predominantly to imply poor treatment candidacy. For example, one presenter argued that "surgery is not ideal because of [the patient's] multiple comorbidities".

Beyond comorbidity burden, a medication list was provided for 21.3% of the cases. Social support (9.3%), functional status (6.7%), cognition (5.3%), nutritional status (4.0%), and mood (1.3%) were reported much less frequently. Falls risk was captured in only one MCC presentation, but none of the case discussions included objective measures of physical function (Table 3, Figure 2).

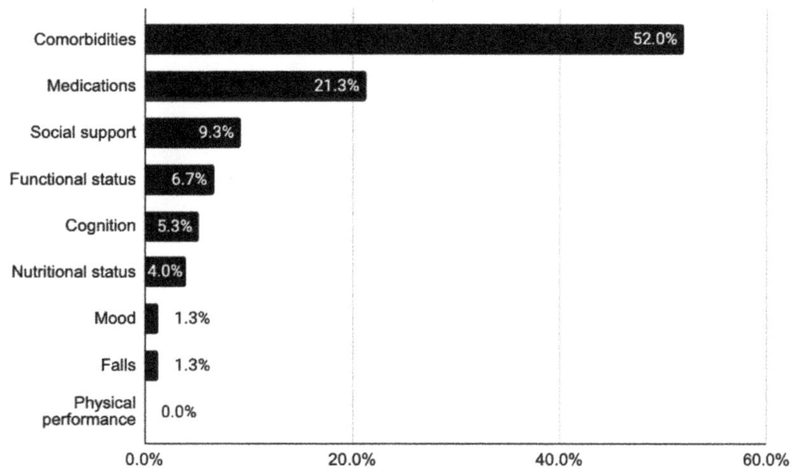

Figure 2. Mentions of GA domains across all case presentations (n = 75).

Interestingly, one (1.3%) of the cases included mention of an assessment by geriatric oncology, specifically quoting their estimate of a patient's five-year survival rate. A comprehensive GA, however, was not discussed during this MCC presentation or discussion.

3.4. Case Presentations by MCC Site

Across the four MCC sites included in this analysis, discussions often included both direct and indirect references to frailty status (Supplementary Table S1). From here on, the sites are labelled as A, B, C, and D, in no particular order. Varying proportions of the sites made explicit mention of frailty or fitness (26.7% of site A, 11.1% of site B, 26.3% of site C, and 15.8% of site D presentations; p-value 0.61). Frailty status was also indirectly implied by reiterating chronological age (53.3% of site A, 11.1% of site B, 36.8% of site C, and 36.8% of site D presentations; p-value 0.072) or by describing overall health (13.3% of site A, 11.1% of site B, 15.8% of site C, and 42.1% of site D presentations; p-value 0.11) and performance status (6.7% of site A, 11.1% of site B, 0% of site C, and 26.3% of site D presentations; p-value 0.069). Although none of the discussions included a validated prediction tool for estimating chemotherapy toxicity or surgical risk, MCC presenters and attendees frequently alluded to projected treatment tolerance across the tumour sites (40% of site A, 22.2% of site B, 15.8% of site C, and 47.4% of site D presentations; p-value 0.14).

Inclusion of GA domains was highly inconsistent. Only comorbidity status was discussed at all sites, albeit with considerable variation (13.3% of site A, 94.4% of site B, 47.4% of site C, and 36.8% of site D presentations; p-value < 0.001). Across the sites, the frequency of more than two GA domains being discussed also varied substantially, with mentions in 13.3% of site A, 83.3% of site B, 5.3% of site C, and 21.2% of site D cases (p-value < 0.001).

3.5. Case Presentations by Presenter Specialty

Of the 71 presentations discussed in the general gastrointestinal, genitourinary, thoracic, and upper gastrointestinal meetings, 22 were led by medical oncologists, 7 by radiation oncologists, and 44 by surgical oncologists. The sum of presenters exceeds the total number of cases as some were jointly presented by multiple specialists. For cases that were jointly presented by physicians of different specialties (for instance, radiation oncology and surgical oncology), any mention of a variable of interest was counted toward each specialty's total. Supplementary Table S2 captures quantitative data from their presentations, stratified by specialty.

Explicit descriptions of patients as frail or fit were included in 22.7%, 28.6%, and 15.9% of the presentations led by medical, radiation, and surgical oncologists, respectively (p-value 0.61). Across the three specialties, chronological age (36.4%, 42.9%, and 34.1%, respectively; p-value 0.94) and projected treatment tolerance (22.7%, 57.1%, and 34.1%, respectively; p-value 0.25) were mentioned more frequently to capture frailty status indirectly. A considerable number of presentations made mention of at least one GA domain (40.9% by medical, 57.1% by radiation, and 61.4% by surgical oncologists; p-value 0.30), but reference to more than two GA domains varied to a greater extent (22.7% by medical, 0% by radiation, 38.6% by surgical oncologists; p-value 0.085). A statistically significant difference in the presenters' inclusion of a patient's performance status was noted, with this variable being mentioned in 27.2% of the cases presented by medical and 4.5% of the cases presented by surgical oncologists, but none of the cases presented by radiation oncologists (p-value 0.019).

3.6. Case Presentations by Presenter Training Level

Of the 71 presentations spanning the four tumour sites included in this analysis, 33 were presented by trainees and 40 by faculty members. As was the case for presenter specialty, the sum of presenters exceeds the total number of cases, as some were jointly presented by trainees and faculty. For this reason, any mention of a variable of interest was counted toward trainee's and faculty's totals. Supplementary Table S3 includes the quantitative data from their presentations, stratified by training level.

Direct mentions of frailty status were included in 21.2% and 17.5% of the presentations led by trainees and faculty members, respectively (p-value 0.77). Trainees and faculty members both offered indirect descriptions of frailty or fitness through chronological age (18.2% and 45.0%, respectively, p-value 0.024), overall health (21.2% and 22.5%, p-value 1.00), performance status (21.2% and 2.5%, p-value 0.019), and projected treatment tolerance (27.3% and 30.0%, p-value 1.00). Interestingly, the only statistically significant differences in mentions of frailty-related variables between training levels were for age and performance status, with the former being mentioned more frequently by faculty and the latter by trainees.

With respect to GA domains, 54.5% of presentations by trainees compared to only 15.0% of presentations by faculty made reference to two or more domains (p-value < 0.001). Regardless of the presenter's training level, comorbidity status was the most frequently mentioned domain.

4. Discussion

This study used a mixed-methods approach to explore the description of frailty considerations and GA domains in MCC case presentations pertaining to individuals aged 75 or older. Although a handful of patients were explicitly described as frail or fit, none of the discussions mentioned a validated assessment tool for identifying or measuring frailty (for instance, the Rockwood Clinical Frailty Scale, Geriatric 8, Vulnerable Elder Survey-13) [15,21]. Instead, presenters tended to focus on surrogate measures to hint at frailty, often with subjective terms based on individual clinicians' perceptions of a patient's appearance, projected treatment tolerance, or overall health. Rather than comprehensively covering different aspects of the GA, comorbidity status was heavily featured, with much less attention paid to the other domains. These trends held true across the tumour board sites, presenter specialties, and training levels. Statistically significant differences, however, were observed between MCC sites for the discussion of at least two GA domains, between presenter specialties for the discussion of performance status, and between presenter training levels for the discussion of age, performance status, and at least two GA domains. Overall, our findings suggest that MCC case presentations disproportionately rely on chronological age and comorbidity burden with a lack of standardized language to define and explore other geriatric considerations relevant to frailty.

It is important to note, however, that chronological age has been previously studied and found to be negatively associated with poor clinical outcomes in oncology. The MACH-NC Collaborative Group, for instance, found that older patients, compared to their younger counterparts, had a statistically significant reduction in potential benefit from concomitant chemotherapy with loco-regional treatment for head and neck cancer [22]. Similarly, Coate et al. found worsening survival with increasing age in the setting of stage III non-small-cell lung cancer [23]. Yet, when performance status, comorbidity burden, and other confounding factors were controlled for in their multivariate model, no difference in survival was identified between age groups after aggressive treatment with curative intent [23]. This finding highlights the importance of not relying on chronological age alone, particularly as mentions of chronological age, depending on how it is discussed, may perpetuate ageism [24,25].

Despite growing recognition of the importance of language, particularly in the care of older adults, only a small body of work to date has delved into the actual words and phrases used in clinical decision making for this demographic [8,13,14,16–19]. At a tertiary hospital in Australia, Lane et al. found a predominance of disease-centred language during MCC case presentations on older adults, who were often depicted using nonobjective, potentially ambiguous descriptors (e.g., "fit", "well", and "good"); their comorbid medical conditions, in contrast, were discussed at greater length with precise medical terminology [8]. A prospective six-centre audit by Lakhanpal et al., also based in Australia, reported comorbidities as the most frequently mentioned geriatric domain (92%), while fewer references were made to other relevant variables, such as functional status with regard to ADLs (50%) and instrumental ADLs (26%) [13]. Two of the presented cases reached a decision to withhold treatment on the basis of advanced age alone [13]. Bolle et al. similarly found limited inclusion of patient-centred information, such as patient values and preferences, in MCCs conducted across five nonacademic hospitals in The Netherlands [14]. In that country, a single-site cross-sectional review by Festen et al. corroborated the poor representation of patient-centred information and the reliance on comorbidity-related information when depicting older individuals [18]. A single-centre study centred around a gynaecological cancer multidisciplinary team in the United Kingdom also noted that disease-specific details appeared to take precedence over patient-related factors, including patient choice [16]. The ensuing skewed discussions give rise to the possibility of age-biased decisions. In their observational study on MCCs at two French centres, Billon et al. concluded that nearly half of the therapeutic decisions for older adults with cancer were "age-adapted" (i.e., driven by age alone) [17]. Finally, Restivo et al. explored how the inclusion of nonmedical characteristics affected treatment decisions and practices at a French cancer centre [19]. They found that patients' age and "likeability", described using terms such as "nice" or "annoying", were the most frequently mentioned variables; inclusion of these characteristics was positively associated with deferred decisions, suggesting that the addition of nonmedical information can serve to remind clinicians of the complexity inherent in caring for older adults [19].

These studies from around the world offer findings that are concordant with the results of our study. Despite the recommendation from the International Society of Geriatric Oncology to tailor treatment decisions to a patient's health status as opposed to their chronological age, prior literature and our work suggest ongoing shortcomings in how older patients and relevant geriatric considerations—beyond age alone—are discussed [26]. The limited incorporation of the GA reflects another critical practice gap. While the use of the GA has been shown to increase the likelihood of cancer treatment completion, lower rates of hospitalization, improve patient-centred communication, and enhance patient satisfaction among older adults, our study reveals skewed, comorbidity-focused representation of the GA domains [27–30].

With our efforts to investigate this significant guideline-practice gap, our study possesses a number of strengths. First, this is the only study, to our knowledge, that compares the language at MCCs across various oncologic specialties and presenter training levels. This may reflect nuances in training practices or team cultures that contribute to heterogeneity in geriatric language use. It may also provide a glimmer of hope that some reporting trends are improving among trainees compared to faculty, since we observed significantly less reporting of age and more reporting of performance status among trainees. Second, this is the only paper to capture mentions of both frailty depictions and GA domains; while Lakhanpal et al. and Bolle et al. also examined the latter, neither examined how patients are described as fit or frail when discussing potential treatment plans [14,18]. Third, we included cases from various tumour sites to increase the generalizability of our results and to capture differences across sites. Fourth, our mixed methods approach enabled us to identify themes and quantify language use, providing a more fulsome picture of the words and phrases included at these meetings. Finally, this is the first study in North America to explore the depiction of older patients and their treatment considerations at MCCs [8,13,14,16–19].

Our findings must be interpreted with caution, however, in the context of our study's limitations. First, the nature of our methodology left potential room for the observer effect, as the MCC presenters were informed in advance of our attendance. Consequently, our involvement, even without any active participation, may have altered how the healthcare providers communicated or behaved during MCC meetings. This may have led to optimistic estimates for our observed outcomes. Second, our data collection relied on field notes compiled by different research team members. To mitigate inter-rater differences, however, we had used a standardized data collection form, and we had undergone trials of joint data collection to ensure similar recording by all research team members. Third, our sample size was modest, with discrepancies between MCCs sites, notably with a small number of head and neck MCCs included due to scheduling challenges. Fourth, we focused exclusively on the discussions at MCCs without extending into post-meeting decisions or outcomes. As a result, the ultimate clinical impact of the language used at these MCCs remains unknown.

There are several potential next steps with significant implications both in terms of clinical practice and research. For future clinical practice, our study highlights the need to mitigate the risk of ageism and improve how older patients are discussed beyond their chronological age. This demographic tended to be depicted using vague and subjective language, which begs the question of how clinicians can be encouraged to incorporate more objective descriptors in hopes of minimizing age-biased decision making [12]. For instance, one wonders whether a checklist comprising the GA domains would be helpful for MCC presenters to review for each geriatric case. This strategy may also help foster more comprehensive discussions that better address elder-relevant priorities, such as the preservation of functional autonomy and quality of life. Similarly, the presence and integration of a geriatrician at MCCs may offer richer conversations about geriatric considerations beyond cancer- or comorbidity-focused variables, although the feasibility of this approach may be dictated by local resources [14,31]. For future research, our study paves the way for further work with larger sample sizes that may reveal even more statistically significant differences between tumour sites, presenter specialties, and training levels. Such efforts could identify training strategies or team cultures and treatment philosophies that could be leveraged, as well as specific areas of weakness to be addressed. Additionally, ongoing research is needed to investigate when and how to consider chronological age at MCCs. As mentioned above, previous studies have identified an association between advanced age and worse treatment outcomes, yet a small but growing body of literature has also raised a concern that age-focused discussions may increase the risk of ageist decision making. Finally, another area to explore would be the ultimate impact of frailty- and geriatric-assessment-informed discussions on management decisions in geriatric oncology; this research could help reinforce the significance of purposeful language use in the collaborative care of older adults with cancer.

5. Conclusions

This study found that MCCs often lack standardized language or objective assessments when describing the fitness and frailty of older adults with cancer. With an over-reliance on chronological age and comorbidity status to characterize a patient's projected treatment tolerance or their overall health, practitioners attending MCCs may be at risk of age-based decision making. By incorporating frailty measurements from validated tools and/or by exploring multiple GA domains during case presentations, MCCs may be able to foster more comprehensive discussions that reflect important geriatric considerations and reduce ageist biases. Future work on the downstream effects of frailty- and GA-informed MCC presentations may further elucidate the role language can play in impacting clinical decisions and outcomes.

Supplementary Materials: The following supporting information can be downloaded at: https://www.mdpi.com/article/10.3390/cancers16081477/s1, Table S1: Presentation of frailty-related descriptors and GA domains by MCC site; Table S2: Presentation of frailty-related descriptors and GA domains by presenter specialty; Table S3: Presentation of frailty-related descriptors and GA domains by presenter training level.

Author Contributions: Conceptualization, S.M.H.A., A.J.H., R.W.J., V.S.K., E.P. and N.P.; methodology, S.M.H.A., A.C., V.S.K., E.P., I.T. and T.T.; formal analysis, S.M.H.A., A.C., V.S.K. and E.P.; writing—original draft preparation, A.C. and V.S.K.; writing—review and editing, S.M.H.A., A.C., A.J.H., R.W.J., V.S.K., E.P., N.P., I.T. and T.T. All authors have read and agreed to the published version of the manuscript.

Funding: This research received funding from the Sinai Health/University Health Network's 2020 Geriatrics Summer Scholars Program.

Institutional Review Board Statement: The study was conducted in accordance with the Declaration of Helsinki and approved by the Research Ethics Board of University Health Network (protocol code 20-586) on 16 December 2020.

Informed Consent Statement: Patient consent was waived as data collection and analysis posed minimal impact to clinical decisions or outcomes. Our research team attended MCCs and recorded data passively without participating in the discussions themselves; the intent was to capture, not influence, the language used to present patient cases, and, notably, there was no direct patient involvement throughout the study. In accordance with the precedent established by prior studies that had similarly involved observing MCC discussions, patient consent was waived.

Data Availability Statement: Restrictions apply to the availability of these data. Data were obtained from University Health Network and are available with permission from the Research Ethics Board of University Health Network.

Conflicts of Interest: The authors declare no conflicts of interest. The funders had no role in the design of the study; in the collection, analyses, or interpretation of data; in the writing of the manuscript; or in the decision to publish the results.

Appendix A

The data collection form below was used by all members of the research team to record variables of interest during MCC presentations pertaining to patients aged 75 or older.

Date:	MCC site:		Presenter's specialty: ☐ MO ☐ RO ☐ SO	
Patient study ID:	Patient age, sex:		Presenter: ☐ Trainee ☐ Staff	
For each case, check off the item(s) mentioned by the presenter (second column) during the MCC presentation and by the audience (third column) during the subsequent discussion.	By presenter	By audience	Notes from presentation	Notes from audience
Cancer-related items				
HPI	☐	☐		
Stage and/or grade (suspected or confirmed)	☐	☐		
Past treatment and modalities	☐	☐		
Proposed treatment intent (curative or palliative)	☐	☐		
Proposed treatment modality—record all ☐ Surgery ☐ Chemotherapy ☐ Radiotherapy ☐ Immunotherapy ☐ Other—please specify	☐	☐		
Non-cancer-related items				
Patient preference and/or goals of care	☐	☐		
Family involvement in decision at hand	☐	☐		
Smoking status and/or alcohol use	☐	☐		
Socioeconomic status (e.g., education, income)	☐	☐		
Living situation	☐	☐		
Employment status	☐	☐		
Race/Ethnicity	☐	☐		
English-/Non-English speaking	☐	☐		
Fitness/Frailty descriptions				
Fit/Vulnerable/Frail	☐	☐		
Active/Inactive	☐	☐		
Independent/Dependent	☐	☐		

Performance status	☐	☐
Mobility	☐	☐
Appearance (e.g., "younger than stated age")	☐	☐
Overall health	☐	☐
Other synonyms—record verbatim in space to the right	☐	☐
GA domains		
Functional status (with explicit mention of ADLs/IADLs)	☐	☐
Performance-based measures (e.g., grip strength, gait speed)	☐	☐
Falls	☐	☐
Comorbidities	☐	☐
Medications	☐	☐
Cognition	☐	☐
Mood	☐	☐
Social activity/support	☐	☐
Nutritional status	☐	☐

Note: "MCC" = multidisciplinary cancer conference, "MO" = medical oncology, "RO" = radiation oncology, "SO" = surgical oncology, "HPI" = history of presenting illness, "ADLs" = activities of daily living, "IADLs" = instrumental activities of daily living.

References

1. Marosi, C.; Köller, M. Challenge of cancer in the elderly. *ESMO Open* **2016**, *1*, e000020. [CrossRef] [PubMed]
2. Sedrak, M.S.; Freedman, R.A.; Cohen, H.J.; Muss, H.B.; Jatoi, A.; Klepin, H.D.; Wildes, T.M.; Le-Rademacher, J.G.; Kimmick, G.G.; Tew, W.P.; et al. Older adult participation in cancer clinical trials: A systematic review of barriers and interventions. *CA Cancer J. Clin.* **2021**, *71*, 78–92. [CrossRef] [PubMed]
3. Mohile, S.G.; Mohamed, M.R.; Xu, H.; Culakova, E.; Loh, K.P.; Magnuson, A.; A Flannery, M.; Obrecht, S.; Gilmore, N.; Ramsdale, E.; et al. Evaluation of geriatric assessment and management on the toxic effects of cancer treatment (GAP70+): A cluster-randomised study. *Lancet* **2021**, *398*, 1894–1904. [CrossRef] [PubMed]
4. Given, B.; Given, C.W. Older adults and cancer treatment. *Cancer* **2008**, *113* (Suppl. 12), 3505–3511. [CrossRef] [PubMed]
5. Hernandez-Torres, C.; Korc-Grodzicki, B.; Hsu, T. Models of Clinical Care Delivery for Geriatric Oncology in Canada and the United States: A Survey of Geriatric Oncology Care Providers. *J. Geriatr. Oncol.* **2022**, *13*, 447–453. [CrossRef] [PubMed]
6. Wright, F.; De Vito, C.; Langer, B.; Hunter, A.; Expert Panel on the Multidisciplinary Cancer Conference Standards. Multidisciplinary cancer conferences: A systematic review and development of practice standards. *Eur. J. Cancer* **2007**, *43*, 1002–1010. [CrossRef]
7. Specchia, M.L.; Frisicale, E.M.; Carini, E.; Di Pilla, A.; Cappa, D.; Barbara, A.; Ricciardi, W.; Damiani, G. The impact of tumor board on cancer care: Evidence from an umbrella review. *BMC Health Serv. Res.* **2020**, *20*, 73. [CrossRef] [PubMed]
8. Lane, H.P.; McLachlan, S.; Philip, J.A.M. "Pretty fit and healthy": The discussion of older people in cancer multidisciplinary meetings. *J. Geriatr. Oncol.* **2019**, *10*, 84–88. [CrossRef] [PubMed]
9. Barthélémy, P.; Heitz, D.; Mathelin, C.; Polesi, H.; Asmane, I.; Litique, V.; Rob, L.; Bergerat, J.-P.; Kurtz, J.-E. Adjuvant chemotherapy in elderly patients with early breast cancer. Impact of age and comprehensive geriatric assessment on tumor board proposals. *Crit. Rev. Oncol. Hematol.* **2011**, *79*, 196–204. [CrossRef] [PubMed]
10. Festen, S.; Kok, M.; Hopstaken, J.S.; van der Wal-Huisman, H.; van der Leest, A.; Reyners, A.K.; de Bock, G.H.; de Graeff, P.; van Leeuwen, B.L. How to incorporate geriatric assessment in clinical decision-making for older patients with cancer. An implementation study. *J. Geriatr. Oncol.* **2019**, *10*, 951–959. [CrossRef] [PubMed]
11. Blanc, M.; Dialla, O.; Manckoundia, P.; Arveux, P.; Dabakuyo, S.; Quipourt, V. Influence of the geriatric oncology consultation on the final therapeutic decision in elderly subjects with cancer: Analysis of 191 patients. *J. Nutr. Health Aging* **2014**, *18*, 76–82. [CrossRef] [PubMed]
12. Kyi, K.; Gilmore, N.; Kadambi, S.; Loh, K.P.; Magnuson, A. Stigmatizing language in caring for older adults with cancer: Common patterns of use and mechanisms to change the culture. *J. Geriatr. Oncol.* **2023**, *14*, 101593. [CrossRef] [PubMed]

13. Lakhanpal, R.; Yoong, J.; Joshi, S.; Yip, D.; Mileshkin, L.; Marx, G.M.; Dunlop, T.; Hovey, E.J.; Della Fiorentina, S.A.; Venkateswaran, L.; et al. Geriatric assessment of older patients with cancer in Australia—A multicentre audit. *J. Geriatr. Oncol.* **2015**, *6*, 185–193. [CrossRef] [PubMed]
14. Bolle, S.; Smets, E.M.A.; Hamaker, M.E.; Loos, E.F.; van Weert, J.C.M. Medical decision making for older patients during multidisciplinary oncology team meetings. *J. Geriatr. Oncol.* **2019**, *10*, 74–83. [CrossRef] [PubMed]
15. Rockwood, K.; Song, X.; MacKnight, C.; Bergman, H.; Hogan, D.B.; McDowell, I.; Mitnitski, A. A global clinical measure of fitness and frailty in elderly people. *CMAJ* **2005**, *173*, 489–495. [CrossRef] [PubMed]
16. Kidger, J.; Murdoch, J.; Donovan, J.L.; Blazeby, J.M. Clinical decision-making in a multidisciplinary gynaecological cancer team: A qualitative study. *BJOG Int. J. Obstet. Gynaecol.* **2009**, *116*, 511–517. [CrossRef] [PubMed]
17. Billon, E.; Tassy, L.; Sarabi, M.; Braticevic, C.; Cecile, M.; Albrand, G.; Terret, C.; Rousseau, F. Use's assessment of geriatric variables in the older patient with cancer's multidisciplinary team meeting. *J. Geriatr. Oncol.* **2020**, *11*, 536–539. [CrossRef] [PubMed]
18. Festen, S.; Nijmeijer, H.; van Leeuwen, B.L.; van Etten, B.; van Munster, B.C.; de Graeff, P. Multidisciplinary decision-making in older patients with cancer, does it differ from younger patients? *Eur. J. Surg. Oncol.* **2021**, *47*, 2682–2688. [CrossRef] [PubMed]
19. Restivo, L.; Apostolidis, T.; Bouhnik, A.D.; Garciaz, S.; Aurran, T.; Julian-Reynier, C. Patients' non-medical characteristics contribute to collective medical decision-making at multidisciplinary oncological team meetings. *PLoS ONE* **2016**, *11*, e0154969. [CrossRef] [PubMed]
20. Mohile, S.G.; Velarde, C.; Hurria, A.; Magnuson, A.; Lowenstein, L.; Pandya, C.; O'Donovan, A.; Gorawara-Bhat, R.; Dale, W. Geriatric assessment-guided care processes for older adults: A delphi consensus of geriatric oncology experts. *J. Natl. Compr. Cancer Netw.* **2015**, *13*, 1120–1130. [CrossRef]
21. Decoster, L.; Van Puyvelde, K.; Mohile, S.; Wedding, U.; Basso, U.; Colloca, G.; Rostoft, S.; Overcash, J.; Wildiers, H.; Steer, C.; et al. Screening tools for multidimentional health problems warranting a geriatric assessment in older cancer patients: An update on SIOG recommendations. *Ann. Oncol.* **2015**, *26*, 288–300. [CrossRef] [PubMed]
22. Pignon, J.P.; le Maître, A.; Maillard, E.; Bourhis, J.; The MACH-NC Collaborative Group. Meta-analysis of chemotherapy in head and neck cancer (MACH-NC): An update on 93 randomised trials and 17,346 patients. *Radiother. Oncol.* **2009**, *92*, 4–14. [CrossRef] [PubMed]
23. Coate, L.E.; Massey, C.; Hope, A.; Sacher, A.; Barrett, K.; Pierre, A.; Leighl, N.; Brade, A.; de Perrot, M.; Waddell, T.; et al. Treatment of the elderly when cure is the goal: The influence of age on treatment selection and efficacy for stage III non-small cell lung cancer. *J. Thorac. Oncol.* **2011**, *6*, 537–544. [CrossRef] [PubMed]
24. Peake, M.D.; Thompson, S.; Lowe, D.; Pearson, M.G. Ageism in the management of lung cancer. *Age Ageing* **2003**, *32*, 171–177. [CrossRef] [PubMed]
25. Freyer, G.; Braud, A.-C.; Chaibi, P.; Spielmann, M.; Martin, J.-P.; Vilela, G.; Guerin, D.; Zelek, L. Dealing with metastatic breast cancer in elderly women: Results from a French study on a large cohort carried out by the "Observatory on elderly patients". *Ann. Oncol.* **2006**, *17*, 211–216. [CrossRef] [PubMed]
26. Boyle, H.; Alibhai, S.; Decoster, L.; Efstathiou, E.; Fizazi, K.; Mottet, N.; Oudard, S.; Payne, H.; Prentice, M.; Puts, M.; et al. Updated recommendations of the International Society of Geriatric Oncology on prostate cancer management in older patients. *Eur. J. Cancer* **2019**, *116*, 116–136. [CrossRef] [PubMed]
27. Kalsi, T.; Babic-Illman, G.; Ross, P.; Maisey, N.; Hughes, S.; Fields, P.E.; Martin, F.C.; Wang, Y.; Harari, D. The impact of comprehensive geriatric assessment interventions on tolerance to chemotherapy in older patients. *Br. J. Cancer* **2015**, *112*, 1435–1444. [CrossRef] [PubMed]
28. Soo, W.K.; King, M.; Pope, A.; Parente, P.; Darzins, P.; Davis, I.D. Integrated geriatric assessment and treatment (INTEGRATE) in older people with cancer planned for systemic anticancer therapy. *J. Clin. Oncol.* **2020**, *38* (Suppl. S15), 12011. [CrossRef]
29. Mohile, S.G.; Epstein, R.M.; Hurria, A.; Heckler, C.E.; Canin, B.; Culakova, E.; Duberstein, P.; Gilmore, N.; Xu, H.; Plumb, S.; et al. Communication with older patients with cancer using geriatric assessment: A cluster-randomized clinical trial from the national cancer institute community oncology research program. *JAMA Oncol.* **2020**, *6*, 196–204. [CrossRef] [PubMed]
30. Singhal, S.; Marwell, J.G.; Khaki, A.R. Geriatric assessment in the older adult with genitourinary cancer: A narrative review. *Front Oncol.* **2023**, *13*, 1124309. [CrossRef] [PubMed]
31. Wildes, T.M.; O'Donovan, A.; Colloca, G.F.; Cheung, K.L. Tumour boards in geriatric oncology. *Age Ageing* **2018**, *47*, 168–170. [CrossRef]

cancers

MDPI

Article

Predictors of Survival, Treatment Modalities, and Clinical Outcomes of Diffuse Large B-Cell Lymphoma in Patients Older Than 70 Years Still an Unmet Medical Need in 2024 Based on Real-World Evidence

Luís Alberto de Pádua Covas Lage [1,2,*], Rita Novello De Vita [1], Lucas Bassolli de Oliveira Alves [1], Mayara D'Auria Jacomassi [1], Hebert Fabrício Culler [1,2], Cadiele Oliana Reichert [2], Fábio Alessandro de Freitas [2], Vanderson Rocha [1,2,3,4], Sheila Aparecida Coelho Siqueira [5], Renata de Oliveira Costa [6,7] and Juliana Pereira [1,2,7]

1 Department of Hematology, Hemotherapy & Cell Therapy, Faculty of Medicine, University of São Paulo (FM-USP), São Paulo 05403000, Brazil; juliana.pereira@hc.fm.usp.br (J.P.)

2 Laboratory of Medical Investigation in Pathogenesis and Directed Therapy in Onco-Immuno-Hematology (LIM-31), Faculty of Medicine, University of São Paulo (FM-USP), São Paulo 05403000, Brazil; fabio.alessandro@alumni.usp.br (F.A.d.F.)

3 Fundação Pró-Sangue, Blood Bank of São Paulo, São Paulo 05403000, Brazil

4 Department of Hematology & Hemotherapy, Churchill Hospital, Oxford University, Oxford OX3 7LE, UK

5 Department of Pathology, Faculty of Medicine, University of São Paulo (FM-USP), São Paulo 05403000, Brazil

6 Department of Hematology & Hemotherapy, Faculty of Medicine, Centro Universitário Lusíada (Unilus), Santos 11045101, Brazil; renatadeoliveiracosta@uol.com.br

7 Department of Hematology & Oncology, Hospital Alemão Oswaldo Cruz (HAOC), São Paulo 05403000, Brazil

* Correspondence: luis.lage@hc.fm.usp.br or luisalberto_lage@yahoo.com.br; Tel.: +55-11-4573-7639

Simple Summary: Here, we assessed clinical outcomes, predictors of survival, and compared responses and toxicities among different therapeutic modalities in a large cohort of older adults with DLBCL. A total of 185 Brazilian patients were included from 2009 to 2020. After a long follow-up, we demonstrated a 5-year OS of 50.2%. The R-MiniCHOP regimen was associated with a lower ORR; however, these patients were more malnourished and had a higher risk on prognostic indexes. Although associated with higher rates of severe neutropenia, the R-CHOP regimen was associated with substantial OS and PFS advantages. We also identified independent prognostic factors associated with poor outcomes, including age $\geq$ 75 years, high LDH, B-symptoms, clinical stage III/IV, neutrophilia, and reduced lymphocyte/monocyte ratio. Although a significant portion of older DLBCL patients are highly fragile and ineligible for enhanced regimens, attenuated protocols promoted remarkably inferior outcomes compared to those achieved by the R-CHOP.

Abstract: Background: Diffuse large B-cell lymphoma (DLBCL) especially affects the older population. Old ($\geq$60 years) and very old age ($\geq$80 years) DLBCL patients often present high-risk molecular alterations, lower tolerability to conventional immunochemotherapy, and poor clinical outcomes. In this scenario, attenuated therapeutic strategies, such as the R-MiniCHOP and R-MiniCHOP of the elderly regimens, have emerged for this particularly fragile population. However, the responses, clinical outcomes, and toxicities of these regimens currently remain poorly understood, mainly because these individuals are not usually included in controlled clinical trials. Methods: This retrospective, observational, and single-center real-world study included 185 DLBCL, NOS patients older than 70 years treated at the largest oncology center in Latin America from 2009 to 2020. We aimed to assess the outcomes, determine survival predictors, and compare responses and toxicities between three different primary therapeutic strategies, including the conventional R-CHOP regimen and the attenuated R-MiniCHOP and R-MiniCHOP of the elderly protocols. Results: The median age at diagnosis was 75 years (70–97 years), and 58.9% were female. Comorbidities were prevalent, including 19.5% with immobility, 28.1% with malnutrition, and 24.8% with polypharmacy. Advanced clinical stage was observed in 72.4%, 48.6% had bulky disease $\geq$7 cm, 63.2% had B-symptoms, and 67.0% presented intermediate–high/high-risk IPI. With a median follow-up of 6.3 years, the estimated 5-year OS and PFS were 50.2% and 44.6%, respectively. The R-MiniCHOP of the elderly regimen had a lower ORR ($p = 0.040$); however, patients in this group had higher rates of unfavorable clinical and laboratory findings, including hypoalbuminemia ($p = 0.001$), IPI ≥ 3 ($p = 0.013$), and NCCN-IPI ≥ 3 ($p = 0.002$). Although associated with higher rates of severe neutropenia ($p = 0.003$), the R-CHOP regimen promoted increased OS ($p = 0.003$) and PFS ($p = 0.005$) in comparison to the attenuated protocols. Additionally, age ≥ 75 years, high levels of LDH, B-symptoms, advanced clinical stage (III/IV), neutrophilia, and low lymphocyte/monocyte ratio were identified as poor prognostic factors in this cohort. Conclusions: In this large and real-life Latin American cohort, we demonstrated that patients with DLBCL, NOS older than 70 years still do not have satisfactory clinical outcomes in 2024, with half of cases not reaching 5 years of life expectancy after diagnosis. Although the conventional R-CHOP offers response and survival advantages over attenuated regimens, its myelotoxicity is not negligible. Therefore, the outcomes reported and the prognostic factors here identified may assist clinicians in the appropriate selection of therapeutic strategies adapted to the risk for old and very old DLBCL patients.

Keywords: diffuse large B-cell lymphoma (DLBCL); old and very old; prognostic factors; clinical outcomes; up-front immunochemotherapy; less intensified regimens

1. Introduction

Diffuse large B-cell lymphoma (DLBCL) is the most common subtype of non-Hodgkin's lymphoma (NHL), accounting for 30–40% of all lymphoid malignancies. It is characterized by the monoclonal proliferation of large and pleomorphic lymphoid B-cells, with a diffuse histopathological growth pattern, and origin in the germinal center (centroblasts) or post-germinal center (immunoblasts) [1,2]. DLBCL has wide clinical and biological diversity, and also a remarkably heterogeneous prognosis [2]. Although it is aggressive in nature, with an expected survival of less than 1 year without treatment, DLBCL is potentially curable with immunochemotherapy based on the R-CHOP (rituximab, cyclophosphamide, hydroxydoxorubicin, vincristine, and prednisone) regimen [3,4]. The R-CHOP regimen has high efficacy; however, up to 30–40% of patients will not respond or will relapse, particularly individuals older than 60 years and with other adverse prognostic factors [3,4].

DLBCL especially affects older adults, with an increasing incidence with advancing age [5,6]. Aging is the main risk factor for the development of cancer, and the prognosis of hematological malignancies is notably worse in older adults with cancer when compared to young individuals [7–9]. DLBCL of old (≥60 years) and very old (≥80 years) patients has numerous particularities, including high-risk genetic–molecular findings, such as a higher frequency of complex karyotype and higher tumor mutational burden, greater association with infection by Epstein–Barr virus (EBV), lower tolerability to conventional immunochemotherapy, higher expression of genes associated with multidrug resistance (MDR), and, consequently, worse clinical outcomes [10].

With a median age above 70 years at DLBCL diagnosis, older adults with cancer usually have comorbidities that preclude the administration of full doses of standard chemotherapy, as well as having altered pharmacodynamics, a greater tendency to drug toxicity, and an increased probability of mortality associated with treatment [11,12]. Older individuals react less effectively to adverse events resulting from polychemotherapy administration, presenting lower therapeutic tolerability. Physiological changes associated with aging predispose to mucositis, higher rates of infectious complications, greater cardiotoxicity, acute renal injury due to reduced clearance of antineoplastic agents, and greater occurrence of anemia, neutropenia, and thrombocytopenia, resulting from the myelosuppressive effect of cytostatic drugs [13,14].

Therefore, when choosing treatment for old and very old age adults with DLBCL, we must consider several factors, including the individual's life expectancy, the chemo sensitivity of their neoplasm, pre-existing comorbidities, and the presence of geriatric syndromes, such as instability, immobility, polypharmacy, neurological impairment, and frailty. To this end, several geriatric scales have been developed, such as the Comprehensive Geriatric Assessment (CGA), which considers the functional, nutritional status, mobility, sensory conditions, cognition and mood, social support, and the environment in which the patient is inserted. However, the application of these scales is sometimes complex and difficult, dependent on a qualified and trained professional, requiring extensive time for its use, constituting little-used and impractical tools [15].

Currently, standard-of-care therapy for DLBCL patients of all ages with early-stage disease (I/II) is based on four to six cycles of R-CHOP-21 followed or not by involved-field radiotherapy (IF-RT) with 30-36 Gy. For those individuals with advanced-stage disease (III/IV), six to eight cycles of R-CHOP-21 are applied; however, for patients with advanced disease and International Prognostic Index (IPI) ≥ 3 (intermediate–high or high-risk), Pola-R-CHP (polatuzumab vedotina, rituximab, cyclophosphamide, hydroxydoxorubicin, and prednisone) has become the current new standard of care [3,16,17]. For octogenarians, old individuals with serious comorbidities, or very frail patients, suggested attenuated and/or non-anthracycline-containing immunochemotherapy regimens include the R-MiniCHOP (R-CHOP with 50% dose reduction of doxorubicin [25 mg/sqm I.V. on D1]), R-MiniCHOP of the elderly (rituximab 375 mg/sqm I.V. on D1, cyclophosphamide 400 mg/sqm I.V. on D1, hydroxydoxorubicin 25 mg/sqm I.V. on D1, vincristine 1 mg [fixed dose] I.V. on D1, and prednisone 40 mg/sqm P.O. on days 1 to 5), R-GEMOX (rituximab, gemcitabine, and oxaliplatin), R-CEOP (rituximab, cyclophosphamide, etoposide, vincristine, and prednisone), R-COMP (rituximab, cyclophosphamide, non-pegylated liposomal doxorubicin, vinblastine, and prednisone), R-GCVP (rituximab, gemcitabine, cyclophosphamide, vincristine, and prednisone), R-CEPP (rituximab, cyclophosphamide, etoposide, procarbazine, and prednisone), and BR (bendamustine plus rituximab) [12,18,19]. Although potentially curable, such attenuated immunochemotherapeutic regimens offer decreased responses and poorer outcomes when compared to the conventional R-CHOP-21. However, we emphasize that older individuals are usually underrepresented in clinical trials and that the balance between efficacy and tolerability of alternative regimens to full-dose R-CHOP is also not well established in the current literature.

The World Health Organization (WHO) estimates 80% of older adults by 2050, and population aging is not only a global demographic trend but is particularly prominent in low- and middle-income countries due to the accelerated demographic shift characterized by the inversion of the age pyramids observed in these locations over the last three decades. Based on this premise, the current study aims to describe clinical and laboratory characteristics, assess outcomes, determine predictors of survival, and compare responses and toxicities between different up-front immunochemotherapeutic regimens based on anthracyclines (conventional [R-CHOP-21] and attenuated [R-MiniCHOP and R-MiniCHOP] of the elderly) in a large cohort of older adults than 70 years with DLBCL, NOS.

2. Material and Methods

2.1. Study Design and Ethical Issues

This is an observational, retrospective, and single-center study carried out at the Instituto do Câncer do Estado de São Paulo (ICESP)/Hospital das Clínicas, Faculty of Medicine, University of São Paulo (HC-FMUSP), Brazil. It was approved by the local Ethics Committee in 2021 (CAAE number: 48897221.2.0000.0068), with the application of the Free and Informed Consent Form (FICF) to all living participants included in the study and with their respective consents. The waiver of the FICF application was obtained for dead patients and with non-recoverable contact. All clinical–demographic, laboratory, pathological, imaging, and therapeutic data were obtained from institutional electronic medical records.

2.2. Patients, Elegibility Criteria, and Staging Procedures

Considering all 2798 patients diagnosed with NHL registered in the ICESP/HC-FMUSP Non-Hodgkin's Lymphoma Database, 1495 patients diagnosed with diffuse large B-cell lymphoma, not otherwise specified (DLBCL, NOS) were initially selected. Of these, 205 (13.7%) were aged $\geq$ 70 years. Finally, 185/205 (90.2%) were included in this study because they presented clinical–demographic and evolutionary data considered satisfactory for survival analysis. Eligibility criteria included age $\geq$ 70 years, patients diagnosed and treated at ICESP/HC-FMUSP from January 2009 to December 2020, and biopsy-proven diagnosis of DLBCL, NOS according to the criteria proposed by the World Health Organization Classification for Lymphoid and Hematopoietic Tissue Neoplasms published in 2016 (WHO-2016) [1]. Patients diagnosed with DLBCL from immunoprivileged sites (primary central nervous system lymphoma [PCNSL] or primary testicular DLBCL), high-grade B-cell lymphoma associated with immunosuppression (human acquired immunodeficiency syndrome [AIDS] or post-transplant lymphoproliferative disorders [PTLD]), primary mediastinal DLBCL (PML), T-cell/histiocyte-rich DLBCL (T/H DLBCL), leg-type DLBCL, and low-grade non-Hodgkin lymphomas with histological transformation to DLBCL were excluded from this analysis.

Clinical–epidemiological, laboratory, and histopathological data accessed at diagnosis included age, gender, ethnicity, Eastern Cooperative Oncology Group (ECOG) performance status, Ann Arbor/Cotswold clinical stage, bone marrow (BM) infiltration, central nervous system (CNS) involvement, bulky disease ($\geq$ 7 cm), B-symptoms, immobility, polypharmacy (regular use of $\geq$ 5 medications), elderly body mass index (E-BMI), and comorbidity profile. Charlson Comorbidity Index (CCI) score was calculated for all patients according to the literature [20,21]. The International Prognostic Index (IPI), Revised International Prognostic Index (R-IPI), and National Comprehensive Cancer Network International Prognostic Index (NCCN-IPI) scores were calculated for all cases as originally described [22–24]. Socio-demographic data, such as educational level and family support, were also obtained from the patients' electronic medical records by a specific researcher. Laboratory variables related to blood cell count (hemoglobin, WBC, neutrophils, lymphocytes, monocytes, neutrophil/lymphocyte ratio [N/Ly], lymphocyte/monocyte ratio [Ly/Mo], and total platelet count), lactic dehydrogenase (LDH), β2-microglobulin, albumin, globulins, and viral serological status for HIV, hepatitis B, and C were also accessed. The lymphoma's cell of origin (COO) was accessed using the Hans immunohistochemical algorithm [25] in all cases with available formalin-fixed paraffin-embedded (FFPE) material.

Date of diagnosis, complete response (CR), disease relapse and progression, first and last cycle of chemotherapy and radiotherapy, date and cause of death, and date of last follow-up were obtained to assess the overall response rate (ORR), complete response (CR), partial response (PR), overall survival (OS), progression-free survival (PFS), and disease-free survival (DFS). At diagnosis, all DLBCL, NOS patients underwent a complete blood count, comprehensive biochemical tests, including renal and hepatic function, and tests for tumor lysis syndrome (TLS), as well as LDH and β2-microglobulin measurements, and serology for HIV, hepatitis B, and C. All patients eligible for anthracycline-based induction regimens underwent transthoracic echocardiography to estimate left ventricular function (LVF).

Staging was carried out with contrast-enhanced computed tomography (CT) scans of the neck, chest, abdomen, and pelvis, or preferably by CT with positron emission with 18-fluorodeoxyglucose (18-FDG-PET-CT). Unilateral BM biopsy with immunohistochemistry (IHC) was performed in all cases not staged with 18-FDG-PET-CT. Patients with gastrointestinal symptoms underwent upper gastrointestinal endoscopy (UGE) and/or colonoscopy with biopsies. Patients with involvement of $\geq$ 2 extranodal sites and intermediate–high or high-risk IPI, as well as those with paranasal sinus involvement, paravertebral mass with foraminal invasion, involvement of kidneys, adrenal glands, testicles, ovaries, or breasts had cerebrospinal fluid (CSF) puncture with chemo cytological analysis as part of the staging procedures to exclude secondary CNS involvement.

2.3. Up-front Therapy, Response Assessment, and Follow-Up

Up-front treatment of newly diagnosed DLBCL, NOS patients older than 70 years included in this study followed the current institutional protocols at the time of diagnosis. The R-CHOP-21 regimen (rituximab 375 mg/sqm I.V. on D1, cyclophosphamide 750 mg/sqm I.V. on D1, hydroxydoxorubicin 50 mg/sqm I.V. on D1, vincristine 1.4 mg/sqm [maximum 2.0 mg] I.V. on D1, and prednisone 100 mg/day P.O. on days 1 to 5) was administered for 4 to 8 cycles with an interval of 21 days to patients aged between 70 and 80 years, ECOG < 2, Karnofsky Performance Status (KPS) > 70, low index of comorbidities, and without severe organic dysfunction ("fit" patients). Variants of this regimen included R-MiniCHOP or modified R-CHOP-21 (standard R-CHOP-21 with reduced doxorubicin dose to 25 mg/sqm I.V. on D1) and R-mini-CHOP-21 of the elderly (rituximab 375 mg/sqm I.V. on D1, cyclophosphamide 400 mg/sqm I.V. on D1, doxorubicin 25 mg/sqm I.V. on D1, vincristine 1 mg fixed dose I.V. on D1, and prednisone 40 mg/sqm P.O. on days 1 to 5). The R-MiniCHOP regimen was administered for 6 to 8 cycles for patients aged between 70 and 80 years, ECOG 2–3, KPS 50–70, or ≥2 relevant clinical comorbidities ("unfit" patients). The R-mini-CHOP-21 of the elderly regimen was administered for 6 cycles for patients aged ≥ 80 years or for those aged between 70 and 80 years, ECOG 3–4, KPS < 50, and/or ≥2 serious clinical comorbidities ("frail" cases). A minority of frail patients were alternatively treated with non-anthracycline-containing regimens, such as the R-CVP regimen (rituximab 375 mg/sqm I.V. on D1, cyclophosphamide 750 mg/sqm I.V. on D1, vincristine 1.4 mg/sqm [maximum 2.0 mg] I.V. on D1, and prednisone 100 mg/day P.O. on days 1 to 5) for 6 to 8 cycles with non-curative intent. The latter was used in patients with absolute contraindications to anthracyclic agents (symptomatic heart failure or left ventricular ejection fraction < 30%), as well as for very frail individuals (ECOG 4, KPS < 50, and with severe organic dysfunctions).

A pre-phase with CVP (cyclophosphamide 300 mg/sqm I.V. on D1, vincristine 1 mg fixed dose I.V. on D1, and prednisone 40 mg/sqm P.O. on days 1 to 7) was used in frail patients, with ECOG > 2 at diagnosis, KPS < 70, involvement of the gastrointestinal tract with risk of perforation or with high tumor burden (bulky ≥ 7 cm), and risk of tumor lysis syndrome (TLS). This cytoreductive regimen was used for 1 cycle given 7–14 days before curative intent immunochemotherapy. Patients with paranasal sinus involvement, paravertebral lesion with foraminal invasion, involvement of kidneys, adrenal glands, testicles, ovaries, breasts, or with involvement of ≥2 extranodal sites and intermediate–high or high-risk IPI received CNS prophylaxis with intrathecal infusion of 12 mg methotrexate and 2 mg dexamethasone during the first 4 cycles of R-CHOP-like chemotherapy. Involved-field radiotherapy (IF-RT) with 30–36 Gy was administered as consolidation therapy for bulky disease (≥7 cm), early-stage disease, or single mass with residual 18-FDG uptake on PET-CT at the end of immunochemotherapy.

Prophylaxis for infection was unified across the three main different treatment regimens and included use of granulocyte growth factors (G-CSFs) for individuals with absolute neutropenia < 1.0×10^9/L, as well as universal prophylaxis for pneumocystosis with trimethoprim–sulfamethoxazole 400/80 mg P.O. per day and secondary prophylaxis for herpes zoster with acyclovir 400 mg P.O. twice per day. Antibacterial prophylaxis with quinolones was not routinely adopted for either treatment group.

Response assessment was performed after the fourth cycle for interim evaluation and after the last cycle of immunochemotherapy or radiotherapy using CT or 18-FDG-PETCT as recommended by Cheson et al [26]. Clinical follow-up was performed every 3 months in the first two years after complete remission, every 4 months in the third year, every 6 months in the fourth year, and annually after the fifth year.

2.4. Histopathological Diagnosis

All cases were diagnosed by two experts in hematopathology and categorized as DLBCL, NOS according to the World Health Organization Classification for Hematopoietic and Lymphoid Tissue Neoplasms published in 2016 (WHO-2016) [1]. The tissue biopsies obtained at diagnosis were kept in formalin-fixed paraffin-embedded (FFPE) material. FFPE sections of 5 µm were displayed on silanized slides and stained with hematoxylin and eosin (HE) for initial analysis. Immunohistochemistry (IHC) was carried out with monoclonal antibodies CD45 (Dako, 2B11+PD7/26, 1/2000, Glostruo, Denmark), pan-B CD20 (Dako, L26, 1/1000), pan-T CD3 (Dako, F7.2.38, 1/500), proliferative marker Ki-67 (Dako, J55, 1/1600), CD10 (Novocastra, S6C6, 1/2000, Newcastle, UK, BCL6 (Abcam, EPR11410-43, 1/500, Boston, MA, USA), and MUM-1/IRF-4 (Abcam, EPR5653, 1/500). The immunohistochemical algorithm proposed by Hans et al was used to determine the cell of origin (COO), analyzing the expression pattern of the markers CD10, BCL6, and MUM-1/IRF-4 [25].

2.5. Statistical Analysis

Data were shown in accordance with the variables evaluated. Categorical variables were presented in absolute (N) and relative (%) values. Numerical variables were presented as measures of central tendency (median), dispersion (min–max range), and position. The median follow-up time was calculated using the reverse Kaplan–Meier method (reverse KM). Analysis of overall survival (OS), progression-free survival (PFS), and disease-free survival (DFS) was performed using the Kaplan–Meier (KM) method, and the log-rank test was used to establish associations between variables and outcomes. The Chi-square test and the Kruskal–Wallis test were applied to assess statistically significant differences in clinical–demographic characteristics and responses between different treatment modalities. OS was considered from the date of diagnosis to death, PFS from the date of diagnosis to disease progression, death, or last follow-up, and DFS from the date of complete response (CR) to disease progression, death, or last follow-up. Data were censored at the last follow-up.

Analysis to determine predictors for outcomes, including those related with OS and PFS, was performed using Cox's semiparametric univariate method. Multivariate analysis using a multi-step Cox's regression model was conducted to determine independent prognostic variables. All variables with a p-value ≤ 0.10 identified in univariate analysis were included in the final model for multivariate analysis. The results were presented in hazard ratio (HR) and 95% confidence interval (95% CI). All analyses were performed using the R-statistical software version 4.1.3 for Windows and a p-value ≤ 0.05 was assigned as statistically significant.

3. Results

3.1. Clinical, Epidemiological, Laboratorial, and Histopathological Findings

The clinical–demographic, laboratory, and pathological findings of the 185 patients with DLBCL, NOS are summarized in Table 1. The median age was 75 years (range: 70–97 years). A total of 109 patients (58.9%) were female, 76.7% (142) were Caucasian, and only 7.6% (7/92) had tertiary education. The median Charlson Comorbidity Index (CCI) score was 6 points (range: 5–10 points), and 63.2% (117) had at least one relevant comorbidity. More than a quarter of the whole cohort (25.4%; 47) had diabetes mellitus, 7% (13) had congestive heart failure, and 6.5% (12) had chronic obstructive pulmonary disease (COPD), as well as cerebrovascular disease (6.5%; 12) or secondary malignancy (6.5%; 12). Synchronous thrombosis at the diagnosis of DLBCL was observed in 11.4% (21) of cases. Immobilism occurred in 19.5% (36) of cases, and polypharmacy, defined as regular use of $\geq$ 5 medications, was observed in 24.8% (46). According to the Karnofsky Performance Status, 56.2% (104) of patients were categorized as "fit" (KPS > 70), 27.6% (51) as "unfit" (KPS 50–70), and 16.2% (30) as "frail" (KPS < 50). The median for body mass index (BMI) was 25.2 (range: 16.1–40.2), with malnutrition (geriatric BMI < 22) occurring in 28.1% (52) and overweight (geriatric BMI > 27) observed in 34.1% (63). Advanced-stage disease (Ann Arbor/Cotswold III/IV) was observed in 72.4% (134), 48.6% (90) had bulky disease $\geq$ 7 cm, 63.2% (117) had B-symptoms, 76.2% (141) had extranodal involvement, and 37.2% (69) had $\geq$ 2 extranodal sites involved by NHL. Bone marrow infiltration was demonstrated in only 3.8% (7) of cases, as well as CNS involvement. Patients with intermediate–high and high-risk NCCN IPI corresponded to the majority of our cohort (88.1%;163), as well as patients with intermediate–high and high-risk IPI, corresponding to 67% (124) of cases.

Table 1. Clinical–demographic and laboratorial characteristics of 185 Brazilian patients with DLBCL, NOS aged ≥ 70 years.

Characteristic	N = 185 (%; 95% CI)
Gender Male Female	 76 (41.1%; 34.3–48.4%) 109 (58.9%; 51.8–65.9%)
Median age (range)	75 years (70–97 years)
Caucasian ethnicity	142 (76.7%; 69.5–81.8%)
≥1 comorbidity	117 (63.2%; 56.2–70.1%)
Immobilism	36 (19.5%; 13.7–25.2%)
Polypharmacy (≥5 drugs)	46 (24.8%; 18.6–30.9%)
Desnutrition (geriatric BMI < 22)	52 (28.1%; 21.6–34.5%)
Categorization according to KPS Fit (KPS > 70) Unfit (KPS 50–70) Frail (KPS < 50)	 104 (56.2%; 46.5–65.8%) 51 (27.6%; 15.3–39.8%) 30 (16.2%; 2.9–29.5%)
B-symptoms	117 (63.2%; 56.2–70.1%)
Bulky disease ≥ 7 cm	90 (48.6%; 41.4–55.7%)
Extranodal involvement	141 (76.2%; 70.0–82.3%)
≥2 extranodal sites	69 (37.2%; 30.2–44.1%)
BM infiltration	7 (3.8%; 1.0–6.5%)
CNS infiltration	7 (3.8%; 1.0–6.5%)
Advanced-stage III or IV	134 (72.4%; 66.0–78.7%)
Intermediate–high/high-risk IPI	124 (67.0%; 60.2–73.7%)
Intermediate–high/high-risk NCCN-IPI	163 (88.1%; 83.4–92.7%)
LDH ≥ 1.5 × UVN	48 (25.9%; 19.5–32.2%)
Hypoalbuminemia (<3.5 g/dL)	52 (28.6%; 22.0–35.1%)—N miss = 3
Hypogammaglobulinemia (<1.5 g/dL)	2 (1.1%; 0.4–1.7%)—N miss = 5
COO according to IHC (Hans algorithm) GCB-like phenotype ABC-like phenotype	N = 109 57 (52.3%; 42.9–61.9%) 52 (47.7%; 38.2–57.2%)

BMI: body mass index; KPS: Karnofsky Performance Status scale; BM: bone marrow; CNS: central nervous system; IPI: International Prognostic Index; NCCN-IPI: National Comprehensive Cancer Network International Prognostic Index; LDH: lactic dehydrogenase; UVN: upper value of normality; COO: cell of origin; IHC: immunohistochemistry; GCB: germinal center B-cell; ABC: activated B-cell; N miss: missing data.

The medians of hemoglobin, total white blood cell (WBC) count, neutrophils, lymphocytes, monocytes, and platelets were 121 g/L, 7.82 × 10^9/L, 5.19 × 10^9/L, 1.30 × 10^9/L, 0.70 × 10^9/L, and 256 × 10^9/L, respectively. The medians of the neutrophil/lymphocyte (N/Ly) and lymphocyte/monocyte (Ly/Mo) ratios were 3.0 and 2.0, respectively. The medians of the patient LDH/control LDH ratio, β2-microglobulin, albumin, and total globulins were 1.0, 3.2 mg/dL, 3.9 g/dL, and 2.8 g/dL, respectively. Anemia occurred in 15.2% (28/184) of cases, leukocytosis in 14.1% (26/184), neutrophilia in 20.1% (37/184), lymphocytosis in 6% (11/184), and monocytosis in 16.3% (30/184). More than a quarter of the whole cohort (25.9%; 48) had a patient LDH/control LDH ratio ≥ 1.5, hypoalbuminemia (<3.5 g/dL) was observed in 28.6% (52/182), and hypogammaglobulinemia (<1.5 g/dL) occurred in only 1.1% (2/180) of cases. Additionally, positivity for HBsAg, total anti-HBc, and anti-HCV occurred in 0% (0/176), 15.9% (28/176), and 4.8% (8/171) of cases, respectively. The immunohistochemical algorithm proposed by Hans et al. could be applied in 58.9% (109) of cases [25]. Of these, 52.3% (57) had a germinal center (GCB)-like phenotype and 47.7% (52) had an activated B-cell (ABC)-like phenotype.

3.2. Up-Front Therapy for Elderly DLBCL, NOS Patients: Modalities, Responses, and Toxicities

Among the 185 DLBCL older than 70 years patients NOS included in this study, 1.6% (3) did not experience any antineoplastic therapy, because they died before starting first-line treatment. Among the 182 (98.4%) effectively treated cases, 57.1% (104) received the R-CHOP-21 regimen as induction, 18.0% (51) received the R-Mini-CHOP/modified R-CHOP-21 regimen, 13.2% (24) received the R-Mini-CHOP-21 of the elderly regimen, and only 1.7% (3) were treated without curative intent with the R-CVP regimen. Cytoreduction based on the CVP regimen was used in 65.9% (120) of treated cases, while CNS prophylaxis with the administration of intrathecal chemotherapy was applied in 50.5% (92) of cases. Seventy-six patients (41.8%) experienced IF-RT as an adjunct to primary therapy.

The overall response rate (ORR) for the whole cohort was 68.1% (95% CI: 60.8–74.8%), with complete response (CR) achieved in 65.9% (95% CI: 58.5–72.7%) and partial response (PR) in 2.2% (95% CI: 0.6–5.5%). Primary refractory disease occurred in 13.2% (95% CI: 8.6–18.9%) of cases, including 1.1% (2) with stable disease (SD) and 12.1% (22) with persistent or progressive disease (PD) at the end of up-front immunochemotherapy. The mortality rate (MR) during first-line therapy was 18.7% (95% CI: 13.3–25.1%). Among these 34 early deaths, 70.6% (24) occurred due to infectious complications, 17.6% (6) were due to disease progression, and in 11.8% (4), the cause of death could not be defined, usually in cases with death registered outside the oncological service of origin. The overall mortality rate (OMR) during all follow-up was 52.4% (97), with disease progression as the main cause of death (56; 57.7%). The early mortality rate (EMR), characterized as the percentage of deaths during the first 100 days after the DLBCL diagnosis, was 9.7% (18), occurring mainly due to infectious complications (10; 55.6%).

Table 2 summarizes the main up-front treatment modalities, clinical–demographic characteristics, responses, and toxicities of each treatment arm. The R-mini-CHOP of the elderly regimen had a lower overall response rate (ORR) (p = 0.040). However, as expected, patients in this group were not only older, but had other unfavorable clinical–laboratory characteristics, including higher rates of hypoalbuminemia (p = 0.001), and higher frequency of cases with IPI $\geq$ 3 (p = 0.013) and NCCN-IPI $\geq$ 3 (p = 0.002). The CCI scores were well balanced between the treatment groups. No differences were observed regarding thrombocytopenia, febrile neutropenia, therapy interruption, and mortality during first-line therapy, although grade 3/4 neutropenia was more common in patients treated with R-CHOP-21 (p = 0.003).

Table 2. Up-front therapy modalities, characteristics, responses, and adverse event profile in 179 Brazilian patients with DLBCL, NOS aged $\geq$ 70 years.

	R-CHOP-21 (N = 104; 95% CI)	R-MiniCHOP (N = 51; 95% CI)	R-Mini-CHOP of the Elderly (N = 24; 95% CI)	p-Value
Median age	73 years	78 years	83 years	0.367 *
CCI score	5.5 points	6.0 points	6.0 points	0.998 *
LDH ratio > 1.5	21 (20.4%; 12.6–28.1%)	16 (31.4%; 18.6–44.1%)	7 (29.2%; 11.0–47.3%)	0.269 **
Albumin < 3.5g/dL	19 (18.8%; 11.2–26.3%)	16 (31.4%; 18.6–44.1%)	13 (54.2%; 34.2–74.2%)	0.001 **
IPI $\geq$ 3	60 (57.7%; 48.1–67.2%)	40 (78.4%; 67.0–89.7%)	19 (79.2%; 62.9–95.4%)	0.013 **
NCCN-IPI $\geq$ 3	83 (79.8%; 72.0–87.5%)	50 (98.0%; 94.1–100%)	24 (100%)	0.002 **

Table 2. *Cont.*

	R-CHOP-21 (N = 104; 95% CI)	R-MiniCHOP (N = 51; 95% CI)	R-Mini-CHOP of the Elderly (N = 24; 95% CI)	*p*-Value
G3/4 neutropenia	103 (99.0%; 97.0–100%)	47 (92.2%; 84.8–99.5%)	20 (83.3%; 68.3–98.2%)	0.003 **
Febrile neutropenia	57 (54.8%; 45.2–64.3%)	27 (52.9%; 39.1–66.6%)	12 (50.0%; 29.9–70.1%)	0.907 **
G3/4 thrombocytopenia	22 (21.2%; 13.3–29.0%)	12 (23.5%; 11.8–35.1%)	9 (37.5%; 18.1–56.9%)	0.238 **
Therapy interruption	13 (12.5%; 6.1–18.8%)	4 (7.8%; 0.4–15.1%)	3 (12.5%; 6.2–18.8%)	0.671 **
Mortality during induction regimen	18 (17.3%; 10.1–24.5%)	10 (19.6%; 8.6–30.5%)	6 (25.0%; 7.7–42.2%)	0.681 **
ORR	75 (72.1%; 63.4–80.7%)	36 (70.6%; 58.1–83.0%)	11 (45.6%; 25.6–65.6%)	0.040 **

CCI: Charlson Comorbidity Index; LDH: lactic dehydrogenase; IPI: International Prognostic Index; NCCN-IPI: National Comprehensive Cancer Network International Prognostic Index; ORR: overall mortality rate; G3/G4: grade 3 or 4—according to the CTCAE version 5.0. * *p*-value was obtained by Kruskal–Wallis test; ** *p*-value was obtained by chi-square test.

3.3. Clinical Outcomes

The median follow-up for the whole cohort was 6.3 years (95% CI: 5.5–6.7 years). The median overall survival (OS) was 5.3 years (95% CI: 2.5–8.8 years), with an estimated 2-year OS of 61.6% (95% CI: 54.1–68.2%) and 50.2% (95% CI: 42.4–57.5%) in 5 years (Figure 1A). The median progression-free survival (PFS) was 3.7 years (95% CI: 2.0–5.8 years), and the estimated 2-year and 5-year PFS were 57.5% (95% CI: 50.0–64.3%) and 44.6% (95% CI: 37.0–51.9%), respectively (Figure 1B). Additionally, the median disease-free survival (DFS) was 9.8 years (95% CI: 5.8—not reached), with an estimated 2-year and 5-year DFS of 79.7% (95% CI: 70.2–84.6%) and 63.4% (95% CI: 52.0–68.2%), respectively (Figure 1C).

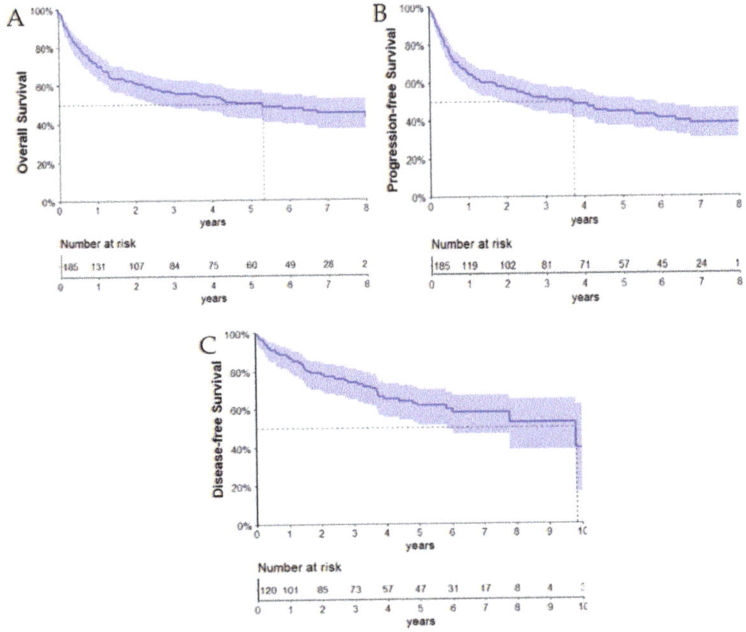

Figure 1. Survival curves for 185 Brazilian patients with DLBCL, NOS aged ≥ 70 years. (**A**) Overall survival, (**B**) progression-free survival, and (**C**) disease-free survival.

Considering the age at diagnosis, 69.7% (129) of cases were diagnosed between 70 and 80 years and 30.3% (56) over 80 years. The median OS was 5.5 years (95% CI: 4.5–6.6 years) for patients aged between 70 and 80 years, and 3.6 years (95% CI: 2.3–4.9 years) for patients over 80 years ($p = 0.05$). The estimated 2-year and 5-year OS were 77.9% (95% CI: 69.2–87.8%) and 64.8% (95% CI: 54.0–77.7%), respectively, for the group aged between 70 and 80 years, and 43.8% (95% CI: 31.0–62.0%) and 32.0% (95% CI: 20.0–51.0%), respectively, for the group aged over 80 years, $p = 0.05$.

Concerning the clinical outcomes stratified by up-front therapeutic modality, the median OS for patients treated with R-CHOP, R-MiniCHOP, and R-MiniCHOP of the elderly were 8.9 years (95% CI: 7.7–10.1 years), 6.0 years (95% CI: 4.4–7.6 years), and 2.9 years (95% CI: 1.2–4.7 years), respectively, $p = 0.003$. The estimated 2-year and 5-year OS were 82.0% (95% CI: 73.9–91.2%) and 71.6% (95% CI: 61.0–84.0%) for the R-CHOP group, 67.5% (95% CI: 51.5–88.4%) and 57.8% (95% CI: 41.0–81.6%) for the R-MiniCHOP group, and 48.1% (95% CI: 24.5–94.1%) and 24.1% (95% CI: 5.1–71.3%) for the R-MiniCHOP of the elderly group, $p = 0.003$ (Figure 2A). The median PFS for patients treated with R-CHOP, R-MiniCHOP, and R-MiniCHOP of the elderly were 5.6 years (95% CI: 4.5–6.7 years), 4.4 years (95% CI: 3.0–5.7 years), and 1.7 years (95% CI: 0.6–2.9 years), respectively, $p = 0.005$. The estimated 2-year and 5-year PFS were 61.1% (95% CI: 51.8–72.2%) and 45.7% (95% CI: 36.2–57.8%) for the R-CHOP group, 56.4% (95% CI: 42.1–75.5%) and 40.7% (95% CI: 26.3–63.1%) for the R-MiniCHOP group, and 20.5% (95% CI: 6.6–63.5%) and 10.2% (95% CI: 1.7–61.3%) for the R-MiniCHOP of the elderly group, $p = 0.005$ [Figure 2B].

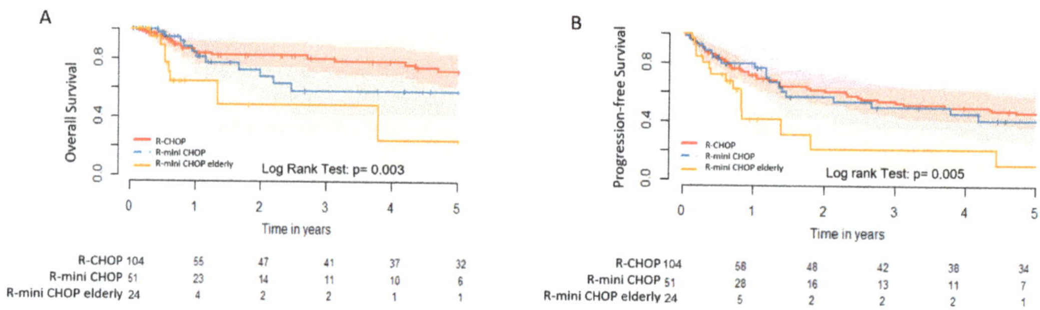

Figure 2. (**A**) OS curve ($p = 0.003$) and (**B**) PFS curve ($p = 0.005$) for 179 treated DLBCL, NOS patients older than 70 years according to up-front immunochemotherapeutic regimen. Red: conventional R-CHOP-21 regimen, blue: R-MiniCHOP-21 regimen, and yellow: R-MiniCHOP of the elderly regimen.

3.4. Prognostic Factors: Univariate and Multivariate Analysis

In the univariate analysis, the variables associated with decreased OS were age $\geq$ 75 years [HR: 2.08, 95% CI: 1.35–3.20, $p = 0.001$], non-Caucasian ethnicity [HR: 1.80, 95% CI: 1.14–2.83, $p = 0.012$], neurologic comorbidity [HR: 2.37, 95% CI: 1.19–4.72, $p = 0.014$], LDH > UVN [HR: 1.60, 95% CI: 1.07–2.41, $p = 0.023$], leukocytosis $\geq 11.0 \times 10^9$/L [HR: 2.61, 95% CI: 1.59–4.28, $p < 0.001$], neutrophilia $\geq 7.0 \times 10^9$/L [HR: 2.32, 95% CI: 1.46–3.67, $p < 0.001$], monocytosis $\geq 1.0 \times 10^9$/L [HR: 2.01, 95% CI: 1.17–3.02, $p < 0.001$], Ly/Mo ratio < median [HR: 2.19, 95% CI: 1.32–3.64, $p = 0.002$], hypoalbuminemia [HR: 1.59, 95% CI: 1.03–2.46, $p = 0.036$], advanced-stage III/IV [HR: 2.36, 95% CI: 1.38–4.04, $p = 0.002$], B-symptoms [HR: 1.89, 95% CI: 1.21–2.93, $p = 0.005$], and involvement of $\geq$ 2 extranodal sites [HR: 2.73, 95% CI: 1.19–6.26, $p = 0.018$].

Predictors for decreased PFS were age $\geq$ 75 years [HR: 2.00, 95% CI: 1.33–3.01, $p = 0.001$], non-Caucasian ethnicity [HR: 1.68, 95% CI: 1.09–2.60, $p = 0.020$], neurologic comorbidity [HR: 2.76, 95% CI: 1.38–5.49, $p = 0.004$], LDH > UVN [HR: 1.48, 95% CI: 1.00–2.17, $p = 0.048$], leukocytosis $\geq 11.0 \times 10^9$/L [HR: 2.26, 95% CI: 1.38–3.69, $p = 0.001$], neutrophilia $\geq 7.0 \times 10^9$/L [HR: 2.09, 95% CI: 1.34–3.27, $p = 0.001$], monocytosis $\geq 1.0 \times 10^9$/L [HR: 1.97, 95% CI: 1.24–2.73, $p = 0.007$], Ly/Mo ratio < median [HR: 2.04, 95% CI: 1.25–3.33,

$p = 0.004$], hypoalbuminemia [HR: 1.50, 95% CI: 1.08–2.27, $p = 0.049$], advanced-stage III/IV [HR: 2.58, 95% CI: 1.53–4.34, $p < 0.001$], B-symptoms [HR: 1.84, 95% CI: 1.21–2.80, $p = 0.004$], and involvement of ≥2 extranodal sites by NHL [HR: 2.38, 95% CI: 1.04–5.45, $p = 0.039$].

In the multivariate analysis, the independent prognostic factors associated with decreased OS in our older DLBCL, NOS cohort were age ≥ 75 years [HR: 2.22, 95% CI: 1.42–3.47, $p = 0.001$], neutrophilia ≥ 7.0×10^9/L [HR: 2.18, 95% CI: 1.23–3.84, $p = 0.007$], Ly/Mo ratio < median [HR: 1.98, 95% CI: 1.18–3.32, $p = 0.010$], and advanced Ann Arbor clinical stage (III/IV) [HR: 2.36, 95% CI: 1.34–4.13, $p = 0.003$]. Similarly, age ≥ 75 years [HR: 2.33, 95% CI: 1.52–3.58, $p < 0.001$], high LDH (>UVN) [HR: 1.09, 95% CI: 1.00–1.18, $p = 0.047$], B-symptoms [HR: 1.62, 95% CI: 1.04–2.52, $p = 0.032$], advanced-stage III/IV [HR: 2.38, 95% CI: 1.38–4.11, $p = 0.002$], neutrophilia ≥ 7.0×10^9/L [HR: 2.25, 95% CI: 1.41–3.59, $p = 0.001$], and low Ly/Mo ratio [HR: 2.08, 95% CI: 1.25–3.46, $p = 0.005$] were independently associated with decreased PFS. Table 3 summarizes the main prognostic factors for OS and PFS identified in our cohort.

Table 3. Main prognostic factors for OS and PFS identified in elderly DLBCL, NOS patients aged ≥ 70 years.

Variable	OS Univariate	OS Multivariate	PFS Univariate	PFS Multivariate
Age ≥ 75 years	HR: 2.08, 95% CI: 1.35–3.20, $p = 0.001$	HR: 2.22, 95% CI: 1.42–3.47, $p = 0.001$	HR: 2.00, 95% CI: 1.33–3.01, $p = 0.001$	HR: 2.33, 95% CI: 1.52–3.58, $p < 0.001$
Non-Caucasian ethnicity	HR: 1.80, 95% CI: 1.14–2.83, $p = 0.012$		HR: 1.68, 95% CI: 1.09–2.60, $p = 0.020$	
Neurologic comorbidity	HR: 2.37, 95% CI: 1.19–4.72, $p = 0.014$		HR: 2.76, 95% CI: 1.38–5.49, $p = 0.004$	
LDH > UVN	HR: 1.60, 95% CI: 1.07–2.41, $p = 0.023$		HR: 1.48, 95% CI: 1.00–2.17, $p = 0.048$	HR: 1.09, 95% CI: 1.00–1.18, $p = 0.047$
Leukocytosis	HR: 2.61, 95% CI: 1.59–4.28, $p < 0.001$		HR: 2.26, 95% CI: 1.38–3.69, $p = 0.001$	
Neutrophilia	HR: 2.32, 95% CI: 1.46–3.67, $p < 0.001$	HR: 2.18, 95% CI: 1.23–3.84, $p = 0.007$	HR: 2.09, 95% CI: 1.34–3.27, $p = 0.001$	HR: 2.25, 95% CI: 1.41–3.59, $p = 0.001$
Monocytosis	HR: 2.01, 95% CI: 1.17–3.02, $p < 0.001$		HR: 1.97, 95% CI: 1.24–2.73, $p = 0.007$	
L/M ratio < median	HR: 2.19, 95% CI: 1.32–3.64, $p = 0.002$	HR: 1.98, 95% CI: 1.18–3.32, $p = 0.010$	HR: 2.04, 95% CI: 1.25–3.33, $p = 0.004$	HR: 2.08, 95% CI: 1.25–3.46, $p = 0.005$
Hypoalbuminemia	HR: 1.59, 95% CI: 1.03–2.46, $p = 0.036$		HR: 1.50, 95% CI: 1.08–2.27, $p = 0.049$	
Ann Arbor CS III/IV	HR: 2.36, 95% CI: 1.38–4.04, $p = 0.002$	HR: 2.36, 95% CI: 1.34–4.13, $p = 0.003$	HR: 2.58, 95% CI: 1.53–4.34, $p < 0.001$	HR: 2.38, 95% CI: 1.38–4.11, $p = 0.002$
B-symptoms	HR: 1.89, 95% CI: 1.21–2.93, $p = 0.005$		HR: 1.84, 95% CI: 1.21–2.80, $p = 0.004$	HR: 1.62, 95% CI: 1.04–2.52, $p = 0.032$
≥2 extranodal sites	HR: 2.73, 95% CI: 1.19–6.26, $p = 0.018$		HR: 2.38, 95% CI: 1.04–5.45, $p = 0.039$	

OS: overall survival, PFS: progression-free survival, HR: hazard ratio; 95% CI: 95% confidence interval, *p*: *p*-value, LDH: lactic dehydrogenase, UVN: upper value of normality, L/M: lymphocyte/monocyte ratio, CS: clinical stage.

4. Discussion

In this study, we reported the main clinical–demographic, laboratory characteristics, clinical outcomes, and survival predictors in a large retrospective cohort of old and very old adults aged over 70 years and with a biopsy-proven diagnosis of DLBCL, NOS treated in a real-life setting in Brazil. We also assessed the response rates and long-term clinical outcomes in this population submitted to different up-front immunochemotherapy strategies based on anthracyclines, aiming to compare the efficacy and toxicity profile between conventional therapy with full-dose R-CHOP-21 and attenuated regimens, such as the R-MiniCHOP and R-MiniCHOP of the elderly. The identification of such prognostic factors and the reporting of these outcomes is essential for a better understanding of the DLBCL behavior in older adults in different geographic areas. Our data reflect the characteristics of one of the largest cohorts of older individuals with DLBCL in Latin America. Currently, the clinical–epidemiological characterization and outcomes of cohorts composed of older adults with DLBCL from North America and Europe are well established in the literature; however, data from Latin America, and particularly South America, are virtually unknown. Additionally, the determination of prognostic factors, response patterns, and toxicity profile reported upon treatment with different up-front immunochemotherapeutic regimens may assist in establishing risk-adapted therapeutic strategies for older adults with DLBCL, NOS.

Although the initial management of DLBCL in older adults (aged $\geq$ 60 years) still remains centered on the R-CHOP-21, an appreciable portion of cases will not be candidates for this regimen due to very old age, poor performance status, or due to severe and limiting comorbidities [3,4,18,27]. Therefore, the primary treatment of DLBCL in old and very old adults is challenging, and to determine the better up-front therapeutic modality, we must weigh the biological aggressiveness of the neoplasm, its high curative potential, and the geriatric vulnerability presented by this population [27]. Given all these particularities, attenuated or low-dose therapeutic strategies based and not based on anthracyclic agents have emerged for the management of unfit or frail older adults with DLBCL. Some of them, particularly non-containing anthracycline regimens, are merely palliative; however, many attenuated regimens are applied with curative intent [12,28]. Two examples of these curative attenuated regimens involve the R-MiniCHOP (or modified R-CHOP, with 50% dose reduction of doxorubicin) and the R-MiniCHOP of the elderly (with approximately 50% dose reduction of all conventional cytotoxic agents) [29]. However, the real impact of these low-dose strategies on the long-term outcomes of older adults with DLBCL is poorly known, mainly because this population is often excluded from prospective and controlled clinical trials. Given this gap in the medical literature, we aimed in this study to address this issue in a real-world scenario.

In our study, the R-MiniCHOP of the elderly regimen showed a significantly decreased overall response rate (ORR) (45.6%) compared to the full-dose R-CHOP (72.1%) and R-MiniCHOP (70.6%), p = 0.040. However, mortality during up-front therapy was not different between patients treated with the three regimens (17.3% for R-CHOP, 19.6% for R-MiniCHOP, and 25.0% for R-MiniCHOP of the elderly, p = 0.681). It is worth mentioning that individuals treated with the R-MiniCHOP of the elderly regimen, in addition to being older (median ages of 73 years for R-CHOP, 78 years for R-MiniCHOP, and 83 years for R-MiniCHOP of the elderly), had numerous unfavorable clinical–biological characteristics, including a higher percentage of malnutrition (p = 0.001), and a higher percentage of individuals with IPI (p = 0.013) and NCCN-IPI (p = 0.002) categorized as intermediate–high and high risk, as demonstrated in Table 2. Certainly, this poor clinical–biological characterization contributed to decreased ORR observed in the arm treated with the R-MiniCHOP of the elderly. Interestingly, severe hematological toxicities, including the occurrence of grade 3/4 thrombocytopenia (p = 0.238) and febrile neutropenia (p = 0.907), did not differ between the three treatment arms. Despite a higher occurrence of grade 3/4 neutropenia in individuals treated with full-dose R-CHOP (p = 0.003), this did not translate into higher rates of febrile neutropenia (p = 0.907), treatment interruption (p = 0.671), or mortality during the induction (p = 0.681). We believe that the universal prophylactic use of white cell growth factors adopted in our cohort based on neutrophil counts < 1.0×10^9/L may have strongly contributed to these favorable results.

Concerning the long-term clinical outcomes, we observed that DLBCL older adults treated with full-dose R-CHOP had benefits in OS and PFS when compared to individuals undergoing the attenuated R-MiniCHOP and R-MiniCHOP of the elderly regimens. The estimated 5-year OS was 71.6% for R-CHOP, 57.8% for R-MiniCHOP, and 24.1% for R-MiniCHOP of the elderly, p = 0.003. Similarly, the estimated 5-year PFS was 45.7% for

R-CHOP, 40.7% for R-MiniCHOP, and only 10.2% for R-MiniCHOP of the elderly, $p = 0.005$. These outcomes obtained in our real-life study are in agreement with those presented by Meguro et al [30]. These authors compared the efficacy of the conventional R-CHOP-21 regimen (n = 69) with the attenuated R-70%CHOP regimen (n = 61) in a retrospective cohort of elderly DLBCL patients from Japan. The R-70%CHOP regimen was applied in older adults aged over 70 years, while full-dose R-CHOP was administered to patients aged between 50 and 69 years. Patients treated with R-70%CHOP had worse 3-year OS (58% vs 68%, $p < 0.05$) and 3-year EFS (45% vs 70%, $p < 0.05$) compared to those treated with full-dose R-CHOP. Furthermore, in this study, patients in the R-70%CHOP arm had similar rates of grade 4 thrombocytopenia and grade 4 anemia compared to those submitted to R-CHOP. However, the full-dose R-CHOP group had a higher frequency of grade 4 leukopenia (76.8% vs 60.7%), although the rates of febrile neutropenia and infection were comparable in both groups [30]. In other words, taking into account the methodological differences, as previously revealed by the Japanese group, we demonstrated in our real-life study that attenuated regimens based on anthracyclic agents were associated with decreased outcomes in DLBCL older adults, and although conventional treatment with R-CHOP was associated with higher rates of severe neutropenia, this adverse event may be easily manageable and was not translated into higher rates of infectious complications or higher mortality.

Due to the increased risk of hematological and cardiac toxicity in older adults treated with full-dose R-CHOP, attenuated varieties of this regimen have been recently evaluated. In this sense, Peyrade et al. prospectively evaluated the efficacy of the R-MiniCHOP of the elderly regimen in a multicenter cohort consisting of 150 DLBCL patients older than 80 years. This regimen was shown to be safe and feasible, with an ORR of 73%, and 2-year PFS and OS estimates of 47% and 59%, respectively [29]. Unlike what was demonstrated by Peyrade et al, in our cohort, the outcomes presented by patients treated with the R-MiniCHOP of the elderly regimen were very poor, with an ORR of 45.6%, and estimated 2-year PFS and OS of only 20.5% and 48.1%, respectively [29]. However, we emphasize that our study was conducted retrospectively in a real-life setting, differently from the study of the Franco-Belgian group, which had a prospective design and included highly selected older patients, where individuals with poor performance status (ECOG $\geq$ 2) or high rates of comorbidities were excluded. The multivariate analysis of the study conducted by Peyrade et al. demonstrated that OS was strongly affected by serum albumin concentrations below 35 g/L (HR: 3.2, 95% CI: 1.4–7.1, $p = 0.0053$) [29]. In our series, 54.2% (13) of patients treated with R-MiniCHOP of the elderly had hypoalbuminemia, which may, at least partially, justify the worse outcomes found in our cohort.

High-level evidence for the management of older adults with DLBCL considered unfit or frail is unavailable in the current medical literature, considering that most prospective studies published to date are single-arm. Therefore, to date, only one meta-analysis has compared the efficacy and safety of different first-line treatments in this population [31]. This meta-analysis included 1839 patients enrolled in 13 clinical trials and demonstrated a PFS advantage for patients treated with the R2CHOP-21 (lenalidomide plus R-CHOP-21) regimen compared to the R-COMP (R-CHOP with non-pegylated liposomal doxorubicin), R-MiniCEOP (with epirubicin replacing doxorubicin), RCHOP-14, and RCHOP-21. No statistically significant differences in ORR, CR, EFS, and OS were demonstrated between the previously mentioned regimens, although the R-COMP regimen promoted lower rates of toxic cardiac events and severe neutropenia [31].

The standard of care for older adults with DLBCL centered on the R-CHOP-21 regimen was established by the Groupe d'Etudes des Lymphomes de l'Adulte (GELA) LNH-98-5, RICOVER-60, LNH03-6B, and UK NCRI R-CHOP14v21 randomized trials, enrolling newly diagnosed DLBCL patients aged between 60 and 80 years. These trials validated the superiority of the R-CHOP regimen versus CHOP polychemotherapy in older adults, with an absolute increase of 13% in OS with the addition of the anti-CD20 monoclonal antibody to the CHOP backbone and demonstrated equivalence in terms of efficacy of the R-CHOP-

21 and R-CHOP-14 regimes. However, these clinical trials did not involve octogenarians and included highly selected patients with ECOG ≤ 1 [32–37]. As shown in Table 4, the full-dose R-CHOP regimen promoted ORR between 83 and 91% in these studies, and 5-year PFS and OS estimates of around 54–73% and 58–69%, respectively. In our real-world study, the ORR of older adults treated with full-dose R-CHOP-21 was lower (72.1%); however, the estimated 5-year OS of this subgroup (71.6%) was similar to that observed in previously reported trials. Our median DFS was quite long (9.8 years); therefore, we believe that our high early mortality rate (17.3% in the R-CHOP regimen) resulting from the poor conditions presented by our patients at diagnosis adversely impacted the ORR of older adults treated with R-CHOP-21; however, once these patients achieved remission, their responses were durable and promoted OS comparable to that described in other international cohorts.

Table 4. Responses and clinical outcomes obtained in the main clinical trials involving newly diagnosed DLBCL older adults.

Modality	Trial	Phase	Treatment	N	ORR %	PFS %	OS %
Anthracycline full dose	LNH98-5 [32]	3	CHOP R-CHOP	399	69 83	30 (5y) 54 (5y)	45 (5y) 58 (5y)
	RICOVER [34]	3	R-CHOP + 2xR R-CHOP + 2xR + RT	166	76 (CR) 78 (CR)	72 (3y) 73 (3y)	77 (3y) 78 (3y)
	UK NCRI [37]	3	R-CHOP14 R-CHOP21	604	91 91	64 (5y)	69 (5y)
	LNH03-6B [35]	3	R-CHOP14 R-CHOP21	602	87 86	60 (3y) 62 (3y)	69 (3y) 72 (3y)
	Corazzelli et al., 2011 [38]	2	R-COMP14	41	73	77 (4y)	67 (4y)
Anthracycline dose attenuated	Peyrade et al., 2011 [29]	2	R-MiniCHOP of the elderly	150	73	47 (2y)	59 (2y)
	ANZINTER3 [39]	3	R-MiniCEOP* R-CHOP	224	81 87	46 (5y) 48 (5y)	63 (5y) 62 (5y)
Non-anthracycline	Park et al., 2016 [40]	2	BR	23	78	5.4 months (median)	10.2 months (median)
	Fields et al., 2014 [41]	2	R-GCVP	62	61.3	50 (2y)	56 (2y)
	Qui-Dan et al., 2018 [42]	2	R-GEMOX	60	49	49 (3y)	65 (3y)

CHOP (cyclophosphamide, doxorubicin, vincristine, and prednisone); R-CHOP (rituximab plus CHOP); R: rituximab; RT: radiotherapy; R-COMP (rituximab, cyclophosphamide, vincristine, liposomal doxorubicin, and prednisone); R-MiniCEOP* (epirubicin); mini-CEOP** (etoposide); BR (bendamustine plus rituximab); R-GCVP (rituximab, gemcitabine, cyclophosphamide, vincristine, and prednisone); R-GEMOX (rituximab, gemcitabine, and oxaliplatin); ORR: overall response rate; PFS: progression-free survival; OS: overall survival.

Regimens containing alternative anthracyclines, such as non-pegylated liposomal formulations of doxorubicin (R-COMP) and epirubicin (R-MiniCEOP), are promising strategies to minimize cardiotoxicity in older adults with DLBCL without substantially compromising therapeutic efficacy [38,39]. For frail patients or those with contraindications to the use of anthracyclic agents, alternative regimens such as R-CEOP (rituximab, cyclophosphamide, etoposide, and prednisone), R-CVP (rituximab, cyclophosphamide, vincristine, and prednisone), BR (bendamustine plus rituximab), or regimens containing gemcitabine (R-GEMOX [rituximab, gemcitabine, and oxaliplatin] and R-GCVP [rituximab, gemcitabine, cyclophosphamide, vincristine, and prednisone]) have been evaluated. Although they are still considered potentially curable, long-term survival usually does not exceed 50%, being lower than that offered by anthracycline-containing regimens [40–43]. In our study, we did not assess the role of such attenuated regimens not based on doxorubicin, although they constitute interesting alternatives for a specific niche of elderly people with newly diagnosed DLBCL.

Despite obtaining satisfactory responses and outcomes in the population of older adults with DLBCL considered "fit" (ECOG $\leq$ 2 and KPS > 70) and treated with the full-dose R-CHOP regimen in our study, with an ORR of 72.1% and estimated 2-year OS and PFS of 82% and 61.1%, respectively, the estimated 5-year OS and PFS for the whole cohort composed of 185 patients older than 70 years were poor, corresponding to 50.2% and 44.6%, respectively. These data reflect that currently, in a real-life context, the up-front treatment of DLBCL in old elderly and very old adults is still an unmet medical need, and therefore clinical outcomes can be improved with the use of new therapeutic approaches focused on target drugs, or through the appropriate selection of cases who are candidates for full-dose regimens. We believe that the low survival expectations of our whole cohort were due to the high proportion of frail patients with severe comorbidities, treated in this context with alternative protocols based on attenuated doses of anthracyclines. Although in our cohort we did not categorize a patient's fitness according to Comprehensive Geriatric Assessment (CGA) recommendations, many individuals were classified as unfit (27.6%) or frail (16.2%) according to the Karnofsky Performance Status (KPS) scale. In addition, the prevalence of other robust markers of geriatric frailty was very high, such as immobility (19.5%), malnutrition (28.1%), and the presence of more than one serious comorbidity (63.2%), making 40.5% (75) of our population ineligible for the full-dose R-CHOP protocol. Table 5 summarizes the main clinical outcomes of old DLBCL patients stratified according to their geriatric vulnerability obtained in other studies, revealing data similar to those demonstrated by us.

Table 5. Clinical outcomes obtained in selected studies involving older adults with DLBCL stratified according to geriatric vulnerability.

Study	Design	N	Median Age	Stratification	Outcomes
Tucci et al., 2015 Italy [15]	Prospective	173	77	Fit 46% Unfit 16% Frail 38%	2-year OS: Fit: 84% Non-fit 47%
Merli et al., 2014 Italy [44]	Prospective	318	Fit 72 Frail 78	Fit 70% Frail 30%	5-year OS: Fit: 71.5% Frail: 23.8% Whole cohort: 28%
Ong et al., 2019 Australia [45]	Retrospective	205	73	Fit 41% Unfit 21% Frail 38%	3-year OS: Fit: 82% Unfit: 60% Frail: 53%
Spina et al., 2012 Italy [46]	Prospective	100	75	Fit 55% Unfit 32% Frail 13%	5-year OS: Whole cohort: 60%
Olivieri et al., 2012 Italy [47]	Prospective	91	74	Fit 59% Unfit 24% Frail 17%	5-year OS: Whole cohort: 46% 5-year EFS: Whole cohort: 31%

Table 5. *Cont.*

Study	Design	N	Median Age	Stratification	Outcomes
Marchesi et al., 2013 Italy [48]	Retrospective	73	78	Fit 29% Unfit 38% Frail 33%	2-year OS: Fit: 58.3% Non-fit: 24.3% 2-year PFS: Fit: 47.2% Non-fit 21.6%
Lage et al., 2024 Brazil (This study)	Retrospective	185	75	* Fit 56.2% Unfit 27.6% Frail 16.2%	5-year OS: Fit: 71.6% Unfit: 57.8% Frail **: 24.1% Whole cohort: 50.2%

* Fitness according to KPS scale; ** Estimated 5-year OS considering just treated cases with anthracycline-containing regimens (three frail cases not treated and three frail cases treated with R-CVP were excluded); OS: overall survival; PFS: progression-free survival.

New therapeutic approaches focused on improving outcomes for older adults with DLBCL involve combining new agents with the conventional R-CHOP regimen. However, to date, such strategies have not demonstrated a high capacity to increase CR and OS in this population compared to conventional immunochemotherapy based on anthracyclines. Although the combination of lenalidomide (15 mg on days 1–14) plus R-CHOP was tested in a phase II study involving 49 fit patients with DLBCL aged 60–80 years demonstrating promising results, including a CR rate of 86%, and 2-year OS and PFS estimates of 92% and 80%, respectively [49], other combinations involving new drugs were unable to improve outcomes in the geriatric population. In this sense, the REMARC trial evaluated the role of maintenance therapy with lenalidomide in elderly DLBCL patients who responded to R-CHOP. In this study, the PFS increase promoted by maintenance with lenalidomide was very slight and no benefit was observed in OS when this therapy was compared to the placebo group [50]. Additionally, the ibrutinib plus R-CHOP combination was tested in a phase III study involving patients with non-GCB DLBCL with a median age of 62 years. The study also failed to meet its primary endpoint (EFS increase) in the whole cohort and in the subgroup of patients older than 60 years, and the ibrutinib + R-CHOP regimen was associated with substantially increased rates of severe adverse events, including febrile neutropenia and infectious complications, as well as higher rates of therapy discontinuation when compared to cases treated with R-CHOP [51].

In the last five years, great progress has been made in the management of relapsed and refractory DLBCL through the incorporation of new therapeutic strategies, such as chimeric antigen receptor T (CAR-T) cell therapy and bispecific monoclonal antibodies (BsMoAbs). Offering promising responses, bispecific antibodies and CAR-T therapies have also proven to be applicable alternatives in elderly and fit patients with DLBCL. In this sense, a recent study conducted by Ram R et al. (2021) compared clinical outcomes between 41 R/R DLBCL patients older than 70 years and 41 younger patients undergoing CAR-T therapy. The authors demonstrated no differences in the incidence of grade ≥ 3 toxicities, such as cytokine release syndrome (CRS) ($p = 0.29$), neurotoxicity ($p = 0.54$), and duration of hospitalization ($p = 0.55$), between younger and older adults. Additionally, response rates were similar between both groups ($p = 0.33$), and older adults achieved satisfactory outcomes, with 12-month OS and PFS of 69% and 32%, respectively [52].

Similarly, the use of anti-CD20/CD3 bispecific monoclonal antibodies has been expanded to older adults with DLBCL. The toxicity of these agents is usually lower than that of CAR-T therapy, which makes them very promising in the geriatric population, including frail individuals. Among these, epcoritamab is of particular interest in patients aged ≥ 60 years, given its subcutaneous administration. A recent trial conducted by Thieblemont et al. (2023), involving 157 patients with R/R DLBCL, with a median age of 64 years and treated with epcoritamab, demonstrated an ORR of 63% and a CR of 39%.

Although CRS occurred frequently, it was usually mild (≤grade 2), being easily manageable in most cases [53]. Another study explored the use of mosunetuzumab as monotherapy for the up-front treatment of old (>60 years) and very old (>80 years) patients who were frail and ineligible for conventional immunochemotherapy. In this study, involving 54 individuals with a median age of 83 years, ORR was 56%, with CR of 43%, and no occurrence of CRS or neurotoxicity ≥ grade 3 [54]. Therefore, we believe that the independent prognostic factors found in our study, combined with the identification of classic biomarkers associated with frailty, such as age ≥ 80 years, malnutrition (albumin < 3.5 g/dL or geriatric BMI < 22), and KPS < 70, may be valuable tools for selecting older adults with DLBCL for new therapies capable of offering promising outcomes, such as those listed above, as well as for attenuated immunochemotherapeutic regimens, such as R-MiniCHOP, R-MiniCHOP of the elderly, and protocols not based on anthracyclines.

Another way to optimize outcomes for older DLBCL patients is based on the systematic use of tools capable of selecting suitable candidates for intensified or attenuated therapeutic approaches, offering personalized strategies adapted to the frailty profile of each individual. In older adults with cancer, the aim of maintaining quality of life can often exceed the aim of promoting a cure or extension of survival. Therefore, Comprehensive Geriatric Assessments (CGAs) can be used for this purpose. CGAs may include assessments of functional status, comorbid medical conditions, cognition, psychological status, social support, nutritional status, and concomitant medications [55]. However, such assessments are quite complex and require a lot of time and are rarely applied in clinical practice. As a result, judging the frailty of older adults with DLBCL has been subjective and based on parameters such as age, comorbidity index, and performance status. Aiming to establish more objective and easier-to-implement parameters, different collaborative groups have proposed adapted CGAs, such as the FIL tool (Italian Lymphoma Foundation) that incorporates the Chronic Illness Rating Scale-Geriatric (CIRS-G), Instrumental Activities of Daily Living (IADL), and Activities of Daily Living (ADL) to categorize patients as fit, unfit, or frail [56]. The FIL tool can assist in the selection of fit and unfit patients for therapies with curative intent and guide clinicians to discuss palliative approaches in frail patients. However, it lacks strong validation in large prospective cohorts and remains little adopted in clinical practice. In our study, we did not apply any tool based on CGAs to stratify the geriatric vulnerability of our patients; however, we categorized our cases into fit, unfit, and frail according to the KPS scale, and we were able to demonstrate OS estimates clearly distinct between individuals with KPS > 70, between 50 and 70, and <50, as well as employing attenuated therapeutic strategies for cases considered unfit or frail according to this scale.

Due to the increasing incidence of chronic diseases with advancing age, approximately 70% of our cohort had one or more comorbidities. A population study conducted in the Netherlands demonstrated a similar prevalence, where 66% of patients with lymphoma aged over 70 years had comorbidities [57]. Additionally, the same group analyzed the severity of comorbidities and showed that patients with NHL and cardiovascular disease had a 3.3 times higher chance of developing treatment toxicity [58]. Interestingly, in our analysis, the presence of cerebrovascular disease was a predictor of worse OS and PFS. We also observed malnutrition in 28.1% of our cases and low albumin levels adversely affected our cohort, as demonstrated in the univariate analysis. Recently, a geriatric nutritional risk index calculated from body weight and serum albumin was an IPI-independent adverse factor predicting OS in older adults with DLBCL [59]. While immobility was observed in almost 20% of our cohort, walking speed has been shown to adversely correlate with survival. With a cumulative risk for the incidence of deep vein thrombosis (DVT) of around 3% in DLBCL patients [60], our cohort presented a rate of 11.4% for thromboembolic events at the diagnosis of DLBCL. Although it appears high, this may be due to the large number of incidental and asymptomatic thrombotic events detected during staging procedures based on CTs and 18-FDG-PETCT. Classically, the prevalence of non-GCB DLBCL increases continuously with age, reaching 40–50% after the age of 60 years, according to data obtained from North American and European cohorts [61,62]. This DLBCL subtype is usually characterized by extranodal involvement, molecular findings associated with immune evasion, the presence of recurrent MYD88 L265P and CD79B mutations, and worse clinical outcomes [63]. Although we accessed the cell of origin of DLBCL in only 109 patients, we found 47.7% (52) of cases with a non-GCB phenotype in our cohort. These data are in agreement with what was previously reported in cohorts of patients from developed countries, despite being a population from another geographic area and with different ancestry.

Here, we also identified that age $\geq$ 75 years, advanced clinical stage III/IV, B-symptoms, high LDH levels, neutrophilia, and low Ly/Mo ratio were independent adverse prognostic factors associated with decreased OS and PFS in adults older than 70 years with DLBCL, NOS. These data are in agreement with those previously reported by other international collaborative groups. Characteristically, advanced age, elevated LDH, and Ann Arbor/Cotswold clinical stage III/IV are listed as variables associated with poor clinical outcomes in robust prognostic indices widely used in clinical practice for the risk stratification of individuals with DLBCL, such as the IPI, R-IPI, and NCCN-IPI [22–24]. The presence of constitutional symptoms, such as fever, weight loss, and night sweats (B-symptoms), indirectly reflects the lymphoma tumor burden, being associated with adverse outcomes in different subtypes of chronic lymphoproliferative disorders [64,65]. Some laboratory parameters, easily accessible to the peripheral blood count, have recently been incorporated into biological prognostic indexes and present a strong association with adverse clinical outcomes in cancer. Absolute neutrophil count has been considered a surrogate marker of inflammation, absolute lymphocyte count reflects host immunity, and absolute monocyte count, as well as the tumor-associated macrophage content, are surrogate markers of the tumor microenvironment. Therefore, some applications derived from these blood cells have been studied, including the neutrophil/lymphocyte ratio and lymphocyte/monocyte ratio, both associated with a poor prognosis in patients with DLBCL [66–68]. The identification of all these prognostic factors is of great importance in identifying older adults with DLBCL with a greater probability of therapeutic failure or early progression and who, consequently, may be candidates for intensified therapeutic strategies and associated with a greater chance of long-term survival, such as the full-dose R-CHOP regimen.

5. Conclusions

In this large and real-life South American cohort, we demonstrated that patients with DLBCL, NOS older than 70 years still do not have satisfactory clinical outcomes in 2024, with half of cases not reaching 5 years of life expectancy after diagnosis. Although the conventional R-CHOP offers response and survival advantages over attenuated regimens, such as R-MiniCHOP and R-MiniCHOP of the elderly, its myelotoxicity is not negligible. However, we highlight that a substantial portion of these individuals present great geriatric vulnerability, being ineligible for the full-dose R-CHOP regimen. This subgroup of patients should be promptly identified at the time of diagnosis and will be candidates for therapeutic strategies adapted to their frailty profile. Therefore, we hope that the outcomes reported, and the prognostic factors identified here, may assist clinicians in the appropriate selection of risk-adapted therapeutic strategies for old and very old DLBCL patients in a real-life setting, due to the fact that Comprehensive Geriatric Assessments are complex and unfeasible tools and are not routinely incorporated into clinical practice.

Author Contributions: Conceptualization, L.A.d.P.C.L. and J.P.; data curation, R.N.D.V.; funding acquisition, not applicable; investigation, L.A.d.P.C.L., R.N.D.V., M.D.J., H.F.C., F.A.d.F. and R.d.O.C.; methodology, L.B.d.O.A., C.O.R. and S.A.C.S.; project administration, L.A.d.P.C.L. and J.P.; validation and supervision, L.A.d.P.C.L., V.R. and J.P.; writing—original draft, R.d.O.C. and L.A.d.P.C.L.; writing—review and editing, L.A.d.P.C.L. and J.P. All authors have read and agreed to the published version of the manuscript.

Funding: This research received no external funding.

Institutional Review Board Statement: The local Ethics Committee (Research Ethic Committee of São Paulo university) approved this study in 2021 under the number CAAE: 48897221.2.0000.0068. All procedures followed were in accordance with the ethical standards of the responsible committees on human experimentation (institutional and national) and with the Helsinki Declaration of 1975, as revised in 2008.

Informed Consent Statement: All participants included in this study signed the Free and Informed Consent Form (FICF).

Data Availability Statement: All data generated and analyzed during this study were included in this published article. The raw data for this study are in possession of the correspondence author and may be fully available in the event of a request to the correspondence author via e-mail.

Conflicts of Interest: The authors declare no conflicts of interest.

References

1. Swerdlow, S.H.; Campo, E.; Pileri, S.A.; Harris, N.L.; Stein, H.; Siebert, R.; Advani, R.; Ghielmini, M.; Salles, G.A.; Zelenetz, A.D.; et al. The 2016 revision of the World Health Organization classification of lymphoid neoplasms. *Blood* **2016**, *127*, 2375–2390. [CrossRef]
2. Alaggio, R.; Amador, C.; Anagnostopoulos, I.; Attygalle, A.D.; Araujo, I.B.O.; Berti, E.; Bhagat, G.; Borges, A.M.; Boyer, D.; Calaminici, M.; et al. The 5th edition of the World Health Organization Classification of Haematolymphoid Tumours: Lymphoid Neoplasms. *Leukemia* **2022**, *36*, 1720–1748. [CrossRef]
3. Sehn, L.H.; Salles, G. Diffuse Large B-Cell Lymphoma. *N. Engl. J. Med.* **2021**, *384*, 842–858. [CrossRef]
4. Poletto, S.; Novo, M.; Paruzzo, L.; Frascione, P.M.M.; Vitolo, U. Treatment strategies for patients with diffuse large B-cell lymphoma. *Cancer Treat. Rev.* **2022**, *110*, 102443. [CrossRef]
5. Martelli, M.; Ferreri, A.J.; Agostinelli, C.; Di Rocco, A.; Pfreundschuh, M.; Pileri, S.A. Diffuse large B-cell lymphoma. *Crit. Rev. Oncol./Hematol.* **2013**, *87*, 146–171. [CrossRef] [PubMed]
6. Kanas, G.; Ge, W.; Quek, R.G.W.; Keeven, K.; Nersesyan, K.; Jon, E.A. Epidemiology of diffuse large B-cell lymphoma (DLBCL) and follicular lymphoma (FL) in the United States and Western Europe: Population-level projections for 2020-2025. *Leuk. Lymphoma* **2022**, *63*, 54–63. [CrossRef] [PubMed]
7. Campisi, J. Aging, cellular senescence, and cancer. *Annu. Rev. Physiol.* **2013**, *75*, 685–705. [CrossRef] [PubMed]
8. Johnstone, S.E.; Gladyshev, V.N.; Aryee, M.J.; Bernstein, B.E. Epigenetic clocks, aging, and cancer. *Science* **2022**, *378*, 1276–1277. [CrossRef]
9. López-Otín, C.; Pietrocola, F.; Roiz-Valle, D.; Galluzzi, L.; Kroemer, G. Meta-hallmarks of aging and cancer. *Cell Metab.* **2023**, *35*, 12–35. [CrossRef]
10. Moccia, A.A.; Thieblemont, C. Curing diffuse large B-cell lymphomas in elderly patients. *Eur. J. Intern. Med.* **2018**, *58*, 14–21. [CrossRef]
11. Chiappella, A.; Castellino, A.; Nicolosi, M.; Santambrogio, E.; Vitolo, U. Diffuse Large B-cell Lymphoma in the elderly: Standard treatment and new perspectives. *Expert Rev. Hematol.* **2017**, *10*, 289–297. [CrossRef]
12. Allen, P. Diffuse Large B-Cell Lymphoma in the Elderly: Current Approaches. *Curr. Oncol. Rep.* **2020**, *22*, 114. [CrossRef]
13. Grann, V.R.; Hershman, D.; Jacobson, J.S.; Tsai, W.Y.; Wang, J.; McBride, R.; Mitra, N.; Grossbard, M.L.; Neugut, A.I. Outcomes and diffusion of doxorubicin-based chemotherapy among elderly patients with aggressive non-Hodgkin lymphoma. *Cancer* **2006**, *107*, 1530–1541. [CrossRef]
14. Caimi, P.F.; Barr, P.M.; Berger, N.A.; Lazarus, H.M. Non-Hodgkin's lymphoma in the elderly. *Drugs Aging* **2010**, *27*, 211–238. [CrossRef]
15. Tucci, A.; Martelli, M.; Rigacci, L.; Riccomagno, P.; Cabras, M.G.; Salvi, F.; Stelitano, C.; Fabbri, A.; Storti, S.; Fogazzi, S.; et al. Comprehensive geriatric assessment is an essential tool to support treatment decisions in elderly patients with diffuse large B-cell lymphoma: A prospective multicenter evaluation in 173 patients by the Lymphoma Italian Foundation (FIL). *Leuk. Lymphoma* **2015**, *56*, 921–926. [CrossRef] [PubMed]
16. Tilly, H.; Morschhauser, F.; Sehn, L.H.; Friedberg, J.W.; Trněný, M.; Sharman, J.P.; Herbaux, C.; Burke, J.M.; Matasar, M.; Rai, S.; et al. Polatuzumab Vedotin in Previously Untreated Diffuse Large B-Cell Lymphoma. *N. Engl. J. Med.* **2022**, *386*, 351–363. [CrossRef] [PubMed]
17. Nastoupil, L.J.; Bartlett, N.L. Navigating the Evolving Treatment Landscape of Diffuse Large B-Cell Lymphoma. *J. Clin. Oncol. Off. J. Am. Soc. Clin. Oncol.* **2023**, *41*, 903–913. [CrossRef]
18. Tavares, A.; Moreira, I. Diffuse large B-cell lymphoma in very elderly patients: Towards best tailored treatment—A systematic review. *Crit. Rev. Oncol. /Hematol.* **2021**, *160*, 103294. [CrossRef] [PubMed]
19. Spinner, M.A.; Advani, R.H. Current Frontline Treatment of Diffuse Large B-Cell Lymphoma. *Oncology* **2022**, *36*, 51–58. [CrossRef] [PubMed]
20. Charlson, M.E.; Pompei, P.; Ales, K.L.; MacKenzie, C.R. A new method of classifying prognostic comorbidity in longitudinal studies: Development and validation. *J. Chronic Dis.* **1987**, *40*, 373–383. [CrossRef]

21. Lin, T.L.; Kuo, M.C.; Shih, L.Y.; Dunn, P.; Wang, P.N.; Wu, J.H.; Tang, T.C.; Chang, H.; Hung, Y.S. The impact of age, Charlson comorbidity index, and performance status on treatment of elderly patients with diffuse large B cell lymphoma. *Ann. Hematol.* **2012**, *91*, 1383–1391. [CrossRef] [PubMed]
22. International Non-Hodgkin's Lymphoma Prognostic Factors Project. A predictive model for aggressive non-Hodgkin's lymphoma. *N. Engl. J. Med.* **1993**, *329*, 987–994. [CrossRef] [PubMed]
23. Sehn, L.H.; Berry, B.; Chhanabhai, M.; Fitzgerald, C.; Gill, K.; Hoskins, P.; Klasa, R.; Savage, K.J.; Shenkier, T.; Sutherland, J.; et al. The revised International Prognostic Index (R-IPI) is a better predictor of outcome than the standard IPI for patients with diffuse large B-cell lymphoma treated with R-CHOP. *Blood* **2007**, *109*, 1857–1861. [CrossRef]
24. Zhou, Z.; Sehn, L.H.; Rademaker, A.W.; Gordon, L.I.; Lacasce, A.S.; Crosby-Thompson, A.; Vanderplas, A.; Zelenetz, A.D.; Abel, G.A.; Rodriguez, M.A.; et al. An enhanced International Prognostic Index (NCCN-IPI) for patients with diffuse large B-cell lymphoma treated in the rituximab era. *Blood* **2014**, *123*, 837–842. [CrossRef]
25. Hans, C.P.; Weisenburger, D.D.; Greiner, T.C.; Gascoyne, R.D.; Delabie, J.; Ott, G.; Müller-Hermelink, H.K.; Campo, E.; Braziel, R.M.; Jaffe, E.S.; et al. Confirmation of the molecular classification of diffuse large B-cell lymphoma by immunohistochemistry using a tissue microarray. *Blood* **2004**, *103*, 275–282. [CrossRef]
26. Cheson, B.D.; Fisher, R.I.; Barrington, S.F.; Cavalli, F.; Schwartz, L.H.; Zucca, E.; Lister, T.A. Recommendations for initial evaluation, staging, and response assessment of Hodgkin and non-Hodgkin lymphoma: The Lugano classification. *J. Clin. Oncol. Off. J. Am. Soc. Clin. Oncol.* **2014**, *32*, 3059–3068. [CrossRef] [PubMed]
27. Di, M.; Huntington, S.F.; Olszewski, A.J. Challenges and Opportunities in the Management of Diffuse Large B-Cell Lymphoma in Older Patients. *Oncol.* **2021**, *26*, 120–132. [CrossRef]
28. Khan, Y.; Brem, E.A. Considerations for the Treatment of Diffuse Large B Cell Lymphoma in the Elderly. *Curr. Hematol. Malig. Rep.* **2019**, *14*, 228–238. [CrossRef]
29. Peyrade, F.; Jardin, F.; Thieblemont, C.; Thyss, A.; Emile, J.F.; Castaigne, S.; Coiffier, B.; Haioun, C.; Bologna, S.; Fitoussi, O.; et al. Attenuated immunochemotherapy regimen (R-miniCHOP) in elderly patients older than 80 years with diffuse large B-cell lymphoma: A multicentre, single-arm, phase 2 trial. *Lancet. Oncol.* **2011**, *12*, 460–468. [CrossRef]
30. Meguro, A.; Ozaki, K.; Sato, K.; Oh, I.; Fujiwara, S.; Hosonuma, R.; Sasazaki, M.; Kikuchi, Y.; Hirata, Y.; Yamamoto, C.; et al. Rituximab plus 70% cyclophosphamide, doxorubicin, vincristine and prednisone for Japanese patients with diffuse large B-cell lymphoma aged 70 years and older. *Leuk. Lymphoma* **2012**, *53*, 43–49. [CrossRef]
31. Wang, Y.; Ren, X.; Huang, K.; Liang, X.; Pu, L.; Hu, L.; Zhai, Z. Comparison of first-line treatments for elderly patients with diffuse large B-cell lymphoma: A systematic review and network meta-analysis. *Front. Immunol.* **2022**, *13*, 1082293. [CrossRef]
32. Coiffier, B.; Lepage, E.; Briere, J.; Herbrecht, R.; Tilly, H.; Bouabdallah, R.; Morel, P.; Van Den Neste, E.; Salles, G.; Gaulard, P.; et al. CHOP chemotherapy plus rituximab compared with CHOP alone in elderly patients with diffuse large-B-cell lymphoma. *N. Engl. J. Med.* **2002**, *346*, 235–242. [CrossRef] [PubMed]
33. Feugier, P.; Van Hoof, A.; Sebban, C.; Solal-Celigny, P.; Bouabdallah, R.; Fermé, C.; Christian, B.; Lepage, E.; Tilly, H.; Morschhauser, F.; et al. Long-term results of the R-CHOP study in the treatment of elderly patients with diffuse large B-cell lymphoma: A study by the Groupe d'Etude des Lymphomes de l'Adulte. *J. Clin. Oncol. Off. J. Am. Soc. Clin. Oncol.* **2005**, *23*, 4117–4126. [CrossRef]
34. Pfreundschuh, M.; Schubert, J.; Ziepert, M.; Schmits, R.; Mohren, M.; Lengfelder, E.; Reiser, M.; Nickenig, C.; Clemens, M.; Peter, N.; et al. Six versus eight cycles of bi-weekly CHOP-14 with or without rituximab in elderly patients with aggressive CD20+ B-cell lymphomas: A randomised controlled trial (RICOVER-60). *Lancet. Oncol.* **2008**, *9*, 105–116. [CrossRef] [PubMed]
35. Delarue, R.; Tilly, H.; Mounier, N.; Petrella, T.; Salles, G.; Thieblemont, C.; Bologna, S.; Ghesquières, H.; Hacini, M.; Fruchart, C.; et al. Dose-dense rituximab-CHOP compared with standard rituximab-CHOP in elderly patients with diffuse large B-cell lymphoma (the LNH03-6B study): A randomised phase 3 trial. *Lancet. Oncol.* **2013**, *14*, 525–533. [CrossRef] [PubMed]
36. Cunningham, D.; Hawkes, E.A.; Jack, A.; Qian, W.; Smith, P.; Mouncey, P.; Pocock, C.; Ardeshna, K.M.; Radford, J.A.; McMillan, A.; et al. Rituximab plus cyclophosphamide, doxorubicin, vincristine, and prednisolone in patients with newly diagnosed diffuse large B-cell non-Hodgkin lymphoma: A phase 3 comparison of dose intensification with 14-day versus 21-day cycles. *Lancet* **2013**, *381*, 1817–1826. [CrossRef]
37. Kühnl, A.; Cunningham, D.; Counsell, N.; Hawkes, E.A.; Qian, W.; Smith, P.; Chadwick, N.; Lawrie, A.; Mouncey, P.; Jack, A.; et al. Outcome of elderly patients with diffuse large B-cell lymphoma treated with R-CHOP: Results from the UK NCRI R-CHOP14v21 trial with combined analysis of molecular characteristics with the DSHNHL RICOVER-60 trial. *Ann. Oncol. Off. J. Eur. Soc. Med. Oncol.* **2017**, *28*, 1540–1546. [CrossRef] [PubMed]
38. Corazzelli, G.; Frigeri, F.; Arcamone, M.; Lucania, A.; Rosariavilla, M.; Morelli, E.; Amore, A.; Capobianco, G.; Caronna, A.; Becchimanzi, C.; et al. Biweekly rituximab, cyclophosphamide, vincristine, non-pegylated liposome-encapsulated doxorubicin and prednisone (R-COMP-14) in elderly patients with poor-risk diffuse large B-cell lymphoma and moderate to high 'life threat' impact cardiopathy. *Br. J. Haematol.* **2011**, *154*, 579–589. [CrossRef]
39. Merli, F.; Luminari, S.; Rossi, G.; Mammi, C.; Marcheselli, L.; Tucci, A.; Ilariucci, F.; Chiappella, A.; Musso, M.; Di Rocco, A.; et al. Cyclophosphamide, doxorubicin, vincristine, prednisone and rituximab versus epirubicin, cyclophosphamide, vinblastine, prednisone and rituximab for the initial treatment of elderly "fit" patients with diffuse large B-cell lymphoma: Results from the ANZINTER3 trial of the Intergruppo Italiano Linfomi. *Leuk. Lymphoma* **2012**, *53*, 581–588. [CrossRef]

40. Park, S.I.; Grover, N.S.; Olajide, O.; Asch, A.S.; Wall, J.G.; Richards, K.L.; Sobol, A.L.; Deal, A.M.; Ivanova, A.; Foster, M.C.; et al. A phase II trial of bendamustine in combination with rituximab in older patients with previously untreated diffuse large B-cell lymphoma. *Br. J. Haematol.* **2016**, *175*, 281–289. [CrossRef]
41. Fields, P.A.; Townsend, W.; Webb, A.; Counsell, N.; Pocock, C.; Smith, P.; Jack, A.; El-Mehidi, N.; Johnson, P.W.; Radford, J.; et al. De novo treatment of diffuse large B-cell lymphoma with rituximab, cyclophosphamide, vincristine, gemcitabine, and prednisolone in patients with cardiac comorbidity: A United Kingdom National Cancer Research Institute trial. *J. Clin. Oncol. Off. J. Am. Soc. Clin. Oncol.* **2014**, *32*, 282–287. [CrossRef]
42. Shen, Q.D.; Zhu, H.Y.; Wang, L.; Fan, L.; Liang, J.H.; Cao, L.; Wu, W.; Xia, Y.; Li, J.Y.; Xu, W. Gemcitabine-oxaliplatin plus rituximab (R-GemOx) as first-line treatment in elderly patients with diffuse large B-cell lymphoma: A single-arm, open-label, phase 2 trial. *Lancet. Haematol.* **2018**, *5*, e261–e269. [CrossRef]
43. Moccia, A.A.; Schaff, K.; Hoskins, P.; Klasa, R.; Savage, K.J.; Shenkier, T.; Gascoyne, R.D.; Connors, J.M.; Sehn, L.H. R-CHOP with Etoposide Substituted for Doxorubicin (R-CEOP): Excellent Outcome in Diffuse Large B Cell Lymphoma for Patients with a Contraindication to Anthracyclines. *Blood* **2009**, *114*, 408. [CrossRef]
44. Merli, F.; Luminari, S.; Rossi, G.; Mammi, C.; Marcheselli, L.; Ferrari, A.; Spina, M.; Tucci, A.; Stelitano, C.; Capodanno, I.; et al. Outcome of frail elderly patients with diffuse large B-cell lymphoma prospectively identified by Comprehensive Geriatric Assessment: Results from a study of the Fondazione Italiana Linfomi. *Leuk. Lymphoma* **2014**, *55*, 38–43. [CrossRef]
45. Ong, D.M.; Ashby, M.; Grigg, A.; Gard, G.; Ng, Z.Y.; Huang, H.E.; Chong, Y.S.; Cheah, C.Y.; Devitt, B.; Chong, G.; et al. Comprehensive geriatric assessment is useful in an elderly Australian population with diffuse large B-cell lymphoma receiving rituximab-chemotherapy combinations. *Br. J. Haematol.* **2019**, *187*, 73–81. [CrossRef] [PubMed]
46. Spina, M.; Balzarotti, M.; Uziel, L.; Ferreri, A.J.; Fratino, L.; Magagnoli, M.; Talamini, R.; Giacalone, A.; Ravaioli, E.; Chimienti, E.; et al. Modulated chemotherapy according to modified comprehensive geriatric assessment in 100 consecutive elderly patients with diffuse large B-cell lymphoma. *Oncol.* **2012**, *17*, 838–846. [CrossRef]
47. Olivieri, A.; Gini, G.; Bocci, C.; Montanari, M.; Trappolini, S.; Olivieri, J.; Brunori, M.; Catarini, M.; Guiducci, B.; Isidori, A.; et al. Tailored therapy in an unselected population of 91 elderly patients with DLBCL prospectively evaluated using a simplified CGA. *Oncol.* **2012**, *17*, 663–672. [CrossRef]
48. Marchesi, F.; Cenfra, N.; Altomare, L.; Dessanti, M.L.; Mecarocci, S.; Cerchiara, E.; Rago, A.; D'Andrea, M.; Tomarchio, V.; Olimpieri, O.M.; et al. A retrospective study on 73 elderly patients (≥75years) with aggressive B-cell non Hodgkin lymphoma: Clinical significance of treatment intensity and comprehensive geriatric assessment. *J. Geriatr. Oncol.* **2013**, *4*, 242–248. [CrossRef]
49. Vitolo, U.; Chiappella, A.; Franceschetti, S.; Carella, A.M.; Baldi, I.; Inghirami, G.; Spina, M.; Pavone, V.; Ladetto, M.; Liberati, A.M.; et al. Lenalidomide plus R-CHOP21 in elderly patients with untreated diffuse large B-cell lymphoma: Results of the REAL07 open-label, multicentre, phase 2 trial. *Lancet. Oncol.* **2014**, *15*, 730–737. [CrossRef]
50. Thieblemont, C.; Tilly, H.; Gomes da Silva, M.; Casasnovas, R.O.; Fruchart, C.; Morschhauser, F.; Haioun, C.; Lazarovici, J.; Grosicka, A.; Perrot, A.; et al. Lenalidomide Maintenance Compared With Placebo in Responding Elderly Patients With Diffuse Large B-Cell Lymphoma Treated With First-Line Rituximab Plus Cyclophosphamide, Doxorubicin, Vincristine, and Prednisone. *J. Clin. Oncol. Off. J. Am. Soc. Clin. Oncol.* **2017**, *35*, 2473–2481. [CrossRef]
51. Younes, A.; Sehn, L.H.; Johnson, P.; Zinzani, P.L.; Hong, X.; Zhu, J.; Patti, C.; Belada, D.; Samoilova, O.; Suh, C.; et al. Randomized Phase III Trial of Ibrutinib and Rituximab Plus Cyclophosphamide, Doxorubicin, Vincristine, and Prednisone in Non-Germinal Center B-Cell Diffuse Large B-Cell Lymphoma. *J. Clin. Oncol. Off. J. Am. Soc. Clin. Oncol.* **2019**, *37*, 1285–1295. [CrossRef]
52. Ram, R.; Grisariu, S.; Shargian-Alon, L.; Amit, O.; Bar-On, Y.; Stepensky, P.; Yeshurun, M.; Avni, B.; Hagin, D.; Perry, C.; et al. Toxicity and efficacy of chimeric antigen receptor T-cell therapy in patients with diffuse large B-cell lymphoma above the age of 70 years compared to younger patients—A matched control multicenter cohort study. *Haematologica* **2022**, *107*, 1111–1118. [CrossRef]
53. Thieblemont, C.; Phillips, T.; Ghesquieres, H.; Cheah, C.Y.; Clausen, M.R.; Cunningham, D.; Do, Y.R.; Feldman, T.; Gasiorowski, R.; Jurczak, W.; et al. Epcoritamab, a Novel, Subcutaneous CD3xCD20 Bispecific T-Cell-Engaging Antibody, in Relapsed or Refractory Large B-Cell Lymphoma: Dose Expansion in a Phase I/II Trial. *J. Clin. Oncol. Off. J. Am. Soc. Clin. Oncol.* **2023**, *41*, 2238–2247. [CrossRef]
54. Olszewski, A.J.; Avigdor, A.; Babu, S.; Levi, I.; Eradat, H.; Abadi, U.; Holmes, H.; McKinney, M.; Woszczyk, D.; Giannopoulos, K.; et al. Mosunetuzumab Monotherapy Continues to Demonstrate Promising Efficacy and Durable Complete Responses in Elderly/Unfit Patients with Previously Untreated Diffuse Large B-Cell Lymphoma. *Blood* **2022**, *140*, 1778–1780. [CrossRef]
55. Balducci, L.; Beghe, C. The application of the principles of geriatrics to the management of the older person with cancer. *Crit. Rev. Oncol. /Hematol.* **2000**, *35*, 147–154. [CrossRef] [PubMed]
56. Tucci, A.; Ferrari, S.; Bottelli, C.; Borlenghi, E.; Drera, M.; Rossi, G. A comprehensive geriatric assessment is more effective than clinical judgment to identify elderly diffuse large cell lymphoma patients who benefit from aggressive therapy. *Cancer* **2009**, *115*, 4547–4553. [CrossRef] [PubMed]
57. van Spronsen, D.J.; Janssen-Heijnen, M.L.; Lemmens, V.E.; Peters, W.G.; Coebergh, J.W. Independent prognostic effect of co-morbidity in lymphoma patients: Results of the population-based Eindhoven Cancer Registry. *Eur. J. Cancer* **2005**, *41*, 1051–1057. [CrossRef] [PubMed]

58. Janssen-Heijnen, M.L.; van Spronsen, D.J.; Lemmens, V.E.; Houterman, S.; Verheij, K.D.; Coebergh, J.W. A population-based study of severity of comorbidity among patients with non-Hodgkin's lymphoma: Prognostic impact independent of International Prognostic Index. *Br. J. Haematol.* **2005**, *129*, 597–606. [CrossRef] [PubMed]
59. Lee, S.; Fujita, K.; Morishita, T.; Negoro, E.; Oiwa, K.; Tsukasaki, H.; Yamamura, O.; Ueda, T.; Yamauchi, T. Prognostic utility of a geriatric nutritional risk index in combination with a comorbidity index in elderly patients with diffuse large B cell lymphoma. *Br. J. Haematol.* **2021**, *192*, 100–109. [CrossRef] [PubMed]
60. Borg, I.H.; Bendtsen, M.D.; Bøgsted, M.; Madsen, J.; Severinsen, M.T. Incidence of venous thromboembolism in patients with diffuse large B-cell lymphoma. *Leuk. Lymphoma* **2016**, *57*, 2771–2776. [CrossRef] [PubMed]
61. Mareschal, S.; Lanic, H.; Ruminy, P.; Bastard, C.; Tilly, H.; Jardin, F. The proportion of activated B-cell like subtype among de novo diffuse large B-cell lymphoma increases with age. *Haematologica* **2011**, *96*, 1888–1890. [CrossRef] [PubMed]
62. Klapper, W.; Kreuz, M.; Kohler, C.W.; Burkhardt, B.; Szczepanowski, M.; Salaverria, I.; Hummel, M.; Loeffler, M.; Pellissery, S.; Woessmann, W.; et al. Patient age at diagnosis is associated with the molecular characteristics of diffuse large B-cell lymphoma. *Blood* **2012**, *119*, 1882–1887. [CrossRef]
63. Reddy, A.; Zhang, J.; Davis, N.S.; Moffitt, A.B.; Love, C.L.; Waldrop, A.; Leppa, S.; Pasanen, A.; Meriranta, L.; Karjalainen-Lindsberg, M.L.; et al. Genetic and Functional Drivers of Diffuse Large B Cell Lymphoma. *Cell* **2017**, *171*, 481–494.e415. [CrossRef]
64. Li, C.; Li, W.; Xu, G.; You, M.; Wu, W.; Kuang, L. Relationship between the absolute lymphocyte count/absolute monocyte count ratio, soluble interleukin 2 receptor level, serum programmed cell death 1 level, and the prognosis of patients with diffuse large B-cell lymphoma. *Ann. Palliat. Med.* **2021**, *10*, 10938–10945. [CrossRef]
65. Yin, T.; Qi, L.; Zhou, Y.; Kong, F.; Wang, S.; Yu, M.; Li, F. CD5+ diffuse large B-cell lymphoma has heterogeneous clinical features and poor prognosis: A single-center retrospective study in China. *J. Int. Med. Res.* **2022**, *50*, 3000605221110075. [CrossRef]
66. Porrata, L.F.; Ristow, K.; Habermann, T.; Inwards, D.J.; Micallef, I.N.; Markovic, S.N. Predicting survival for diffuse large B-cell lymphoma patients using baseline neutrophil/lymphocyte ratio. *Am. J. Hematol.* **2010**, *85*, 896–899. [CrossRef] [PubMed]
67. Rambaldi, A.; Boschini, C.; Gritti, G.; Delaini, F.; Oldani, E.; Rossi, A.; Barbui, A.M.; Caracciolo, D.; Ladetto, M.; Gueli, A.; et al. The lymphocyte to monocyte ratio improves the IPI-risk definition of diffuse large B-cell lymphoma when rituximab is added to chemotherapy. *Am. J. Hematol.* **2013**, *88*, 1062–1067. [CrossRef]
68. Li, Z.M.; Huang, J.J.; Xia, Y.; Sun, J.; Huang, Y.; Wang, Y.; Zhu, Y.J.; Li, Y.J.; Zhao, W.; Wei, W.X.; et al. Blood lymphocyte-to-monocyte ratio identifies high-risk patients in diffuse large B-cell lymphoma treated with R-CHOP. *PLoS ONE* **2012**, *7*, e41658. [CrossRef] [PubMed]

cancers

MDPI

Review

The Role of Radiotherapy in Octogenarian Cancer Patients

Aneta Lebiedzińska [1,2,*], Ewa Wasilewska-Teśluk [1,2], Agnieszka Sopel [1,2] and Sergiusz Nawrocki [1,2]

[1] Department of Oncology, Collegium Medicum, University of Warmia and Mazury in Olsztyn, Aleja Wojska Polskiego 37, 10-228 Olsztyn, Poland
[2] Department of Radiotherapy, Clinical Hospital of the Ministry of Internal Affairs and Administration with the Warmia-Mazury Oncology Centre, 10-228 Olsztyn, Poland
* Correspondence: aneta.lebiedzinska@uwm.edu.pl; Tel.: +48-89-539-88-60

Simple Summary: The number of cancer patients aged 80 years and older is steadily increasing worldwide, creating new challenges for oncology. This review is based on recent literature and summarizes current knowledge about the role of radiotherapy in elderly patients. Older individuals are often under-represented in clinical trials, resulting in limited data to guide optimal treatment decisions. Nevertheless, radiotherapy remains one of the most effective and well-tolerated cancer treatments, both for curative and palliative purposes. Technological progress, including modern radiotherapy techniques, has improved treatment precision and reduced side effects, allowing the use of shorter and more convenient treatment schedules. This paper emphasizes the importance of individualized treatment planning and comprehensive geriatric assessment to ensure both safety and efficacy. It also highlights the need for further studies and the development of clinical guidelines to optimize radiotherapy for this growing group of elderly cancer patients.

Abstract: The use of radiotherapy in oncology patients aged 80 years and older represents a significant clinical challenge due to the limited availability of prospective data and the under-representation of this age group in clinical trials. Most existing evidence originates from retrospective analyses of small patient cohorts. Radiotherapy remains a cornerstone of cancer treatment, providing both curative and palliative benefits. Technological advances, including intensity-modulated radiotherapy (IMRT) and stereotactic body radiotherapy (SBRT), have significantly improved treatment precision, reduced toxicity, and enabled the adoption of hypofractionated regimens. These shortened treatment schedules are particularly advantageous for older patients, reducing the burden of prolonged therapy while maintaining therapeutic efficacy. Comprehensive Geriatric Assessment (CGA) plays a crucial role in optimizing treatment decisions for octogenarian patients by addressing their clinical, functional, and psychosocial needs. However, the routine use of CGA remains limited due to logistical and time constraints. Despite these challenges, current evidence suggests that radiotherapy is generally well tolerated in this population, with acceptable toxicity profiles even among frail patients. As the global population of individuals aged 80 years and older continues to increase, the development of specific clinical guidelines tailored to this demographic has become essential. There is an urgent need for prospective studies providing robust evidence regarding the efficacy, safety, and tolerability of radiotherapy in older adults. This review aims to summarize the current state of knowledge on the role of radiotherapy in patients aged 80 years and older and to highlight the need for evidence-based, individualized oncologic care for this growing patient population.

Keywords: radiotherapy; octogenarians; older adults; overall survival; toxicity; cancer

 https://doi.org/10.3390/cancers17233758

1. Introduction

The population of people over 80, called octogenarians, increases in size in the demographic structure of numerous societies worldwide [1].

According to the projections of the Statistics Poland, the number of people in Poland aged 80 and older will systematically increase. In 2020, the population of people in this age group was about 1.7 million, which constituted 4.4% of the total population. By 2050, this number is expected to increase to about 3.5 million, which will constitute 10.4% of the entire population. This means that in 2050, every tenth inhabitant of Poland will be 80 or older. The latest Statistics Poland data on life expectancy in 2023 in Poland showed that the average life expectancy was increasing. It was 74.7 years in men and 82 in women [2].

According to the International Agency for Research on Cancer, globally, the number of new cancer cases could increase by 77% by 2050, reaching 35 million annually [3].

Most tumors are diagnosed in people over 65 years of age [4].

The projections indicate a significantly aging population, an increase in the incidence of neoplastic disease, which will significantly impact the health care system and other socio-economic aspects.

The specificity of oncological treatment in the group of geriatric patients requires special attention. Comorbidities, reduced physiological reserve, general condition and a potentially higher risk of toxicity of various oncological treatment methods currently pose a great challenge related to the selection of an optimal therapy in such patients.

Radiotherapy, along with surgery and systemic treatment, is one of the primary treatment modalities for tumors. This method uses ionizing radiation to destroy tumor cells. The biological effect of ionizing radiation is DNA damage that may lead to cell death. Such effects are associated with cellular radiosensitivity and occur both in tumor cells and in normal tissue cells. Tumor cells, due to their high ability to divide and impaired repair mechanisms, are more sensitive to radiation than healthy cells. Radiotherapy is one of the key elements of oncological therapy, used both in radical and palliative treatment. As technology advances and radiotherapy becomes more precise, this treatment modality is safe, even for patients at advanced age.

Being a non-invasive local treatment method and with great potential for therapy individualization, radiotherapy may be a particularly attractive treatment option for patients. However, the question of the effectiveness, tolerability and safety of irradiation treatment in older adults remains important as they are often excluded or constitute a low percentage of patients participating in randomized clinical trials.

The aim of the study was to provide an up-to-date overview of the use of radiotherapy in geriatric patients with neoplastic diseases, with particular emphasis on patients over 80 years of age.

2. Materials and Methods

The review article was prepared based on an analysis of publications retrieved from available scientific databases, including PubMed, Scopus, and Web of Science, with particular emphasis on studies published over the past 20 years. The literature review included clinical and experimental studies addressing the role, efficacy, and tolerability of radiotherapy in older adults. Only peer-reviewed articles written in English and relevant to the topic were included. The collected data were critically analyzed and synthesized to present the current state of knowledge, highlight technological advances, and identify gaps requiring further research. The literature review was conducted in accordance with the PRISMA

2020 guidelines [5], as illustrated in Figure 1. The following keywords were used during the record search: geriatric radiotherapy, elderly patients, cancer. Inclusion criteria was original research articles on radiotherapy and oncology.

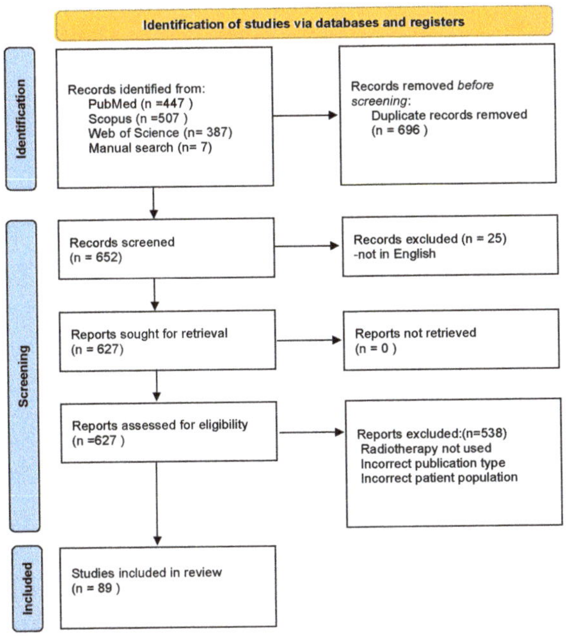

Figure 1. PRISMA 2020 search strategy.

Exclusion criteria was case reports, letters to the editor, commentaries. This study focuses on cancers of the breast, lung, prostate, colorectal cancer, head and neck cancers, and glioblastoma with particular consideration of metastases to the central nervous system.

3. Discussion

3.1. Breast Cancer

Patients who have breast cancer after 80 years of age usually experience a less aggressive course of the disease, but they are clinically diagnosed at more advanced stages of the disease than younger women, which is related to the lack of screening in this age group. Histologically, luminal cancers are more common [6,7]. Their incidence increases with age, while the percentage of basal-like breast cancer in older women decreases [8]. Over 80% of breast cancer cases occurring in women between 80 and 84 express the estrogen receptor (ER), compared to 60% in younger patients [9]. The luminal A subtype is often associated with a better prognosis [10]. It is characterized by slower progression and an indolent course. The presence of hormone receptors, i.e., the ER and PR (progesterone receptor) is not only an indicator of a better prognosis, but it also indicates a good response to hormone therapy [11]. Bastiaannet et al. studied a group of >120,000 women and showed that the percentage of surgery in early breast cancer in the group below 80 years of age was >93% and in the group of octogenarians, the average was 74%. The following age groups receive RT: 75–79 (86.3%), 80–84 (70.8%), 85–89 (35.9%), 90+ (14.6%) [12]. In 2020, Bertolo et al. published the results of an analysis of 97 radically treated women aged 80 and older. The control group consisted of patients aged 65–75 years. They observed that the use of radiotherapy was reduced in the group over 80. In the octogenarian group, 51.5% of patients underwent breast-conserving surgery (BCS) and 33% underwent radiotherapy [7]. In 2024, Fonseca et al. published a meta-analysis including almost 40,000 patients over 70 with breast cancer. The median age was 77.6 years. In the whole group of patients, 44.77% had clinical stage II of breast cancer (CS II) and 29.65% had CS III. BCS was performed in 32.92% and radiotherapy was used in 40.3% of the patients. The authors analyzed 17 studies published in the years 2013–2023. The analysis yielded only 3 studies in which the median age was over 80 years with the total of only 172 women. This shows how little knowledge is currently available regarding this subpopulation. The overwhelming majority of the patients had CS II or CS III cancers, and radiotherapy was implemented in 3 to 25% of the groups. No data on the use of geriatric assessment were available in any of the studies included in the meta-analysis [13].

It is currently accepted that in radical treatment, the standard of management should not deviate from generally accepted principles of breast cancer treatment. According to the SIOG (International Society of Geriatric Oncology) guidelines on the use of radiotherapy for patients >70 years of age as of 2014, candidates for postoperative WBRT (whole-breast radiotherapy) after BCS for invasive cancer and high-risk DCIS (ductal carcinoma in situ) should be in a good general condition (fit). Patients aged 50 and older who do not require lymph node irradiation, are candidates for shortened treatment regimens. Post-mastectomy irradiation should be considered in older patients with pT3-4 tumors or with ≥4 tumor-positive axillary nodes [14]. Postoperative whole-breast radiotherapy is the standard of care for all able-bodied patients following breast-conserving surgery. A combination of BCS and WBRT was associated with a two-fold reduction in recurrence even in older patients, although the absolute 10-year reduction in the risk of locoregional or distant recurrence was found to be lower in women ≥70 years of age and was 8.8% compared to younger women (17.7%) [15]. In older patients, shorter treatment courses using higher fractional doses [hypofractionation (HF)] constitute an alternative to WBRT. Studies evaluating different HF-RT regimens after BCS revealed that HF regimens offered similar local control rates, and comparable toxicity [16,17]. Due to the reduced treatment time, shortened irradiation regimens are an attractive form of therapy, especially for older patients, for whom the distance between the radiotherapy center and their place of residence often constitutes an obstacle in the implementation of treatment. Currently, shortened dose fractionation regimens are recommended both for older and younger patients, which stays in line with the results of the FAST-Forward study. However, patients older than 80 years constituted only 3% of the group [18].

When planning radiotherapy, special emphasis should be placed on the need for modern 3D and 4D planning methods with the use of cardiac protective treatment techniques, deep inspiration breath hold technique, which facilitates limiting the doses in the heart and is an important factor in the group of older patients at a higher risk of ischemic heart disease. In case of post-mastectomy radiotherapy, data are insufficient to suggest that survival gains might include women >70 years of age [19]. A 2014 meta-analysis by the Early Breast Cancer Trialists' Collaborative Group (EBCTCG) revealed that post-mastectomy radiotherapy reduced 20-year breast cancer mortality by 7.9% in patients with three or fewer positive nodes and by 9.3% in patients with four or more positive nodes [20]. The role of RT in patients with three or fewer positive lymph nodes remains a topic of debate [21].

Accelerated partial breast irradiation (APBI) combines the administration of a higher fractional dose, short treatment duration, and a small target volume limited to the tumor bed. IORT (intraoperative radiotherapy with electrons) is an attractive option in older women because it may be administered as a single dose. Two randomized trials on APBI were published. The TARGIT-A study included 3451 patients with the minimum follow-up of 4 years for 1010 patients and 5 years for 611 patients. The absolute difference in local recurrence at 5 years was statistically significant and was 2% higher in the IORT group (3.3%) compared to the WBRT group (1.3%). Grade 3 toxicity was lower in IORT subjects (0.5% vs. 2.1%). Patients older than 74 accounted for about 8% of the participant [21–23]. The ELIOT study included 1305 patients up to 75 years of age with T1–T2 breast cancer (max. up to 2.5 cm) pretreated with BCS. They were randomly assigned to groups receiving postoperative whole-breast irradiation or a single dose (21 Gy) of IORT. The local recurrence rate was 4.4% in the IORT group and 0.4% in the WBRT group with the median follow-up of 5.8 years [24]. The EORTC study compared WBRT with or without an additional radiation dose per tumor bed. The reduction in the risk of local recurrence after the addition of radiation boost was not statistically significant in patients aged 60 years and older. Therefore, boost was recommended in this age group only for patients at a higher risk of relapse [25]. In patients older than 70 with a tumor <2 cm, positive hormone receptors, after BCS, supplementary radiotherapy may be discontinued if a minimum of 5 years of hormone therapy is planned [26]. A meta-analysis conducted by the EBCTCG showed that post-BCS RT reduced the recurrence rate, but the absolute benefit in the older, lower-risk group receiving endocrine therapy was limited [15,20]. The CALGB 9343 study showed that, in women over 70 years of age, the local recurrence rate after 12 years was 10% without radiotherapy compared to 2% with radiotherapy. However, it did not affect the overall survival (OS) [27].

According to current guidelines of the National Comprehensive Cancer Network (NCCN, version 6.2024), it is recommended to consider the omission of radiotherapy after BCS if adjuvant endocrine therapy is planned and patients meet the following criteria: age $\geq$ 70 years, HR+, HER2-negative, cN0, pT1 and age $\geq$65 years, HR+, HER2-negative, pN0, tumor $\leq$ 3 cm in diameter [28].

The preliminary results of a phase III EUROPE study were published in 2025. The study was conducted in a group of patients >70 years of age undergoing BCS for early luminal A breast cancer. The authors compared endocrine therapy and RT in the context of the quality of life after 2 years of follow-up. Patients after RT reported a better quality of life compared to patients undergoing endocrine therapy. Adverse reactions were reported more frequently after endocrine therapy (85% vs. 67%). Endocrine therapy was discontinued in 12% of the patients due to adverse reactions. The study presented preliminary data. The authors suggested that RT might constitute an alternative to several years of endocrine therapy in a certain group of patients. Patients over 80 years of age accounted for 26–28% of the study group [29].

In 2021, joint recommendations were published by two scientific societies, the European Society of Breast Cancer Specialists (EUSOMA) and the SIOG for patients >70 years of age. Whole-breast radiotherapy after breast-conserving surgery remains the standard of care for most older patients and reduces the risk of disease recurrence by half. The benefit of radiotherapy in the group of elderly patients with positive hormone receptors and low-grade cancer is moderate.

WBRT remains the standard of care for older post-BCS patients. The omission of radiotherapy in low-risk patients may be safe and justified (level 1 recommendation). In patients over 60 years of age, it is recommended to use an additional dose of radiation (boost) only in the group at a higher risk of relapse (level 1).

Hypofractionated regimens are recommended (40 Gy in 15 fractions over 3 weeks, or 42.5 Gy in 16 fractions over 3.5 weeks, or 26 Gy in 5 fractions over 1 week) (level 4). Partial breast irradiation (PBI) is recommended in women $\geq$50 years of age with grade 1–2 tumors, pN0, HER2-negative, hormone receptors positive, $\leq$30 mm in diameter, and radial margins

≥1 mm (level 4). The role of post-mastectomy RT in patients with one to three positive lymph nodes remains controversial [30].

The use of radiotherapy in the old patient with breast cancer are presented in Table 1.

Table 1. Summary of radiotherapy in breast cancer patients.

References	Radiotherapy Approach	Outcomes/Tolerability	Guidelines
Fonseca et al. [13]	Meta-analysis of RT in >70 yrs	In >80 yrs RT used in only 3–25%; no geriatric assessment	Need for improved evaluation of older adults
Murray Brunt et al. [18]	Post-BCS RT; hypofractionation	Comparable control and toxicity; ≥80 yrs = 3% of cohort	Recommended HF-RT 26 Gy/5 fractions
McGale et al. [20]	Post-mastectomy RT (PMRT)	Limited data in >70; 20-year mortality reduction 9.3% with ≥4 nodes	Standard for ≥4 positive nodes
Vaidya et al. [22,23] Veronesi et al. [24]	Partial RT (APBI, IORT) vs. WBRT	Higher recurrence with IORT (3.3% vs. 1.3%), lower toxicity	Boost recommended only for high-risk ≥60 yrs
Huges et al. [26,27]	RT omission after BCS in >70 yrs	12-year recurrence 10% without RT vs. 2% with RT; no OS difference	RT may be omitted in ER+ with endocrine therapy
Rashmi et al. [28]	Criteria for RT omission after BCS	RT omission possible: ≥70 yrs, HR+, HER2−, pT1, cN0	NCCN v6.2024
Meattini et al. [29]	RT vs. endocrine therapy	Better QoL after RT; ≥80 yrs = 26–28%	RT as alternative to long-term endocrine therapy
Biganzoli et al. [30]	RT after BCS; HF and PBI	RT halves recurrence risk; may be omitted in low-risk	EUSOMA–SIOG 2021

3.2. Lung Cancer

Lung cancer is the leading cause of cancer death in the world [31]. Surgical treatment remains the gold standard in the treatment of NSCLC stages I and II. Huang et al. [32] conducted a study in the Chinese population including a group of 7861 patients older than 80. The authors showed that lobectomy could be used in patients aged 80–85 years if the general condition of the patient allowed. Li et al. carried out a study in a group of patients >80 with the tumor size up to 4 cm and pleural infiltration. They reported that the results of wedge resection were comparable to those following anatomical resection. Multivariate analysis showed no significant differences in cancer-specific survival (CSS) or overall survival between both surgical groups [33]. Radiotherapy is widely used in patients with lung cancer in both non-small cell lung cancer (NSCLC) and small cell lung cancer (SCLC). It may be successfully implemented in patients over 80 years of age. The study conducted in a group of octogenarians with stage IA non-small cell lung cancer revealed that surgery with lymph node dissection provided better OS outcomes than radiotherapy. The 1-, 3- and 5-year OS rates were 90.0%, 76.9%, 59.9% for surgery and 86.0%, 54.3%, 28.0% in the radiotherapy group, respectively. CSS survival was superior in the surgical group compared with the radiotherapy group. However, in the discussion section, the authors emphasized a possible impact of the negative selection in case of the group qualified for RT. Factors such as perioperative mortality, general condition or comorbidities were not analyzed, and they could have a significant impact on the selection of treatment modality and the results obtained [34]. Robinson et al. compared lobe resection (lobectomy or pneumonectomy) with stereotactic radiotherapy (SBRT) in stage I NSCLC patients. The overall survival (OS, 63.5% vs. 29.6%) was greater for lobe resection, although specific survival rates were comparable (CSS, 81.3% vs. 75.3%). Elderly patients, at the median age of 76 years and more internally burdened patients were eligible for SBRT, while in case of surgery, the median age was 66. Total postoperative mortality was 1.9%, including the

30-day mortality of 1.5% [35]. High postoperative mortality was also found in the study by Stokes et al. in patients >80 years of age: 30 days: 3.03%; 90 days: 3.67%. Differences in the 30- and 90-day post-treatment mortality between surgery and SBRT increased depending on age, with the largest differences in favor of SBRT being observed in patients over 70 years of age [36]. An attempt to conduct a randomized SABRTooth trial in patients with stage I NSCLC comparing surgery in patients at an increased risk of complications and SBRT was discontinued due to the lack of recruitment. The median age was >75 years in the group. A significant proportion of patients randomly assigned to the surgical group refused the procedure and chose SBRT [37].

Stereotactic radiotherapy is an effective treatment modality in patients over 80 with early-stage non-small cell lung cancer. The most benefits were noted in patients with KPS (Karnofsky Performance status) ≥70 [38]. Those observations were confirmed by a retrospective analysis of patients aged ≥80 diagnosed with early-stage non-small cell lung cancer (T1-T2b) treated with SBRT. The study evaluated treatment effectiveness by analyzing indicators such as local recurrence-free survival (LRFS), regional recurrence-free survival (RRFS), progression-free survival (PFS), and overall survival (OS). The average age in the group was 85 years. The three-year survival rates were: OS—65.3%, PFS—58%, RRFS—73.9% and LRFS—85.3%. Multivariate analysis showed that tumor size, general condition, histological type, and pre-treatment C-reactive protein (CRP) value had a significant impact on OS results [39].

Several retrospective subgroup analyses of randomized trials evaluated the effects of concurrent radiochemotherapy (CRT) in elderly patients compared to younger patients, yielding inconsistent results. Subgroup analyses of several phase I-III studies conducted by the Radiation Therapy Oncology Group (RTOG) on radiotherapy alone, sequential CRT, and concurrent CRT showed that concurrent CRT did not improve outcomes and was associated with greater toxicity in patients >70 years of age [40,41]. A total of 12,641 patients with CS III were analyzed. Radiotherapy alone compared to CRT was associated with poorer OS. Age >70 years was a negative prognostic factor. The obtained results may have been influenced by the lack of comprehensive geriatric assessment prior to qualification for treatment.

In elderly patients with advanced CS III disease, radiotherapy as monotherapy is often considered as a radical treatment. Low toxicity and long-lasting local effects, including good symptom control, mean that it may be successfully used in older patients. Pergolizzi et al. conducted a study in a group of 40 patients with CS IIIA and the median age of 77 years (75–83). They used RT as monotherapy at a median dose of 60 Gy (range 54–64 Gy), 2.0 Gy per fraction. In the study, 3-year OS was achieved at the level of 18%. Mild esophagitis was observed in 70%. Two patients experienced clinical radiation pneumonia [42]. Geinitz et al. observed reduced esophageal tolerability in older patients treated with chest irradiation [43]. Lonardi et al. evaluated the total dose of 50 Gy (1.8–2.0 Gy per fraction) in a similar group of patients with CS IIIA/B aged 75–85. A 2-year OS was reached at the level of 10%. However, it should be emphasized that the applied total dose of 50 Gy was suboptimal [44].

Carbon ion radiotherapy (CIRT) is effective and safe for octogenarians with locally advanced non-small cell lung cancer. It is an advanced form of hadron therapy using high-energy carbon ions, offering higher biological effectiveness than photons and protons and therefore providing an effective treatment option for radioresistant and hypoxic tumors. However, the availability of this method is very low. Hayashi et al. examined 32 patients over 80 years of age who were treated with carbon ion radiotherapy only. Patients in CS IIA, IIB, IIIA and IIIB were included in the study. The CIRT dose was 72.0 Gy and the median follow-up was 33.1 months. All patients completed CIRT therapy. No Grade ≥4 toxicity was observed. The rate of 2-year local control (LC) was 83.5%, progression-free survival was 46.7% and the overall survival was 68.0% [45]. (Table 2).

A meta-analysis comparing proton therapy (PT) and photon therapy showed that the use of proton therapy at the early stage of NSCLC remained controversial and the evidence was insufficient to determine its superiority over photon therapy. As regards the effectiveness, no significant differences in 1-year OS, 3-year OS, and 3-year PFS were determined between PT and RT. In the case of toxicity, no significant difference was observed in treatment-related adverse events and radiation pneumonia [46].

In limited disease (LD) small cell lung cancer, the best treatment results are obtained with concurrent radiochemotherapy. However, patients >70 are rarely eligible for clinical trials with this treatment. A retrospective assessment of the therapeutic effectiveness and safety of CRT in elderly patients (≥75 years of age) with LD small cell lung cancer was published in 2024 by Ayako Shiono et al. They showed that no significant differences in PFS or OS occurred between the concurrent and sequential CRT groups. Concurrent treatment is more difficult to perform and more toxic. Sequential CRT may be considered as the treatment of choice for such patients [47]. The CONVERT study established hyperfractionated irradiation at 45 Gy/21 days with platinum-based chemotherapy as the standard of care. Patients over 80 years of age experienced greater toxicity (Grade ≥3). The number of patients was low, which makes it difficult to draw final conclusions. Considering that probably the healthiest group of octogenarians was chosen, the need for caution in offering CRT in this age group was suggested [48].

Prophylactic cranial irradiation (PCI) was found not to improve the 2-year OS and should not be used routinely in a group of patients >70 and lung tumor size >5 cm [49].

Table 2. Summary of radiotherapy in lung cancer patients.

Reference	Radiotherapy Approach	Outcomes/Tolerability	Guidelines/Authors' Comments
Bei et al. [39]	SBRT (T1–T2b) in ≥80 yrs	3-yr: OS 65.3%, PFS 58%, RRFS 73.9%, LRFS 85.3%	SBRT effective; incorporate geriatric assessment and biomarkers
Pergolizzi et al. [42]	RT monotherapy (median 60 Gy, 2.0 Gy/fx)—stage IIIA, median age 77	3-yr OS 18%; mild esophagitis 70%;	Definitive RT monotherapy is a radical option for selected patients
Lonardi et al. [44]	RT 50 Gy (1.8–2.0 Gy/fx)—stage IIIA/B (75–85 yrs)	2-yr OS 10%; total dose considered suboptimal	Consider higher/definitive doses in fit patients
Hayashi et al. [45]	CIRT (carbon ions) for locally advanced NSCLC in >80 yrs	All completed therapy; no ≥G4 toxicity; 2-yr LC 83.5%, PFS 46.7%, OS 68%	CIRT safe and effective but with very limited availability
He et al. [46]	Proton therapy vs. photon RT in early-stage NSCLC	No significant differences in 1- and 3-yr OS or 3-yr PFS; similar toxicity	Evidence insufficient to claim superiority of proton therapy in early-stage disease
Shiono et al. [47]	LD-SCLC: concurrent vs. sequential CRT in ≥75 yrs	No PFS/OS differences; concurrent more toxic	Offer concurrent CRT in fit octogenarians
Christodoulou et al. [48]	LD-SCLC: standard hyperfractionation 45 Gy/21 days + platinum chemo	In >80 yrs higher ≥G3 toxicity; small sample	PCI should not be routine in this subgroup
Kim et al. [49]	PCI in >70 yrs with tumor >5 cm	No 2-yr OS improvement; not recommended routinely	

3.3. Prostate Cancer

In 2040, the estimated incidence of prostate cancer (PC) in the world will be 2.43 million new cases. The number of patients over the age of 80 will double and reach approximately 0.5 million new cases [1]. Patients whose life expectancy is >10 years should be eligible for radical prostatectomy, so the treatment modality is not a preferred one in the octogenarian group. Radiotherapy occupies an important role in this age group. (Table 3).

In low-risk patients with the expected survival of <10 years, the "watch and wait" or active surveillance strategy should be considered [50]. Patients in higher-risk groups with the life expectancy <10 years should receive ADT (Androgen Deprivation Therapy) to alleviate disease symptoms [50]. Geriatric assessment facilitates appropriate qualification for the treatment of older adults with prostate cancer. A better understanding of the role of active surveillance for less aggressive disease also contributes to the individualization of care [51]. The evaluation of the benefits of the applied management strategy, active or conservative treatment and the probability of death due to any cause within 10 and 15 years may be estimated using the PREDICT Prostate tool. An 80-year-old patient with comorbidities has about a 15% chance of surviving 10 years regardless of cancer. The respective percentage in an 85-year-old patient is about 4% [52]. Comorbidities in patients >75 should be a relative contraindication to aggressive treatment in low-risk PC [53]. Nguyen et al. analyzed the oncological results of a small, multicenter cohort of 65 elderly patients at risk (>80 years) with comorbidities requiring treatment, treated with 3D radiation (45 Gy to the pelvis; and 69.5 Gy to the prostate). The authors observed the 5-year OS rate of 77% [54]. Okonogi et al. compared the use of IMRT (Intensity-Modulated Radiation Therapy) at a dose of 78 Gy (+ADT) for the median duration of 17 months in 23 patients >80 years compared to 171 younger patients in the intermediate- or high-risk group. The 3-year OS of 92% was achieved compared to 99.4% in the group <80. However, the small size of the groups did not allow binding conclusions to be drawn [55]. In 2023, Le Tuo el al. published the results of their research in a group of 107 patients >80. In the study group, 72.9% of patients had high-risk cancer, and 27.1% had intermediate-risk prostate cancer. The median follow-up was 97 months. The median dose was 78 Gy. Almost the entire group, i.e., 97.2% of patients, received androgen deprivation therapy. The 5-year OS was 91.4% and 10-year OS was 67.2%. Selected patients over 80 years of age with localized prostate cancer were confirmed to benefit from radiotherapy in combination with ADT. The rate of gastrointestinal (GI) and genitourinary (GU) toxicity was acceptable [56].

IMRT and advanced variant, VMAT (Volumetric Modulated Arc Therapy), in which beam intensity modulation occurs simultaneously with the rotation of the machine around the patient, are commonly used in the treatment of prostate cancer, as they are associated with a lower risk of Grade 3 rectal complications compared to 3D EBRT (external beam radiotherapy) and allow for a reduction in exposure time. These techniques are well suited for hypofractionation.

Hypofractionation with the 5-week 62 Gy regimen is equivalent to the conventional fractionation regimen (80 Gy for 8 weeks) in terms of acute and late toxicity. In a study including 168 individuals, the patients were randomly assigned to receive hypofractionated radiotherapy (62 Gy in 20 fractions over 5 weeks, 4 fractions per week) versus conventional fractionated radiotherapy (80 Gy in 40 fractions over 8 weeks) using the conformal technique for the prostate and seminal vesicles. No differences were observed as regards the frequency or severity of genitourinary toxicity and late gastrointestinal toxicity (GI) between both treatment regimens [57].

Hypofractionation is increasingly used in the treatment of PC, which is important in this group of patients due to the shortening of therapy duration [58]. (Table 3). In the phase III of HYPO-RT-PC study, acute toxicity was shown to be higher with ultrahypofractionation compared to conventional fractionation. The analysis of the quality of life reported by patients showed that ultrahypofractionation was tolerated as well as conventional fractionation. The dosage regimen of 78.0 Gy in 39 fractions, 5 days per week for 8 weeks was compared to ultrahypofractionation (42.7 Gy in 7 fractions, 3 days per week for 2.5 weeks). However, patients >75 were not eligible for the study [59]. A British phase III CHHIP study recruited 3216 men with stage T1b-T3a disease who were randomly assigned to receive 74 Gy in 37 fractions, 57 Gy in 19 fractions, or 60 Gy in 30 fractions (moderately hypofractionated). After 5 years of observation, it was shown that the 60 Gy regimen was not inferior to the 74 Gy regimen and was therefore recommended for use in clinical practice. The study included patients >80 years of age, but the median age of the whole group was 69 years. The dose of 60 Gy was the preferred regimen for the >69 age group. The assessment of late toxicity at 10 years confirmed no differences in three study arms [60].

Brachytherapy (BRT) is effective and safe treatment for men with early localized prostate cancer. Low Dose-Rate Brachytherapy (LDR) has high prostate cancer disease control but worse impact on urinary symptoms. High Dose-Rate Brachytherapy (HDR) provides comparable disease control with less urinary toxicity [61] The role of BRT in old adult patients with low-risk PC and the life expectancy below 10 years is controversial. Li et al. investigated acute toxicities, especially those requiring admission to the emergency department within 30 days following BRT. Age > 75 years was found to be an independent adverse risk factor for acute toxicity [62]. Age > 80 years in BRT patients was found to be an independent risk factor for late genitourinary toxicity ($G \geq 2$) but the group of >80 consisted of only 35 patients out of a total of 1492 participants [63].

Table 3. Prostate Cancer—Radiotherapy in Old Adults.

Reference	Radiotherapy Approach	Outcomes/Tolerability	Guidelines/Authors' Comments
Nguyen et al. [54]	3D-RT: pelvis 45 Gy + prostate 69.5 Gy in >80 with comorbidities	5-year OS 77%.	RT is feasible for selected octogenarians
Okonogi et al. [55]	IMRT 78 Gy + ADT; >80 vs. younger in intermediate/high-risk	3-year OS 92% (>80) vs. 99.4% (<80); small sample limits conclusions	IMRT + ADT feasible in old adults; larger studies needed
Le Tuo et al. [56]	RT (median 78 Gy) + ADT in >80; 72.9% high-risk; 27.1% intermediate-risk	5-year OS 91.4%, 10-year OS 67.2%; acceptable GI/GU toxicity; 97.2% received ADT	Selected >80 with localized PC benefit from RT + ADT
Arcangeli et al. [57]	Hypofractionation 62 Gy/20 fx vs. conventional 80 Gy/40 fx (3D conformal)	No differences in GU frequency/severity or late GI toxicity	HF offers shorter treatment with comparable toxicity—valuable in older adults
Fransson et al. [59]	Ultra-hypofractionation 42.7 Gy/7 fx vs. conventional 78 Gy/39 fx.	Higher acute toxicity with ultra-HF; QoL similar; >75 yrs not eligible	Use caution extrapolating to >75; evidence in the oldest is limited
Syndicus et al. [61]	74 Gy/37 fx vs. 60 Gy/30 fx vs. 57 Gy/19 fx (moderate HF)	60 Gy non-inferior to 74 Gy; no late-toxicity differences at 10 yrs	60 Gy/30 fx recommended in practice, suitable for well-selected older adults

3.4. Colorectal Cancer

In octogenarians, colorectal cancers occur more commonly on the right side. They secrete the CEA marker, cT3/T4 tumors are more common, but they less commonly metastasize to the lymph nodes [64].

Patients >80 are more likely to undergo life-saving surgery. They have lower survival rates and experience higher treatment toxicity [65]. A multivariate analysis of the Japanese population demonstrated that age over 80 was an unfavorable prognostic factor for the overall survival [64]. Similar observations were described for the population of Israel [66].

Chen et al. conducted a meta-analysis of 21 studies including a total of 13,790 patients with colorectal cancer qualified for surgery at the age of 80 and older. The authors observed a high incidence of general postoperative complications, a high incidence of postoperative internal complications, high in-hospital mortality and lower survival rates. Hospital mortality in patients aged 80 was 4-fold higher than in patients aged <80. Subgroup analysis revealed that bowel obstruction, respiratory failure, cardiac events, vascular and neurological complications occurred more frequently in patients aged 80 [67]. The EURECCA study showed a significant variation in the 5-year relative survival between different European countries in patients >80 with rectal cancer. The study showed differences in qualification for preoperative radiotherapy in patients with stages I–III. The percentage of preoperative radiotherapy in CS I-III patients ranged from 7.9% to 28.9% [68].

Qualification for radiochemotherapy of rectal cancer should be based on the use of geriatric scales. A study by Pasetto et al. was conducted in a group of 36 patients >70 (70–82) with CS II and III qualified for preoperative radiochemotherapy. They were assessed with the Charlston scale (from 0–2 points). The patients received 3D radiation at a total dose of 50.4 Gy (45 Gy/25 fractions over 5 weeks to the pelvis, followed by 5.4 Gy/3 fractions as tumor boost) with 5FU chemotherapy, which was discontinued in 13 patients (36%) due to toxicity. Surgery was performed in 32 individuals after 6 weeks. The median PFS was not achieved during the observation of 37 months [69]. (Table 4).

In the study by Margalit et al., 36 patients were enrolled at the median age of 79.0 years (range 75–87 years). Mild or no comorbidities were noted in 53%, and moderate or severe comorbidities were noted in 47% of the patients. Overall, 58% of patients were treated with preoperative CRT, while 33% of patients underwent postoperative CRT. Although 92% of the patients received the planned dose of radiotherapy, 25% required a break in RT treatment and 11% were hospitalized. Dose reduction, treatment interruption, or the discontinuation of chemotherapy were necessary in 33% of cases. A total of 39% of patients completed ≥4 months of adjuvant chemotherapy and 17% completed treatment as planned. The majority of older adults patients with rectal cancer required early termination of treatment, discontinuation, or cytostatic dose reduction. These data suggest that caution is necessary with further intensification of combination therapy for rectal cancer in older adults patients who require the aggressive treatment of comorbidities. Preoperative treatment was better tolerated than the postoperative one [70]. For older patients who are not eligible for chemotherapy, short radiotherapy with deferred surgery is beneficial for unresectable or borderline resectable tumors at diagnosis. In patients with a complete response after short radiotherapy, the "watch and wait" option is possible, especially important in older and frail patients [71,72]. The 5 × 5 Gy regimen with deferred surgery may be routinely used to treat older patients who are not eligible for chemotherapy for both unresectable and early-stage tumors prior to planned resection [73]. No differences in local effectiveness were observed between the 5 × 5 Gy regimen with consolidation chemotherapy and long-term chemoradiotherapy. Nevertheless, improvement in overall survival and lower acute toxicity levels were in favor of the 5 × 5 Gy regimen with consolidation chemotherapy [74]. Long-term results of the 8-year follow-up indicated the equivalence of both methods of treatment [75].

Table 4. Rectal Cancer—Radiotherapy & Outcomes in Older Adults.

Reference	Radiotherapy Approach	Outcomes/Tolerability	Guidelines/Authors' Comments
Pasetto et al. [69]	Preop CRT: 3D RT 50.4 Gy (45 Gy/25 fx + 5.4 Gy/3 fx boost) + 5-FU	In >70 (70–82): chemo stopped in 36%; surgery after 6 weeks in 32/36; median PFS not reached at 37-month follow-up	Use geriatric scales (Charlson 0–2) for selection
Margalit et al. [70]	Pre- vs. postoperative CRT in old adults	92% received planned RT dose; 25% required a break, 11% hospitalized; 33% needed dose-mod/cessation of chemo; only 17% completed as planned. Preop better tolerated than postop	Avoid intensification without aggressive comorbidity management; prefer preop CRT when feasible
Socha et al. [71] Beets et al. [72]	Short-course RT 5 × 5 Gy with deferred surgery; "watch & wait" after complete response	Beneficial for unresectable/borderline-resectable and frail/chemo-ineligible; W&W feasible after CR—important in frail older adults	Consider 5 × 5 Gy + delay as organ-sparing strategy in older chemo-ineligible patients
Bujko et al. [73]	5 × 5 Gy with delay surgery also for early-stage cases prior to planned resection when chemo-ineligible	May be used routinely in this population	Standard option for older chemo-ineligible in unresectable and early-stage pre-resection settings

3.5. Head and Neck Cancer

The basic treatment modalities in patients with squamous cell carcinoma of the head and neck region include surgery, radiotherapy and radiochemotherapy. Qualifying patients for specific treatment options, a comprehensive assessment of overall condition is essential. Patients with head and neck cancers, regardless of age, are often cachectic and frail due to difficulties with oral intake or lifestyle-related factors.

Retrospective analysis of 260 elderly patients showed the following data concerning patients divided into age groups. Patients >80 accounted for 26% (61 individuals). The patients were qualified for surgery, RT or CRT. Patients >80 preferred RT as their primary treatment. Over half of the patients who started RT eventually discontinued the treatment. No significant difference was noted in the overall survival between the groups, regardless of the selected treatment method [76]. Older adults experienced greater acute and late toxicity as treatment was intensified. In particular, the addition of chemotherapy to radiotherapy increased toxicity and decreased therapy tolerability [77]. A meta-analysis of 19,805 patients included in 107 randomized trials concerning chemotherapy in squamous cell carcinoma of the head and neck (MACH-NC) showed that radiochemotherapy (CRT) improved the overall survival with locally advanced cancer. In contrast, age contributed to the deterioration of the treatment results in patients >70 years of age. Caution was advised in qualifying patients for combination therapy [78]. (Table 5).

Radiotherapy as monotherapy may be effective and well-tolerated by the older adults. Chronological age is not a contraindication to radical radiotherapy. Zachariah et al. retrospectively analyzed patients aged 80 years and older who received palliative or radical radiotherapy alone. A total of 203 patients aged 80–94 years were enrolled in the radiotherapy group, out of which 50 were treated for head and neck cancer. A complete response was achieved by 65% of patients treated for HNC. Response to treatment was observed in 81% of palliative patients. The toxicity profile was acceptable. Mucositis was the most common adverse reaction and occurred in 38%. Grade 3 dermatitis was reported in 2% of patients and treatment was discontinued in only 2 patients [79]. Wasil et al. analyzed 183 patients >80 who underwent radical or palliative radiotherapy. The majority of patients completed the planned treatment (77%). Treatment interruptions were required during radiotherapy. They were reported in 36% of the treated patients. Radiotherapy may be safely used in the elderly both when aiming for full recovery and during palliative treatment [80]. Desai et al. conducted a retrospective analysis of 34 patients who were ≥80 years of age at diagnosis, treated between 2012 and 2016. Demographic, clinical and treatment data were collected. Patients who received 3D-RT had the OS of 23 months, while patients undergoing single-modality RT had the OS of 8.5 months [81].

Table 5. Head and Neck Cancer—Radiotherapy in Older Adults.

Reference	Radiotherapy Approach	Outcomes/Tolerability	Guidelines/Authors' Comments
Kim et al. [76]	Retrospective analysis (26% >80); comparison: surgery, RT, CRT	>80 preferred RT; >50% discontinued treatment; no OS difference between modalities	Individualized treatment selection necessary
Lacas et al. [78]	CRT vs. RT in squamous cell HNC	CRT improved OS in locally advanced disease; >70 yrs—worse outcomes	Avoid CRT in older adults; favor RT alone or less toxic regimens
Zachariah et al. [79]	Radical or palliative RT in ≥80	CR in 65% of HNC; 81% response in palliative	RT is effective and well tolerated in ≥80; age not a contraindication for radical RT
Wasil et al. [80]	Radical/palliative RT in >80	77% completed RT; 36% required interruptions; overall safe	RT feasible and effective both in radical and palliative settings in older adults
Desai et al. [81]	3D-RT vs. single-modality RT in ≥80	3D-RT: OS 23 months; single-modality RT: OS 8.5 months	Advanced techniques (3D-RT) improve OS and are well tolerated in the older adults

3.6. Glioblastoma

The older adults with glioblastoma multiforme (GBM) represent a clinical challenge for neurosurgeons and oncologists. However, data on treatment outcomes in patients over 80 years of age undergoing surgical treatment are limited. Abdullah et al. performed a retrospective analysis of factors that might affect the OS of patients over 80 undergoing surgical treatment. The expression of oncogenic immunohistochemical markers (EGFR, p53, IDH1) and the cell proliferation index (Ki-67) were analyzed. The median overall survival was 4.2 months in the group of 58 patients over 80 who had undergone surgery. A statistically significant correlation between overall survival and Karnofsky performance status was demonstrated. Patients who received radiochemotherapy or radiotherapy were characterized by a significantly longer survival compared to patients who did not receive any postoperative adjuvant therapy. Longer overall survival was observed in patients without EGFR or p53 expression. In the octogenarian population, a benefit in terms of the overall survival was observed in patients with higher preoperative performance status (KPS), who received postoperative adjuvant therapy and in whom p53 expression was undetected. The results may be useful in making decisions regarding the treatment of patients with glioblastoma multiforme in the group of octogenarians and also confirm the key role of EGFR and p53 expression in oncogenesis, especially in the context of advanced age [82].

In 2024, Malmström et al. published a meta-analysis of data obtained from three clinical trials: Nordic, NOA-08 and CE.6. The meta-analysis included a total of 1277 people at the median age of >70 (range 60–90 years) [83]. Nordic and NOA-08 studies compared temozolomide (TMZ) therapy with RT in patients over 60 and 65 years of age. The Nordic study showed the superiority of TMZ compared to standard RT. Moreover, hypofractionated RT was shown to improve the overall survival compared to standard RT in patients >70 [84]. The NOA-08 study compared TMZ and RT and showed TMZ equivalence compared to standard RT [85].

In the CE.6 study, patients with glioma aged >65 had better OS in case of hypofractionated RT (40 Gy/15 fractions) with adjuvant TMZ compared to RT as monotherapy [86] (Table 6). The meta-analysis showed that the coexistence of hypertension, diabetes and/or stroke deteriorated survival rates in patients treated with TMZ. The prognostic factors influencing the OS included: the scope of resection, general condition according to the WHO, age, and the use of glucocorticosteroids. It was confirmed that the methylation state of the MGMT promoter was a predictive factor of response to TMZ [83].

Particular attention as regards the subpopulation of the elderly was attributed to the use of shortened irradiation treatment regimens. (Table 6). A study included 100 GBM individuals aged >60 who were postoperatively randomly assigned to receive standard radiotherapy (60 Gy in 30 fractions over 6 weeks) or a shorter course of radiotherapy (40 Gy in 15 fractions over 3 weeks). The overall survival was the primary endpoint of the study. The overall survival was comparable and equaled 5.1 months for standard RT versus 5.6 months for 40 Gy. The probability of surviving 6 months was also similar and equaled 44.7% for standard RT compared to 41.7% in the hypofractionated arm. As regards patients who completed RT as planned, 49% of patients (standard RT) compared to 23% required an increased post-treatment corticosteroid dose. The study confirmed the effectiveness of the regimen involving hypofractionation [87]. Another study in a group of elderly patients, in a poorer general condition, with newly diagnosed glioma, compared short-term radiotherapy of 25 Gy in 5 daily fractions for 1 week to the 40 Gy radiotherapy regimen in 15 fractions for 3 weeks. Short-term radiotherapy was not inferior to commonly used radiotherapy. The median PFS was 4.2 months in both arms. The median overall survival was 7.9 months in the 25 Gy arm and 6.4 months in the 40 Gy arm. The quality of life was comparable in both groups. A short radiotherapy regimen may be recommended as a treatment option for old adults and/or frail patients with newly diagnosed glioblastoma multiforme [88].

Single-agent TMZ chemotherapy may constitute an alternative to RT. This was confirmed by the results of the phase III NOA-8 study in a group of 373 patients with confirmed anaplastic astrocytoma or glioblastoma multiforme, aged >65 years, and with the Karnofsky score of at least 60. A study was conducted to compare single-agent chemotherapy (100 mg/m^2 of temozolomide, administered on days 1–7 of a cycle, 1 week of treatment, 1 week off treatment) to radiotherapy alone at a dose of 60.0 Gy, administered for 6–7 weeks in 30 fractions of 1.8–2.0 Gy. The overall survival was the primary endpoint. The median overall survival was 8.6 months in the temozolomide group compared to 9.6 months in the radiotherapy group. The methylation of the MGMT promoter was associated with longer overall survival. The most common Grade 3–4 adverse reactions associated with TMZ included hematologic and hepatic toxicity. Infections and thromboembolic events were more frequently observed in the chemotherapy group [85]. Octogenarians may be difficult to qualify for the irradiation of the CNS (central nervous system) metastases from other primary foci.

Nieder et al. presented examples of treatment (surgery, radiosurgery, radiotherapy, systemic therapy) and supportive care in patients >80 years of age with CNS metastases. In the selected group, survival after radiosurgery was longer than after whole-brain radiotherapy. The authors emphasized that, in order to optimize the results, prospective studies focused on octogenarians were necessary [89].

Stadlbauer et al. conducted a retrospective analysis in a group of 94 patients >80 with CNS metastases undergoing whole-brain radiotherapy. The authors proposed an assessment of the survival score based on fitness status, the number of CNS lesions (single or multiple), and the assessment of extracranial disease (present or absent). The median survival was 2.0 months in the whole group. Depending on the score obtained, the patients were assigned to one of 3 groups: poor prognosis (7 points), where all patients died within 2 months and should be qualified for best supportive care (BSC). The intermediate prognosis group obtained 10 points. Those patients also had an unfavorable prognosis with the median survival of 2.0 months and the 3-month OS of 25% and the 6-month survival rate of 13%. BSC was also the best choice in the group. Irradiation at a dose of 5 × 4 Gy should be considered only in selected cases.

In the group of good prognosis (13–17 points), the survival of 6 months was achieved by 50%, and 12 months—by 27% of patients. The authors recommended the following irradiation regimens: RT 5 × 4 Gy; 10 × 3 Gy; 20 × 2 Gy. This simple clinical tool may be useful in clinical practice [90].

Chen et al. presented a retrospective study suggesting that whole-brain RT was associated with increased toxicity compared to SBRT in patients >70 years of age and patients >80 years of age (21% of the study group) with brain metastases. The median OS calculated from the time of the diagnosis of brain metastases was 4.3 months in patients receiving whole-brain RT and 14.4 months in patients receiving SBRT. Patients receiving SBRT were characterized by better tolerability of the treatment. However, such results could be influenced by the selection of patients receiving a given therapy resulting from the stage of the underlying primary disease, the volume of intracranial disease or the general condition. The age >80 was not found to have an impact on the greater toxicity of the treatment [91].

Table 6. Glioblastoma & CNS Metastases—Radiotherapy in Older Adults.

Reference	Radiotherapy Approach	Outcomes/Tolerability	Guidelines/Authors' Comments
Perry et al. [86]	HF-RT 40 Gy/15 fx + adjuvant TMZ vs. RT alone in ≥65 with glioma	Better OS for HF-RT + TMZ vs. RT alone	Combine HF-RT + TMZ for fit older adults
Roa et al. [88]	Very short RT 25 Gy/5 fx (1 wk) vs. 40 Gy/15 fx (3 wks) in elderly/frail newly diagnosed GBM	Non-inferior: median PFS 4.2 mo both arms; median OS 7.9 mo (25 Gy) vs. 6.4 mo (40 Gy); QoL comparable	25 Gy/5 fx is a recommended option for older adults/frail
Nieder et al. [89]	CNS metastases in ≥80: SRS vs. WBRT; other modalities (surgery, systemic, BSC)	SRS associated with longer survival than WBRT in selected cases; need for octogenarian-focused prospective data	Prefer SRS when feasible; individualize by disease burden and performance status
Stadlbauer et al. [90]	WBRT in ≥80 with brain metastases: propose survival score (fitness, lesion number, extracranial disease)	Median OS 2.0 mo; score 7 (poor) → all died ≤2 mo (BSC recommended); score 10 → OS 2 mo, 3-mo OS 25%, 6-mo 13% (also BSC favored); score 13–17 → 6-mo 50%, 12-mo 27%; suggested RT: 5 × 4 Gy/10 × 3 Gy/20 × 2 Gy	Simple clinical score aids WBRT vs. BSC decision and fractionation choice
Chen et al. [91]	WBRT vs. SRS in >70 (including >80 = 21%)	Median OS from brain mets diagnosis: 4.3 mo (WBRT) vs. 14.4 mo (SRS); better tolerability with SRS; age >80 not linked to higher toxicity; selection bias likely	Favor SRS when feasible (limited volume/lesions); avoid routine WBRT in toxicity-sensitive

4. Conclusions

The subject of radiotherapy in the group of octogenarians is currently little understood. The data are mainly based on retrospective analyses of small groups of patients.

Treatment recommendations are often extrapolated from other age groups due to the underrepresentation of older adults in clinical trials. Treatment should bring a real benefit to the patient, be well tolerated and organizationally feasible. A significant use of geriatric scales is emphasized to facilitate decision making regarding the choice of the type of therapy for an individual patient. A particular role is attributed to Comprehensive Geriatric Assessment (CGA), which is used to assess various domains regarding the patient, i.e., the clinical, functional, mental, emotional, and social domain. The introduction of CGA as a standard in the assessment of patients allows the individual adjustment of therapy, increasing the effectiveness of treatment and minimizing the risk of side effects. Currently, the CGA scale is rarely used in clinical practice due to its difficulty, complexity and time-consuming nature [13,92]. (Figure 2).

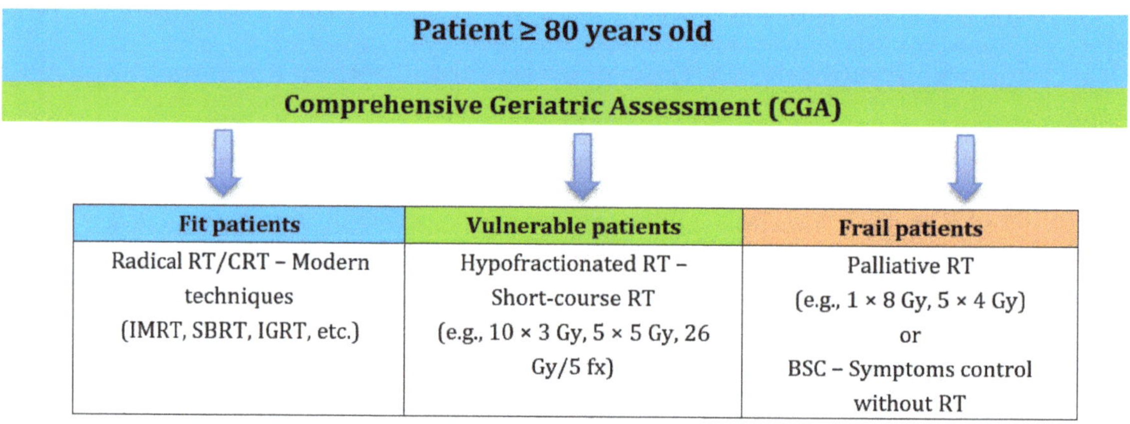

Figure 2. Conceptual overview of radiotherapy decision-making in octogenarian cancer patients.

It is necessary to develop new, simple geriatric assessment tools that facilitate the individualization of treatment. We need to develop research on biomarkers and predictors of treatment tolerance in this population. It is also essential to improve communication with the patient and their family regarding the nature of the disease, the treatment process, clear presentation of risks and benefits and finally the making of informed decisions.

Radiotherapy is an effective and safe method of tumor treatment.

SBRT or hypofractionation RT is effective, safe, well tolerated, and leads to a reduction in the total treatment time. These approaches can be used in the treatment of breast, lung, prostate, and rectal cancers, gliomas.

Combined-modality therapy should be reserved for carefully selected patients due to its toxicity, duration, and the adaptive challenges associated with a prolonged therapeutic process.

The benefit of adjuvant therapies with respect to local recurrence or overall survival in this group is uncertain.

The primary limitation of this review stems from its dependence on retrospective data, which are subject to selection bias and may therefore impact the reliability of the findings.

Prospective clinical trials are needed to provide robust scientific evidence on the effectiveness, tolerability, and safety of radiotherapy in late old adults oncological patients, particularly in those with breast, prostate, or rectal cancer. There is a lack of prospective research, including long-term studies assessing distant treatment outcomes. Nevertheless, in this patient population it appears challenging to design and conduct studies that reliably achieve their intended objectives and generate robust data, due in part to factors such as competing mortality and the fact that octogenarians constitute only approx. 10% of all cancer patients populations.

The aging of societies and the increase in the number of patients with neoplastic diseases mean that oncologists more and more commonly face the dilemma of making therapeutic decisions in patients in this age group. It is necessary to constantly expand the knowledge of the oncological treatment, including the late elderly, i.e., individuals older than 80 years of age.

Author Contributions: Conceptualization, A.L., E.W.-T. and S.N.; resources, A.L., E.W.-T., A.S., S.N.; writing—original draft preparation, A.L., E.W.-T., A.S.; writing—review and editing, S.N. All authors have read and agreed to the published version of the manuscript.

Funding: Funded by the Minister of Science under "the Regional Initiative of Excellence Program".

Data Availability Statement: No new data were created or analyzed in this study.

Conflicts of Interest: The authors declare no conflicts of interest.

References

1. Cancer Tomorrow. Available online: https://gco.iarc.who.int/tomorrow/en/dataviz/tables?cancers=27&age_start=16 (accessed on 23 January 2025).
2. Potyra, M.; Góral-Radziszewska, K.; Waśkiewicz, K.; Gawińska-Drużba, E. *Statistical Analyses*; 2024; ISSN 1507-1340. Available online: www.stat.gov.pl (accessed on 23 January 2025).
3. IARC—International Agency for Research on Cancer. Available online: https://www.iarc.who.int/ (accessed on 28 January 2025).
4. Pallis, A.G.; Fortpied, C.; Wedding, U.; Van Nes, M.C.; Penninckx, B.; Ring, A.; Lacombe, D.; Monfardini, S.; Scalliet, P.; Wildiers, H. EORTC Elderly Task Force Position Paper: Approach to the Older Cancer Patient. *Eur. J. Cancer* **2010**, *46*, 1502–1513. [CrossRef]
5. Page, M.J.; McKenzie, J.E.; Bossuyt, P.M.; Boutron, I.; Hoffmann, T.C.; Mulrow, C.D.; Shamseer, L.; Tetzlaff, J.M.; Akl, E.A.; Brennan, S.E.; et al. The PRISMA 2020 Statement: An Updated Guideline for Reporting Systematic Reviews. *BMJ* **2021**, *372*, n71. [CrossRef]
6. Tesarova, P. Breast Cancer in the Elderly—Should It Be Treated Differently? *Rep. Pract. Oncol. Radiother.* **2012**, *18*, 26–33. [CrossRef]
7. Bertolo, A.; Rosso, C.; Voutsadakis, I.A. Breast Cancer in Patients 80 Years-Old and Older. *Eur. J. Breast Health* **2020**, *16*, 208–212. [CrossRef]
8. Jenkins, E.O.; Deal, A.M.; Anders, C.K.; Prat, A.; Perou, C.M.; Carey, L.A.; Muss, H.B. Age-Specific Changes in Intrinsic Breast Cancer Subtypes: A Focus on Older Women. *Oncologist* **2014**, *19*, 1076–1083. [CrossRef]
9. Anderson, W.F.; Katki, H.A.; Rosenberg, P.S. Incidence of Breast Cancer in the United States: Current and Future Trends. *J. Natl. Cancer Inst.* **2011**, *103*, 1397–1402. [CrossRef] [PubMed]
10. Tsoutsou, P.G.; Vozenin, M.C.; Durham, A.D.; Bourhis, J. How Could Breast Cancer Molecular Features Contribute to Locoregional Treatment Decision Making? *Crit. Rev. Oncol. Hematol.* **2017**, *110*, 43–48. [CrossRef] [PubMed]
11. Van der Leij, F.; van Werkhoven, E.; Bosma, S.; Linn, S.C.; Rutgers, E.J.; van de Vijver, M.J.; Bartelink, H.; Elkhuizen, P.H.M.; Scholten, A. Low Risk of Recurrence in Elderly Patients Treated with Breast Conserving Therapy in a Single Institute. *Breast* **2016**, *30*, 19–25. [CrossRef]
12. Bastiaannet, E.; Liefers, G.J.; De Craen, A.J.M.; Kuppen, P.J.K.; Van De Water, W.; Portielje, J.E.A.; Van Der Geest, L.G.M.; Janssen-Heijnen, M.L.G.; Dekkers, O.M.; Van De Velde, C.J.H.; et al. Breast Cancer in Elderly Compared to Younger Patients in the Netherlands: Stage at Diagnosis, Treatment and Survival in 127,805 Unselected Patients. *Breast Cancer Res. Treat* **2010**, *124*, 801–807. [CrossRef] [PubMed]
13. Fonseca, V.C.; Sidiropoulou, Z. Geriatric Breast Cancer: Staging, Molecular Surrogates, and Treatment. A Review & Meta-Analysis. *Aging Dis.* **2024**, *15*, 1602–1618.
14. Kunkler, I.H.; Audisio, R.; Belkacemi, Y.; Betz, M.; Gore, E.; Hoffe, S.; Kirova, Y.; Koper, P.; Lagrange, J.L.; Markouizou, A.; et al. Review of Current Best Practice and Priorities for Research in Radiation Oncology for Elderly Patients with Cancer: The International Society of Geriatric Oncology (SIOG) Task Force. *Ann. Oncol.* **2014**, *25*, 2134–2146. [CrossRef] [PubMed]

15. Darby, S.; McGale, P.; Correa, C.; Taylor, C.; Arriagada, R.; Clarke, M.; Cutter, D.; Davies, C.; Ewertz, M.; Godwin, J.; et al. Effect of Radiotherapy after Breast-Conserving Surgery on 10-Year Recurrence and 15-Year Breast Cancer Death: Meta-Analysis of Individual Patient Data for 10,801 Women in 17 Randomised Trials. *Lancet* **2011**, *378*, 1707–1716. [CrossRef] [PubMed]
16. Whelan, T.J.; Pignol, J.-P.; Levine, M.N.; Julian, J.A.; MacKenzie, R.; Parpia, S.; Shelley, W.; Grimard, L.; Bowen, J.; Lukka, H.; et al. Long-Term Results of Hypofractionated Radiation Therapy for Breast Cancer. *N. Engl. J. Med.* **2010**, *362*, 513–520. [CrossRef]
17. Haviland, J.S.; Owen, J.R.; Dewar, J.A.; Agrawal, R.K.; Barrett, J.; Barrett-Lee, P.J.; Dobbs, H.J.; Hopwood, P.; Lawton, P.A.; Magee, B.J.; et al. The UK Standardisation of Breast Radiotherapy (START) Trials of Radiotherapy Hypofractionation for Treatment of Early Breast Cancer: 10-Year Follow-up Results of Two Randomised Controlled Trials. *Lancet Oncol.* **2013**, *14*, 1086–1094. [CrossRef]
18. Murray Brunt, A.; Haviland, J.S.; Wheatley, D.A.; Sydenham, M.A.; Alhasso, A.; Bloomfield, D.J.; Chan, C.; Churn, M.; Cleator, S.; Coles, C.E.; et al. Hypofractionated Breast Radiotherapy for 1 Week Versus 3 Weeks (FAST-Forward): 5-Year Efficacy and Late Normal Tissue Effects Results from a Multicentre, Non-Inferiority, Randomised, Phase 3 Trial. *Lancet* **2020**, *395*, 1613. [CrossRef]
19. Smith, B.D.; Haffty, B.G.; Hurria, A.; Galusha, D.H.; Gross, C.P. Postmastectomy Radiation and Survival in Older Women with Breast Cancer. *J. Clin. Oncol.* **2006**, *24*, 4901–4907. [CrossRef] [PubMed]
20. McGale, P.; Taylor, C.; Correa, C.; Cutter, D.; Duane, F.; Ewertz, M.; Gray, R.; Mannu, G.; Peto, R.; Whelan, T.; et al. Effect of Radiotherapy after Mastectomy and Axillary Surgery on 10-Year Recurrence and 20-Year Breast Cancer Mortality: Meta-Analysis of Individual Patient Data for 8135 Women in 22 Randomised Trials. *Lancet* **2014**, *383*, 2127–2135. [CrossRef]
21. Kunkler, I.H.; Canney, P.; van Tienhoven, G.; Russell, N.S. Elucidating the Role of Chest Wall Irradiation in "intermediate-Risk" Breast Cancer: The MRC/EORTC SUPREMO Trial. *Clin. Oncol.* **2008**, *20*, 31–34. [CrossRef]
22. Vaidya, J.S.; Joseph, D.J.; Tobias, J.S.; Bulsara, M.; Wenz, F.; Saunders, C.; Alvarado, M.; Flyger, H.L.; Massarut, S.; Eiermann, W.; et al. Targeted Intraoperative Radiotherapy versus Whole Breast Radiotherapy for Breast Cancer (TARGIT-A Trial): An International, Prospective, Randomised, Non-Inferiority Phase 3 Trial. *Lancet* **2010**, *376*, 91–102. [CrossRef]
23. Vaidya, J.S.; Wenz, F.; Bulsara, M.; Tobias, J.S.; Joseph, D.J.; Keshtgar, M.; Flyger, H.L.; Massarut, S.; Alvarado, M.; Saunders, C.; et al. Risk-Adapted Targeted Intraoperative Radiotherapy Versus Whole-Breast Radiotherapy for Breast Cancer: 5-Year Results for Local Control and Overall Survival from the TARGIT-A Randomised Trial. *Lancet* **2014**, *383*, 603–613. [CrossRef]
24. Veronesi, U.; Orecchia, R.; Maisonneuve, P.; Viale, G.; Rotmensz, N.; Sangalli, C.; Luini, A.; Veronesi, P.; Galimberti, V.; Zurrida, S.; et al. Intraoperative Radiotherapy versus External Radiotherapy for Early Breast Cancer (ELIOT): A Randomised Controlled Equivalence Trial. *Lancet Oncol.* **2013**, *14*, 1269–1277. [CrossRef] [PubMed]
25. Bartelink, H.; Maingon, P.; Poortmans, P.; Weltens, C.; Fourquet, A.; Jager, J.; Schinagl, D.; Oei, B.; Rodenhuis, C.; Horiot, J.C.; et al. Whole-Breast Irradiation With or Without a Boost for Patients Treated with Breast-Conserving Surgery for Early Breast Cancer: 20-Year Follow-up of a Randomised Phase 3 Trial. *Lancet Oncol.* **2015**, *16*, 47–56. [CrossRef]
26. Hughes, K.S.; Schnaper, L.A.; Bellon, J.R.; Cirrincione, C.T.; Berry, D.A.; McCormick, B.; Muss, H.B.; Smith, B.L.; Hudis, C.A.; Winer, E.P.; et al. Lumpectomy plus Tamoxifen With or Without Irradiation in Women Age 70 Years or Older with Early Breast Cancer: Long-Term Follow-up of CALGB 9343. *J. Clin. Oncol.* **2013**, *31*, 2382–2387. [CrossRef] [PubMed]
27. Hughes, K.S.; Schnaper, L.A.; Berry, D.; Cirrincione, C.; McCormick, B.; Shank, B.; Wheeler, J.; Champion, L.A.; Smith, T.J.; Smith, B.L.; et al. Lumpectomy plus Tamoxifen with or without Irradiation in Women 70 Years of Age or Older with Early Breast Cancer. *N. Engl. J. Med.* **2004**, *351*, 971–977. [CrossRef] [PubMed]
28. Rashmi Kumar, N.; Schonfeld, R.; Gradishar, W.J.; Lurie, R.H.; Moran, M.S.; Abraham, J.; Abramson, V.; Aft, R.; Agnese, D.; Allison, K.H.; et al. *NCCN Guidelines Version 6.2024 Breast Cancer*; NCCN: Plymouth Meeting, PA, USA, 2024.
29. Meattini, I.; De Santis, M.C.; Visani, L.; Scorsetti, M.; Fozza, A.; Meduri, B.; De Rose, F.; Bonzano, E.; Prisco, A.; Masiello, V.; et al. Single-Modality Endocrine Therapy versus Radiotherapy after Breast-Conserving Surgery in Women Aged 70 Years and Older with Luminal A-like Early Breast Cancer (EUROPA): A Preplanned Interim Analysis of a Phase 3, Non-Inferiority, Randomised Trial. *Lancet Oncol.* **2025**, *26*, 37–50. [CrossRef]
30. Biganzoli, L.; Battisti, N.M.L.; Wildiers, H.; McCartney, A.; Colloca, G.; Kunkler, I.H.; Cardoso, M.J.; Cheung, K.L.; de Glas, N.A.; Trimboli, R.M.; et al. Updated Recommendations Regarding the Management of Older Patients with Breast Cancer: A Joint Paper from the European Society of Breast Cancer Specialists (EUSOMA) and the International Society of Geriatric Oncology (SIOG). *Lancet Oncol.* **2021**, *22*, e327–e340. [CrossRef]
31. Bray, F.; Laversanne, M.; Sung, H.; Ferlay, J.; Siegel, R.L.; Soerjomataram, I.; Jemal, A. Global Cancer Statistics 2022: GLOBOCAN Estimates of Incidence and Mortality Worldwide for 36 Cancers in 185 Countries. *CA Cancer J. Clin.* **2024**, *74*, 229–263. [CrossRef] [PubMed]
32. Huang, W.; Deng, H.Y.; Xu, K.; Lin, M.Y.; Li, P.; Yuan, C.; Zhou, Q. Initial Treatment of Early-Stage Small-Sized Non-Small Cell Lung Cancer for Octogenarians: A Population-Based Study. *Updates Surg.* **2022**, *74*, 1461–1470. [CrossRef]
33. Li, S.; Ge, Y.; Ma, R.; Wang, J.; Ma, T.; Sun, T.; Feng, S.; Zhang, C.; Zhang, H. Comparison of Wedge Resection and Anatomical Lung Resection in Elderly Patients with Early-Stage Nonsmall Cell Lung Cancer With Visceral Pleural Invasion: A Population-Based Study. *Thorac. Cancer* **2025**, *16*, 15532. [CrossRef]

34. Ni, L.; Lin, G.; Zhang, Z.; Sun, D.; Liu, Z.; Liu, X. Surgery versus Radiotherapy in Octogenarians with Stage Ia Non-small Cell Lung Cancer: Propensity Score Matching Analysis of the SEER Database. *BMC Pulm. Med.* **2022**, *22*, 411. [CrossRef]
35. Robinson, C.G.; Dewees, T.A.; El Naqa, I.M.; Creach, K.M.; Olsen, J.R.; Crabtree, T.D.; Meyers, B.F.; Puri, V.; Bell, J.M.; Parikh, P.J.; et al. Patterns of Failure after Stereotactic Body Radiation Therapy or Lobar Resection for Clinical Stage I Non-Small-Cell Lung Cancer. *J. Thorac. Oncol.* **2013**, *8*, 192–201. [CrossRef]
36. Stokes, W.A.; Bronsert, M.R.; Meguid, R.A.; Blum, M.G.; Jones, B.L.; Koshy, M.; Sher, D.J.; Louie, A.V.; Palma, D.A.; Senan, S.; et al. Post-Treatment Mortality After Surgery and Stereotactic Body Radiotherapy for Early-Stage Non-Small-Cell Lung Cancer. *J. Clin. Oncol.* **2018**, *36*, 642–651. [CrossRef]
37. Franks, K.N.; McParland, L.; Webster, J.; Baldwin, D.R.; Sebag-Montefiore, D.; Evison, M.; Booton, R.; Faivre-Finn, C.; Naidu, B.; Ferguson, J.; et al. SABRTooth: A Randomised Controlled Feasibility Study of Stereotactic Ablative Radiotherapy (SABR) with Surgery in Patients with Peripheral Stage I Nonsmall Cell Lung Cancer Considered to Be at Higher Risk of Complications from Surgical Resection. *Eur. Respir. J.* **2020**, *56*, 2000118. [CrossRef]
38. Cassidy, R.J.; Patel, P.R.; Zhang, X.; Press, R.H.; Switchenko, J.M.; Pillai, R.N.; Owonikoko, T.K.; Ramalingam, S.S.; Fernandez, F.G.; Force, S.D.; et al. Stereotactic Body Radiotherapy for Early-Stage Non-Small-Cell Lung Cancer in Patients 80 Years and Older: A Multi-Center Analysis. *Clin. Lung Cancer* **2017**, *18*, 551–558.e6. [CrossRef]
39. Bei, Y.; Murakami, N.; Nakayama, Y.; Kae, O.; Kashihara, T.; Raturi, V.P.; Okamoto, H.; Takahashi, K.; Inaba, K.; Igaki, H.; et al. Stereotactic Body Radiation Therapy for Early-Stage Non–Small-Cell Lung Cancer in Octogenarians and Older: An Alternative Treatment. *J. Radiat. Res.* **2020**, *61*, 586. [CrossRef]
40. Movsas, B.; Scott, C.; Sause, W.; Byhardt, R.; Komaki, R.; Cox, J.; Johnson, D.; Lawton, C.; Dar, A.R.; Wasserman, T.; et al. The Benefit of Treatment Intensification Is Age and Histology-Dependent in Patients with Locally Advanced Non-Small Cell Lung Cancer (NSCLC): A Quality-Adjusted Survival Analysis of Radiation Therapy Oncology Group (RTOG) Chemoradiation Studies. *Int. J. Radiat. Oncol. Biol. Phys.* **1999**, *45*, 1143–1149. [CrossRef]
41. Werner-Wasik, M.; Scott, C.; Cox, J.D.; Sause, W.T.; Byhardt, R.W.; Asbell, S.; Russell, A.; Komaki, R.; Lee, J.S. Recursive Partitioning Analysis of 1999 Radiation Therapy Oncology Group (RTOG) Patients with Locally-Advanced Non-Small-Cell Lung Cancer (LA-NSCLC): Identification of Five Groups with Different Survival. *Int. J. Radiat. Oncol. Biol. Phys.* **2000**, *48*, 1475–1482. [CrossRef]
42. Pergolizzi, S.; Santacaterina, A.; De Renzis, C.; Settineri, N.; Gaeta, M.; Frosina, P.; Russi, E.G.; Altavilla, G. Older People with Non Small Cell Lung Cancer in Clinical Stage IIIA and Co-Morbid Conditions: Is Curative Irradiation Feasible? Final Results of a Prospective Study. *Lung Cancer* **2002**, *37*, 201–206. [CrossRef] [PubMed]
43. Geinitz, H.; Zimmermann, F.B.; Molls, M. Radiotherapy of the Elderly Patient. Radiotherapy Tolerance and Results in Older Patients. *Strahlenther. Onkol.* **1999**, *175*, 119–127. [CrossRef] [PubMed]
44. Lonardi, F.; Coeli, M.; Pavanato, G.; Adami, F.; Gioga, G.; Campostrini, F. Radiotherapy for Non-Small Cell Lung Cancer in Patients Aged 75 and over: Safety, Effectiveness and Possible Impact on Survival. *Lung Cancer* **2000**, *28*, 43–50. [CrossRef] [PubMed]
45. Hayashi, K.; Yamamoto, N.; Nakajima, M.; Nomoto, A.; Ishikawa, H.; Ogawa, K.; Tsuji, H. Carbon-Ion Radiotherapy for Octogenarians with Locally Advanced Non-Small-Cell Lung Cancer. *Jpn. J. Radiol.* **2021**, *39*, 703. [CrossRef]
46. He, J.; Liu, Y.; Zhang, X.; Li, B.; Yang, L.; Wang, H.; Wang, S.; Yu, J.; Wang, L. Comparison of Proton Therapy and Photon Therapy for Early-Stage Non-Small Cell Lung Cancer: A Meta-Analysis. *Biomark. Res.* **2024**, *12*, 90. [CrossRef]
47. Shiono, A.; Imai, H.; Endo, S.; Katayama, K.; Sato, H.; Hashimoto, K.; Miura, Y.; Okazaki, S.; Abe, T.; Mouri, A.; et al. A Retrospective Evaluation of Therapeutic Efficacy and Safety of Chemoradiotherapy in Older Patients (Aged ≥75 Years) with Limited-Disease Small Cell Lung Cancer: Insights from Two Institutions and Review of the Literature. *Radiol. Oncol.* **2024**, *58*, 432–443. [CrossRef] [PubMed]
48. Christodoulou, M.; Blackhall, F.; Mistry, H.; Leylek, A.; Knegjens, J.; Remouchamps, V.; Martel-Lafay, I.; Farré, N.; Zwitter, M.; Lerouge, D.; et al. Compliance and Outcome of Elderly Patients Treated in the Concurrent Once-Daily Versus Twice-Daily Radiotherapy (CONVERT) Trial. *J. Thorac. Oncol.* **2019**, *14*, 63–71. [CrossRef]
49. Kim, T.G.; Pyo, H.; Ahn, Y.C.; Noh, J.M.; Oh, D. Role of Prophylactic Cranial Irradiation for Elderly Patients with Limited-Disease Small-Cell Lung Cancer: Inverse Probability of Treatment Weighting Using Propensity Score. *J. Radiat. Res.* **2019**, *60*, 630–638. [CrossRef]
50. Cornford, P.; van den Bergh, R.C.N.; Briers, E.; Van den Broeck, T.; Brunckhorst, O.; Darraugh, J.; Eberli, D.; De Meerleer, G.; De Santis, M.; Farolfi, A.; et al. EAU-EANM-ESTRO-ESUR-ISUP-SIOG Guidelines on Prostate Cancer—2024 Update. Part I: Screening, Diagnosis, and Local Treatment with Curative Intent. *Eur. Urol.* **2024**, *86*, 148–163. [CrossRef]
51. Droz, J.P.; Albrand, G.; Gillessen, S.; Hughes, S.; Mottet, N.; Oudard, S.; Payne, H.; Puts, M.; Zulian, G.; Balducci, L.; et al. Management of Prostate Cancer in Elderly Patients: Recommendations of a Task Force of the International Society of Geriatric Oncology. *Eur. Urol.* **2017**, *72*, 521–531. [CrossRef]
52. Predict Prostate. Available online: https://prostate.predict.cam/ (accessed on 24 January 2025).

53. Daskivich, T.J.; Chamie, K.; Kwan, L.; Labo, J.; Palvolgyi, R.; Dash, A.; Greenfield, S.; Litwin, M.S. Overtreatment of Men with Low-Risk Prostate Cancer and Significant Comorbidity. *Cancer* **2011**, *117*, 2058–2066. [CrossRef] [PubMed]
54. Nguyen, T.D.; Azria, D.; Brochon, D.; Poortmans, P.; Miller, R.C.; Scandolaro, L.; Majewski, W.; Krengli, M.; Abacioglu, U.; Moretti, L.; et al. Curative External Beam Radiotherapy in Patients over 80 Years of Age with Localized Prostate Cancer: A Retrospective Rare Cancer Network Study. *Crit. Rev. Oncol. Hematol.* **2010**, *74*, 66–71. [CrossRef] [PubMed]
55. Okonogi, N.; Katoh, H.; Kawamura, H.; Tamaki, T.; Kaminuma, T.; Murata, K.; Ohkubo, Y.; Takakusagi, Y.; Onishi, M.; Sekihara, T.; et al. Clinical Outcomes of Helical Tomotherapy for Super-Elderly Patients with Localized and Locally Advanced Prostate Cancer: Comparison with Patients under 80 Years of Age. *J. Radiat. Res.* **2015**, *56*, 889–896. [CrossRef]
56. Le, T.; Armstrong, S.; Shakespeare, T.P. Outcomes of Dose-Escalated IMRT and ADT in Octogenarians with Prostate Cancer. *J. Med. Imaging Radiat. Oncol.* **2023**, *67*, 539–545. [CrossRef]
57. Arcangeli, G.; Fowler, J.; Gomellini, S.; Arcangeli, S.; Saracino, B.; Petrongari, M.G.; Benassi, M.; Strigari, L. Acute and Late Toxicity in a Randomized Trial of Conventional versus Hypofractionated Three-Dimensional Conformal Radiotherapy for Prostate Cancer. *Int. J. Radiat. Oncol. Biol. Phys.* **2011**, *79*, 1013–1021. [CrossRef]
58. Qureshy, S.A.; Diven, M.A.; Ma, X.; Marciscano, A.E.; Hu, J.C.; McClure, T.D.; Barbieri, C.; Nagar, H. Differential Use of Radiotherapy Fractionation Regimens in Prostate Cancer. *JAMA Netw. Open* **2023**, *6*, E2337165. [CrossRef]
59. Fransson, P.; Nilsson, P.; Gunnlaugsson, A.; Beckman, L.; Tavelin, B.; Norman, D.; Thellenberg-Karlsson, C.; Hoyer, M.; Lagerlund, M.; Kindblom, J.; et al. Ultra-Hypofractionated Versus Conventionally Fractionated Radiotherapy for Prostate Cancer (HYPO-RT-PC): Patient-Reported Quality-of-Life Outcomes of a Randomised, Controlled, Non-Inferiority, Phase 3 Trial. *Lancet Oncol.* **2021**, *22*, 235–245. [CrossRef] [PubMed]
60. Syndikus, I.; Griffin, C.; Philipps, L.; Tree, A.; Khoo, V.; Birtle, A.J.; Choudhury, A.; Ferguson, C.; O'Sullivan, J.M.; Panades, M.; et al. 10-Year Efficacy and Co-Morbidity Outcomes of a Phase III Randomised Trial of Conventional vs. Hypofractionated High Dose Intensity Modulated Radiotherapy for Prostate Cancer (CHHiP; CRUK/06/016). *J. Clin. Oncol.* **2023**, *41*, 304. [CrossRef]
61. Morton, G.; Vigneault, E.; Barkati, M.; Helou, J.; Niazi, T.; Robinson, J.; Loblaw, D.; Tseng, C.; Chung, H.; Delouya, G.; et al. A Randomized Phase II Trial of High Dose-Rate (HDR) and Low Dose-Rate (LDR) Brachytherapy as Monotherapy in Localized Prostate Cancer: Analysis of Initial Arms of Canadian Cancer Trials Group PR19 (NCT02960087). *Radiother. Oncol.* **2025**, *212*, 111124. [CrossRef]
62. Li, B.; Kirshenbaum, E.J.; Blackwell, R.H.; Gange, W.S.; Saluk, J.; Zapf, M.A.C.; Kothari, A.N.; Flanigan, R.C.; Gupta, G.N. Thirty-Day Hospital Revisits After Prostate Brachytherapy: Who Is at Risk? *Prostate Int.* **2019**, *7*, 68–72. [CrossRef]
63. Yamazaki, H.; Masui, K.; Suzuki, G.; Shimizu, D.; Aibe, N.; Yamada, K.; Fujihara, A.; Shiraishi, T.; Okihara, K.; Ukimura, O.; et al. Radiotherapy for Elder Patients Aged ≥80 with Clinically Localized Prostate Cancer—Brachytherapy Enhanced Late GU Toxicity Especially in Elderly. *Clin. Transl. Radiat. Oncol.* **2020**, *25*, 67–74. [CrossRef] [PubMed]
64. Kotake, K.; Asano, M.; Ozawa, H.; Kobayashi, H.; Sugihara, K. Tumour Characteristics, Treatment Patterns and Survival of Patients Aged 80 Years or Older with Colorectal Cancer. *Colorectal Dis.* **2015**, *17*, 205–215. [CrossRef]
65. Kunitake, H.; Zingmond, D.S.; Ryoo, J.; Ko, C.Y. Caring for Octogenarian and Nonagenarian Patients with Colorectal Cancer: What Should Our Standards and Expectations Be? *Dis. Colon Rectum.* **2010**, *53*, 735–743. [CrossRef]
66. Goldvaser, H.; Shroitman, N.K.; Ben-Aharon, I.; Purim, O.; Kundel, Y.; Shepshelovich, D.; Shochat, T.; Sulkes, A.; Brenner, B. Octogenarian Patients with Colorectal Cancer: Characterizing an Emerging Clinical Entity. *World J. Gastroenterol.* **2017**, *23*, 1387–1396. [CrossRef] [PubMed]
67. Chen, B.; Yu, W.; Ma, Y.; Xu, P.; Yao, Q.; Sun, Q.; Ren, J.; Wang, D. Evaluation of the Safety and Efficacy of Perform Enterectomy in Colorectal Cancer Patients Aged 80 or Older. A Meta-Analysis and a Systematic Review. *Int. J. Colorectal Dis.* **2023**, *38*, 1–13. [CrossRef] [PubMed]
68. Claassen, Y.H.M.; Vermeer, N.C.A.; Iversen, L.H.; van Eycken, E.; Guren, M.G.; Mroczkowski, P.; Martling, A.; Cazador, A.C.; Johansson, R.; Vandendael, T.; et al. Treatment and Survival of Rectal Cancer Patients over the Age of 80 Years: A EURECCA International Comparison. *Br. J. Cancer* **2018**, *119*, 517–522. [CrossRef]
69. Pasetto, L.M.; Friso, M.L.; Pucciarelli, S.; Basso, U.; Falci, C.; Bortolami, A.; Toppan, P.; Agostini, M.; Rugge, M.; Serpentini, S.; et al. Rectal Cancer Neoadjuvant Treatment in Elderly Patients. *Anticancer Res.* **2006**, *26*, 3913–3923.
70. Margalit, D.N.; Mamon, H.J.; Ancukiewicz, M.; Kobayashi, W.; Ryan, D.P.; Blaszkowsky, L.S.; Clark, J.; Willett, C.G.; Hong, T.S. Tolerability of Combined Modality Therapy for Rectal Cancer in Elderly Patients Aged 75 Years and Older. *Int. J. Radiat. Oncol. Biol. Phys.* **2011**, *81*, e735–e741. [CrossRef]
71. Socha, J.; Bujko, K. A Watch-and-Wait Strategy or Local Excision in Complete Clinical Responders after Radiation for Early-Stage Rectal Cancer. *Lancet Healthy Longev.* **2022**, *3*, e807–e808. [CrossRef]
72. Beets, G.L.; Figueiredo, N.L.; Habr-Gama, A.; Van De Velde, C.J.H. A New Paradigm for Rectal Cancer: Organ Preservation: Introducing the International Watch & Wait Database (IWWD). *Eur. J. Surg. Oncol.* **2015**, *41*, 1562–1564. [CrossRef]
73. Bujko, K.; Partycki, M.; Pietrzak, L. Neoadjuvant Radiotherapy (5 × 5 Gy): Immediate versus Delayed Surgery. *Recent Results Cancer Res.* **2014**, *203*, 171–187. [CrossRef] [PubMed]

74. Bujko, K.; Wyrwicz, L.; Rutkowski, A.; Malinowska, M.; Pietrzak, L.; Kryński, J.; Michalski, W.; Oledzki, J.; Kuśnierz, J.; Zajac, L.; et al. Long-Course Oxaliplatin-Based Preoperative Chemoradiation versus 5 × 5 Gy and Consolidation Chemotherapy for CT4 or Fixed CT3 Rectal Cancer: Results of a Randomized Phase III Study. *Ann. Oncol.* **2016**, *27*, 834–842. [CrossRef]
75. Ciseł, B.; Pietrzak, L.; Michalski, W.; Wyrwicz, L.; Rutkowski, A.; Kosakowska, E.; Cencelewicz, A.; Spałek, M.; Polkowski, W.; Jankiewicz, M.; et al. Long-Course Preoperative Chemoradiation versus 5 × 5 Gy and Consolidation Chemotherapy for Clinical T4 and Fixed Clinical T3 Rectal Cancer: Long-Term Results of the Randomized Polish II Study. *Ann. Oncol.* **2019**, *30*, 1298–1303. [CrossRef]
76. Kim, H.; Kim, S.D.; Shim, Y.J.; Lee, S.Y.; Sung, M.W.; Kim, K.H.; Hah, J.H. Is There Any Age Cutoff to Treat Elderly Patients with Head and Neck Cancer? Comparing with Septuagenarians and Octogenarians. *J. Korean Med. Sci.* **2016**, *31*, 1300–1306. [CrossRef]
77. VanderWalde, N.A.; Fleming, M.; Weiss, J.; Chera, B.S. Treatment of Older Patients with Head and Neck Cancer: A Review. *Oncologist* **2013**, *18*, 568–578. [CrossRef]
78. Lacas, B.; Carmel, A.; Landais, C.; Wong, S.J.; Licitra, L.; Tobias, J.S.; Burtness, B.; Ghi, M.G.; Cohen, E.E.W.; Grau, C.; et al. Meta-Analysis of Chemotherapy in Head and Neck Cancer (MACH-NC): An Update on 107 Randomized Trials and 19,805 Patients, on Behalf of MACH-NC Group. *Radiother. Oncol.* **2021**, *156*, 281–293. [CrossRef] [PubMed]
79. Zachariah, B.; Balducci, L.; Venkattaramanabalaji, G.V.; Casey, L.; Greenberg, H.M.; DelRegato, J.A. Radiotherapy for Cancer Patients Aged 80 and Older: A Study of Effectiveness and Side Effects. *Int. J. Radiat. Oncol. Biol. Phys.* **1997**, *39*, 1125–1129. [CrossRef]
80. Wasil, T.; Lichtman, S.M.; Gupta, V.; Rush, S. Radiation Therapy in Cancer Patients 80 Years of Age and Older. *Am. J. Clin. Oncol.* **2000**, *23*, 526–530. [CrossRef]
81. Desai, P.A.; Saksena, A.; Miller, F.R.; Karnad, A.B.; Cervantez, S.R. Head and Neck Cancer in Octogenarians: A Single Center Experience. *J. Clin. Oncol.* **2018**, *36*, e18044. [CrossRef]
82. Abdullah, K.G.; Ramayya, A.; Thawani, J.P.; Macyszyn, L.; Martinez-Lage, M.; O'Rourke, D.M.; Brem, S. Factors Associated with Increased Survival after Surgical Resection of Glioblastoma in Octogenarians. *PLoS ONE* **2015**, *10*, e0127202. [CrossRef] [PubMed]
83. Malmström, A.; Oppong, F.B.; O'Callaghan, C.J.; Wick, W.; Laperriere, N.; Gorlia, T.; Weller, M.; Henriksson, R.; Mason, W.; Platten, M.; et al. Prognostic Factors for Overall Survival in Elderly Patients with Glioblastoma: Analysis of the Pooled NOA-08 and Nordic Trials with the CCTG-EORTC (CE.6) Trial. *Neurooncol. Adv.* **2024**, *6*, vdae211. [CrossRef]
84. Malmström, A.; Grønberg, B.H.; Marosi, C.; Stupp, R.; Frappaz, D.; Schultz, H.; Abacioglu, U.; Tavelin, B.; Lhermitte, B.; Hegi, M.E.; et al. Temozolomide versus Standard 6-Week Radiotherapy versus Hypofractionated Radiotherapy in Patients Older than 60 Years with Glioblastoma: The Nordic Randomised, Phase 3 Trial. *Lancet Oncol.* **2012**, *13*, 916–926. [CrossRef] [PubMed]
85. Wick, W.; Platten, M.; Meisner, C.; Felsberg, J.; Tabatabai, G.; Simon, M.; Nikkhah, G.; Papsdorf, K.; Steinbach, J.P.; Sabel, M.; et al. Temozolomide Chemotherapy Alone versus Radiotherapy Alone for Malignant Astrocytoma in the Elderly: The NOA-08 Randomised, Phase 3 Trial. *Lancet Oncol.* **2012**, *13*, 707–715. [CrossRef]
86. Perry, J.R.; Laperriere, N.; O'Callaghan, C.J.; Brandes, A.A.; Menten, J.; Phillips, C.; Fay, M.; Nishikawa, R.; Cairncross, J.G.; Roa, W.; et al. Short-Course Radiation plus Temozolomide in Elderly Patients with Glioblastoma. *N. Engl. J. Med.* **2017**, *376*, 1027–1037. [CrossRef]
87. Roa, W.; Brasher, P.M.A.; Bauman, G.; Anthes, M.; Bruera, E.; Chan, A.; Fisher, B.; Fulton, D.; Gulavita, S.; Hao, C.; et al. Abbreviated Course of Radiation Therapy in Older Patients with Glioblastoma Multiforme: A Prospective Randomized Clinical Trial. *J. Clin. Oncol.* **2004**, *22*, 1583–1588. [CrossRef] [PubMed]
88. Roa, W.; Kepka, L.; Kumar, N.; Sinaika, V.; Matiello, J.; Lomidze, D.; Hentati, D.; De Castro, D.G.; Dyttus-Cebulok, K.; Drodge, S.; et al. International Atomic Energy Agency Randomized Phase III Study of Radiation Therapy in Elderly and/or Frail Patients with Newly Diagnosed Glioblastoma Multiforme. *J. Clin. Oncol.* **2015**, *33*, 4145–4150. [CrossRef]
89. Nieder, C.; Andratschke, N.H.; Grosu, A.L. How We Treat Octogenarians with Brain Metastases. *Front. Oncol.* **2023**, *13*, 1213122. [CrossRef]
90. Stadlbauer, A.; Rades, D.; Delikanli, C.; Schild, S.E.; Kristiansen, C.; Tvilsted, S.; Janssen, S. The First Survival Score for Patients Aged ≥80 Years Irradiated for Brain Metastases. *Biology* **2022**, *11*, 1434. [CrossRef]
91. Chen, L.; Shen, C.; Redmond, K.J.; Page, B.R.; Kummerlowe, M.; Mcnutt, T.; Bettegowda, C.; Rigamonti, D.; Lim, M.; Kleinberg, L. Use of Stereotactic Radiosurgery in Elderly and Very Elderly Patients with Brain Metastases to Limit Toxicity Associated with Whole Brain Radiation Therapy. *Int. J. Radiat. Oncol. Biol. Phys.* **2017**, *98*, 939–947. [CrossRef] [PubMed]
92. Ocanto, A.; Cantero, R.; Morera, R.; Ramírez, R.; Rodríguez, I.; Castillo, K.; Couñago, F.; Samper, P. Results of Radical Treatment of Locally Advanced Rectal Cancer in Geriatric and Non-Geriatric Patients. *Rep. Pract. Oncol. Radiother.* **2025**, *30*, 54–61. [CrossRef] [PubMed]

cancers

MDPI

Review

Geriatric Assessment and Management, Prehabilitation and Rehabilitation for Older Aldults with Non-Colorectal Digestive Cancers

Amélie Aregui [1,*,†], Janina Estrada [2,†], Madeleine Lefèvre [1], Anna Carteaux-Taieb [3], Geoffroy Beraud-Chaulet [4,5], Pascal Hammel [6], Virginie Fossey-Diaz [1,7] and Thomas Aparicio [8]

1 Paris Nord Oncogeriatrics Coordination Unit, Bretonneau and Saint Louis Hospitals, AP-HP, 75018 Paris, France
2 Geriatric Out-Patient Unit, Bretonneau Hospital, AP-HP, 75018 Paris, France
3 Department of Digestive and Endocrine Surgery, Saint-Louis Hospital, AP-HP, 75010 Paris, France
4 Geriatrics Departement, Paul Brousse Hospital, AP-HP, 94800 Villejuif, France
5 Oncogériatric Department, Gustave Roussy Institut, 94800 Villejuif, France
6 Medical Oncology Department, Paul Brousse Hospital, AP-HP, Université Paris Saclay, 94800 Villejuif, France
7 Geriatrics Departement, Bretonneau Hospital, AP-HP, 75018 Paris, France
8 Gastroenterology Department, Saint Louis Hospital, AP-HP, Université Paris Cité, 75010 Paris, France
* Correspondence: amelie.aregui@aphp.fr
† These authors contributed equally to this work.

Simple Summary: Digestive cancers are common among older adults, yet their management can be more challenging in this population given the physiological differences between older and younger patients. That is why geriatricians now work with cancer specialists to help in the decision process and identify patient frailties. Through a global assessment, including lifestyle, muscle function, nutrition, and psychological well-being, geriatricians can help build a tailored treatment. This may involve, depending on the chosen treatments, preparing patients for the surgery and improving their postoperative recovery, or mitigating the side effects of chemotherapy and other therapies. However, geriatrician contributions in the management of non-colorectal cancers (oesophagus, stomach, liver, pancreas, or biliary tract cancers) is not as well-known as in colon or rectal cancer. This paper aims to summarize current research on the geriatric management of non-colorectal digestive cancers: how it can be done and how it can improve treatment outcomes and patients' quality of life.

Abstract: Background: The incidence of cancer in older patients is high, reaching 2.3 million world-wide in 2018 for patients aged over 80. Because the characteristics of this population make therapeutic choices difficult, co-management between geriatricians and other cancer specialists has gradually become essential. Methods: This narrative review aims to synthesize current data on the contribution of geriatric assessment in the management of elderly patients with non-colorectal digestive cancers. Oncogeriatric assessment is multi-domain, including the evaluation of co-morbidities, autonomy, nutrition, cognition, mood, and functional assessment. Results: Oncogeriatric parameters are predictive of mortality and adverse events. In the peri-operative phase of non-colorectal digestive cancer surgical management, geriatric management can assist in the decision-making process, identify frailties, and arrange a specific and personalized trimodal preoperative rehabilitation program, including nutritional management, adapted physical activity, and psychological care. Its aim is to limit the risks of confusion and of decompensation of comorbidities, mainly cardio-respiratory, which is associated with the highest morbidity in biliary-pancreatic surgery for older adults, facilitate recovery of previous autonomy when

https://doi.org/10.3390/cancers17091589

possible, and shorten hospital stay. For metastatic cancers, or during multimodal management, such as peri-operative chemotherapy for localized gastric cancers or pre-operative radio-chemotherapy for oesophageal or rectal cancers, specific assessment of the tolerance of chemotherapy is necessary. Neuropathic toxicity and chemobrain have a greater impact on elderly patients, with an increased loss of autonomy. Joint geriatric management can reduce the rate of grade 3–5 adverse effects of chemotherapy in particular and improve quality of life. Conclusions: Co-management between geriatricians and other specialties should be encouraged wherever possible.

Keywords: geriatric comprehensive assessment; non-colorectal digestive cancer; older adults; treatment tolerance; quality of life

1. Introduction

In 2018, 13.3% of newly diagnosed cancer cases involved patients aged 80 and over, amounting to 2.3 million new cases globally across all cancer types. Given the demographic shift towards an aging population and the heightened incidence of cancer with advancing age, this statistic is anticipated to escalate to 6.9 million by 2050, constituting 21.5% of newly diagnosed cancers [1]. The importance of non-colorectal digestive cancers is far from negligible, since stomach, liver, and oesophageal cancers are among the 10 most frequently diagnosed cancers worldwide, and stomach, liver, oesophageal, and pancreatic cancers are among the top 10 leading causes of cancer deaths [2]. The aging process is associated with a decline in 10-year net survival, the observed survival if cancer is the only cause of death, highlighting the need for further investigation. Multiple factors likely contribute to this decline, including delayed diagnosis in older patients and limitations imposed by comorbidities. For instance, constraints on diagnostic explorations such as contrast injections in cases of renal failure or general anaesthesia before endoscopic ultrasound guided fine needle biopsy in pancreatic cancer may play a role [3]. Cognitive impairment, prevalent in the geriatric population, further disrupts the continuum of care, leading to missed appointments and lapses in follow-up.

Optimal treatment selection poses another challenge. The SAGE Prospective Multicenter Cohort survey revealed an underrepresentation of older patients in therapeutic trials focused on colorectal cancer [4]. This underrepresentation extends to non-colorectal cancers, complicating the decision-making process. Given the inherent heterogeneity of this population, some robust individuals may receive treatments similar to that of younger patients, while more fragile patients may require tailored interventions. Given the generally poor prognosis of non-colorectal digestive cancers (accounting for 26% of cancer-related deaths [2]), and even lower among older adults, we have chosen to search the literature for the particularities of this population and any specific management. Considering the small number of patients in this sub-population in the literature, and the fact that the same specialist manages each cancer, we decided to group them together. Unlike colorectal cancers, the lack of specific recommendations for non-colorectal digestive cancer in older adults adds to the complexity of treatment decision making [5,6].

Consequently, navigating through this intricate decision-making process is crucial, aiming to provide the best possible care for the patient without undertreating them, while preserving autonomy and quality of life. Given these unique challenges, collaboration between geriatricians and other specialized healthcare professionals has gradually become mandatory.

This narrative review aims to describe geriatric assessment and its contribution to the management of older adults with non-colorectal digestive cancers.

2. Methods

A literature search was conducted on PubMed and Google Scholar, encompassing English-language articles published between January 2000 and 2024. The references in the identified articles were also reviewed to find additional publications of interest.

The keywords used were geriatric assessment, elderly, older patients, digestive cancer, hepatobiliary-pancreatic cancer, oesophagogastric cancer, prehabilitation, rehabilitation, fast-track surgery, systemic treatments, chemotherapy, cognitive disorders.

Articles were included in the review based on relevancy and publication types.

3. Oncogeriatric Evaluation Specific to the Non-Colorectal Digestive Cancers, Decision Support

3.1. *Identifying Frail Patients*

While the ECOG PS (PS adapted to the older adults, mainly by adapting references to the ability to work) scale offers a comprehensive assessment of general condition, its applicability for older patients is not universal, and it lacks sensitivity in predicting loss of autonomy [5].

For individuals above 70 years, the International Society of Geriatric Oncology (SIOG) recommends utilizing the G8 score, validated by the Oncodage study [6], and advocates for an in-depth geriatric assessment when the score is less than or equal to 14. The modified G8, although more specific and capable of targeting patients with abnormal geriatric assessments, particularly by incorporating considerations of heart disease, which are crucial for pancreatic and hepatobiliary surgery, is underused in routine clinical practice [7].

3.2. *Comprehensive Geriatric Assessment (CGA)*

The CGA aims to identify pivotal factors and comorbidities influencing the balance between curative and palliative care. This in-depth evaluation encompasses the patient's overall condition, autonomy, nutritional, cognitive, and thymic status, along with an assessment of comorbidities, functional abilities, and the social environment [8]. The geriatrician uses different scales for each of these domains during a lengthy consultation. Geriatricians have access to multiple assessment scales, leading to a lack of standardization in geriatric data collection for clinical trials. This variability contributes to the absence of specific recommendations for non-colorectal digestive cancer management in older adults. To resolve the matter, tools such as the Geriatric Core Dataset have been developed, through a Delphi consensus process, aiming to standardize geriatric data collection in clinical trials and facilitate comparisons across studies [9].

3.2.1. Loss of Autonomy and the Role of the Caregiver

Autonomy, which demonstrates significant heterogeneity within this population, is evaluated according to SIOG recommendations through the Activity of Daily Living (ADL, six items: washing, dressing, walking, toileting, eating, continence evaluation) and the Instrumental Activity of Daily Living (IADL, eight items: ability to use telephone, shopping, food preparation, housekeeping, laundry, mode of transportation, responsibility for own medications, ability to handle finances). Patients are considered dependent if they require assistance with at least one of these items, with IADLs being more sensitive and displaying earlier impacts. They appear to predict treatment feasibility and chemotherapy toxicity [10]. Impaired ADL and IADL are also associated with unscheduled hospitalization and early three-month mortality [11].

After open digestive, hepatobiliary, or gastrointestinal surgery, the decline in ADL is evident irrespective of age, with a more pronounced decline after the age of 80 [12].

The geriatrician, when assessing autonomy, also explores available resources such as the presence of a caregiver at home or nearby, which influences the patient's quality of life [13]. This aspect is crucial, especially in cases of memory disorders, for detecting adverse effects of systemic treatments and ensuring therapy adherence. The Zarit scale should be employed to assess caregiver burden, aiming to mitigate its impact on the caregiver's health [14].

In case of absence of a caregiver or in the event of caregiver exhaustion, it is essential to consider the introduction of professional help at the home.

3.2.2. Malnutrition

Malnutrition is intricately linked to cancer, inflammation, hyper-catabolism, digestive tract damage, and co-morbidities. The 2023 Nutriage study revealed that approximately half of the patients referred to a oncogeriatrician had lost more than 5% of their body weight in the last 6 months [15]. In particular, the prevalence of malnutrition in oesogastric and digestive cancers among a population with a median age of 63 is approximately 55% (pancreas 54%, liver 55%, oesophagogastric 53%) [16,17].

The prevalence of malnutrition increases with age [18] and is higher in digestive cancers. In the study by Poisson et al., involving patients referred to an oncogeriatrician, mortality at 6 months was 20.5%, and cachexia increased the risk of mortality independently of age. Its prevalence is estimated at 52% [19]. In a 2021 review, researchers found a significant link between nutritional status and higher intermediate- and long-term mortality [20].

Symptoms associated with undernutrition differ somewhat in older patients, with loss of appetite, difficulty chewing, dry mouth, and fatigue, but less nausea and vomiting than in younger patients [18,21]. Following weight loss, regaining their initial weight is harder for older individuals than their younger counterpart, even over the long term [22]. Managing malnutrition in older adults can be challenging, but evidence shows that oral nutritional supplements help prevent weight loss, even in pancreatic cancer patients [23]. Measuring resting energy expenditure could aid in the selection of personalized treatment, considering that cancer is associated with dysfunctions in energy homeostasis. An increase in resting energy expenditure can lead to weight loss and is associated with a higher risk of early chemotherapy-limiting toxicity in older cancer patients [24].

3.2.3. Walking and Muscle Function

Changes in body composition associated with aging, characterized by increased fat mass and diminished lean mass, coupled with weight loss and muscle mass reduction, contribute to impaired walking, compromised balance, and a decline in autonomy. Current recommendations for nutritional assessment by oncogeriatricians emphasize the investigation of sarcopenia. Sarcopenia is linked to a 6-month mortality rate of 23% in an all-cancer population averaging 83 years of age (comprising 10.2% non-colorectal digestive cancers and 15% colorectal cancers) [15]. In cancers of the oesophagogastric junction, sarcopenia becomes more prevalent as patients age. Its persistence even after intensive renutrition during neoadjuvant chemotherapy is correlated with heightened mortality and could be considered as a criterion for determining the appropriateness of surgical management [25].

Beyond muscle mass, muscle density may also influence functionality. Walking speed has been correlated with mortality after the age of 65 and is associated with frailty, with a threshold of 1 m per second (m/s) for older cancer patients [26,27]. Specifically, in non-colorectal digestive cancers, the Panesage cohort revealed, through multivariate analysis, that a gait speed below 0.8 m/s is correlated with treatment adaptations compared to reference management [28]. Notably, the gait speed of 1.09 m/s in patients selected by oncologists to receive bi-chemotherapy for bronchial cancer exceeds the frailty threshold, indicating an intuitive consideration of this motor parameter by oncologists [29].

Gait disorders elevate the risk of falls and impede autonomy, requiring consideration in the selection of therapies, especially concerning chemotherapy neurotoxicity. Considering fall's impact on morbidity and mortality, onco-geriatricians must identify sedentary lifestyles, analyse motor functions, and assess muscle mass. Comorbidities such as diabetes or a narrow lumbar canal, which could intensify the consequences of neurotoxicity, should be documented. Physical activity, even in older cancer patients, has been demonstrated to alleviate fatigue. In pancreatic cancer, physical activity not only enhances quality of life but also tends to improve overall survival [30].

3.2.4. Cognitive Disorders

Cognitive disorders show an age-associated increase and are not consistently diagnosed, particularly in their early stages. These disorders may delay the diagnosis of cancer [31] and elevate mortality rates [32]. Although the period following a cancer diagnosis is not ideal for exhaustive cognitive testing, screening for pre-existing or cancer-related neurocognitive disorders is imperative due to their impact on cancer management. The Montreal Cognitive Assessment (MOCA) scale appears to be the most suitable tool for screening patients for cognitive disorders [33]. In the surgical context, memory disorders are a risk factor for postoperative confusion, which, in turn, is associated with postoperative complications, prolonged length of stay, and increased mortality [34–36]. Cognitive disorders also function as risk factors for poor chemotherapy tolerance.

Evaluating initial cognitive functioning is crucial, as certain cognitive issues are linked directly to cancer itself—through inflammation and fatigue—or indirectly through depressive symptoms. Various systemic treatments, whose specific impact on cognition is challenging to discern due to multiple influencing factors, also exhibit cognitive effects [37]. The concept of "chemobrain", defining cognitive impairment associated with chemotherapy, has been extensively studied in adjuvant breast cancer, where 70% of patients report memory complaints during or after chemotherapy [38].

To date, there are no recommendations for adapting or selecting chemotherapies based on pre-existing cognitive impairment. A study involving patients with a median age of 77 awaiting first-line chemotherapy, including 42.9% with digestive cancer, revealed MMSE deterioration in 18.7% of patients. Factors associated with the risk of MMSE alteration during treatment included initial abnormal MMSE, altered Mini Nutritional Assessment (MNA), pain, and alteration of the QLQC30 quality of life questionnaire [39]. The cognitive functions affected by cancer treatments primarily involve memory, concentration, information processing speed, and executive functions. Cognitive disorders or memory complaints may evolve spontaneously after cancer treatment or persist over the long term, and cognitive rehabilitation can assist in managing them [40]. Studies investigating the effects of immunotherapy on cognitive status are also underway [41].

Finally, the detection of sensory disorders is essential to ensure proper understanding of shared information and contributes to mitigating postoperative delirium.

3.2.5. Thymic Assessment

Depression is a common occurrence in oncogeriatrics, with a prevalence of 28.4% based on an assessment of over 1000 patients averaging 80 years old [42]. However, it is frequently under-diagnosed [43]. Several geriatric parameters, including polypharmacy, comorbidities, and functional status, are independently associated with the occurrence of depression. Notably, pancreatic cancer stands out among cancers with one of the highest rates of depression, estimated at around 40% [42].

3.2.6. Impact of Comorbidities

Various scoring systems are available for assessing comorbidities, including the Charlson score (with different versions) and the CIRS-G. To standardize geriatric assessments, it is currently recommended to perform at least one assessment using the modified Charlson score [9]. When evaluating postoperative complications and causes of mortality in pancreatic and biliary surgery, impaired cardiorespiratory function and its management emerge as crucial factors.

After hepatic resection, mortality tends to be higher in older patients, primarily due to cardiorespiratory complications, as opposed to hepatic complications, which do not exhibit significant age-related differences [44]. Additionally, there is an increased risk of cardiorespiratory complications associated with pancreatic surgery [45,46].

3.2.7. Therapeutics in Onco-Geriatrics: Limiting Polypharmacy, Iatrogenesis, and Drug Interactions

Age-related changes in body composition, as well as alterations in renal and hepatic function, modify the pharmacokinetics and risk of adverse effects of various molecules. Investigating potential drug interactions is imperative, given the frequent use of polypharmacy in this population. The prevalence of polypharmacy in the older patients varies widely, ranging from 13 to 92%, depending on the definition and characteristics of the studied population [47]. In the Panesage study, where polypharmacy is defined as taking $\geq$5 active ingredients per day, it was found to be 69% [27]. Collecting information about all the molecules taken by a patient necessitates specific interrogation, including inquiries about various prescriptions and self-medication practices, such as phytotherapy. The STOPP-START tool can aid in determining whether all prescribed medications are indicated or if any should be reconsidered [48].

Pharmaceutical reconciliation is advantageous when possible to limit iatrogenic effects resulting from drug interactions [49]. The impact of polypharmacy in older people with cancer on mortality is not clear but it is well established on morbidity [47]. Polypharmacy has been linked to a higher number of falls, drug interactions, and unplanned hospitalizations [50].

At the conclusion of the comprehensive geriatric assessment, clinicians obtain key elements to guide treatment decisions, but also to assess prognosis. Various geriatric parameters, such as the G8 score (prognostic of overall survival) [51], walking speed before therapeutic decision (predicting frailty with a threshold at 1 m/s) [27], and autonomy assessment by Activities of Daily Living (ADL) (predicting overall survival and postoperative complications) [10] offer valuable prognostic insights. Furthermore, scores combining oncological and geriatric parameters facilitate the estimation of short-term mortality risk, prompting considerations about the appropriateness of cancer-specific treatments when the risk is exceptionally high [52].

The geriatrician's role involves continuous monitoring of the patient throughout their care journey, in collaboration with the organ specialist. Changes in geriatric parameters may necessitate specific adjustments in both geriatric and oncological interventions.

4. Support for Surgical Care

4.1. Preoperative Optimization

4.1.1. Prognostic Evaluation of Surgical Risks Through Geriatric Assessment

Older adults and more comorbid patients face an elevated risk of complications during oncological surgery. The likelihood of experiencing a geriatric event (confusion, dehydration, falls, fractures, pressure sores) is correlated with the risk of specific complications, with higher occurrences observed in gastric or pancreatic surgeries compared to other abdominal locations [53].

4.1.2. Prehabilitation

The Emergence of Prehabilitation

The importance of preoperative functional status in influencing postoperative recovery is now firmly established. It has been demonstrated that pre-therapeutic gait speed is a predictor of frailty [27]. In a study involving nearly 200 patients aged over 70 undergoing abdominal cancer surgery, superior pre-operative physical performance was associated with a reduced risk of severe complications and a lower rate of discharge to a rehabilitation ward compared to a return home [54]. Sarcopenic patients, as defined by the consensus of the European Working Group on Sarcopenia in Older People, are at a higher risk of postoperative complications and increased mortality following abdominal surgery [55].

These findings highlighted the need for preoperative interventions aimed at enhancing patients' functional reserve, improving tolerance to the physiological stress of major surgery, and reducing the risks of postoperative complications, and give rise to the concept of prehabilitation [56].

What Type of Prehabilitation?

Prehabilitation typically consists of three components: physical exercise, nutritional support, and measures to reduce anxiety. While these components can be applied individually, a meta-analysis on patients with oesophagogastric cancer revealed that multimodal prehabilitation significantly reduced overall complication rates compared to standard care, unlike unimodal prehabilitation [57]. These findings align with broader research on abdominal and colorectal cancer surgeries [56,58,59].

The implementation of these three components remains highly heterogeneous and minimally validated, particularly for non-colorectal digestive cancers in older patients as most available data originate from studies on colorectal cancer or, more broadly, abdominal cancers.

The three components of prehabilitation are:

1. Adapted physical activity

Initiating prehabilitation requires an initial assessment, including estimation of the intensity of current physical activity in METs (Metabolic Equivalent of Task), and measurements of muscle mass and function. This assessment helps define a personalized program with specific improvement objectives.

The physical activity component typically includes three approaches, which may be used individually or in combination: Aerobic Exercises (AE), Resistance Training (RT), and Inspiratory Muscle Training (IMT). Before major abdominal surgery, a potential clinical advantage is observed when combining AE and IMT [60].

The optimal frequency, intensity, and modalities (autonomous, partially supervised, or fully supervised) remains unknown. Professional supervision, when feasible, may enhance the positive effects of exercise [61] but the optimal frequency, intensity, and modalities (autonomous, partially supervised, or fully supervised) remains unknown.

2. Nutritional management

Nutritional management aims to prevent or address undernutrition and promote anabolism. This primarily involves a high-protein, high-calorie diet with food fortification and oral nutritional supplements. The various options for taking oral nutritional supplements must be explained to ensure patient compliance. Enteral nutrition is preferred if oral intake is insufficient, as it prepares the digestive tract for resumption of feeding and is less prone to complications other than inhalation pneumonitis. In cases of cognitive impairment or risk of inhalation, artificial nutrition may not be recommended. If the digestive tract is non-functional, or if enteral nutrition fails, parenteral nutrition is recommended. The European Society for Clinical Nutrition and Metabolism recommends perioperative immuno-nutrition for patients scheduled for upper gastrointestinal cancer surgery to reduce the risk of postoperative infection and length of stay [62].

3. Psychological care

Anxiety and depression are prevalent among cancer patients, especially as age advances. Symptoms of depression in older patients can be less apparent than in younger patients but have a negative impact on post-operative follow-up, including length of stay, recovery, pain, and quality of life. Psychological care is therefore essential and should be considered alongside physical and nutritional status [63]. Psychological management can also serve as motivational support for patients undergoing lifestyle changes. Despite this, few studies focus on the psychological component of prehabilitation. A 2015 review of psychological prehabilitation before cancer surgery indicates that it improves quality of life and physical symptoms, with some studies showing sustained benefits at 1-year post-surgery. Some studies even suggest that psychological care may enhance immune function [64]. More recently, a 2022 literature review showed a trend towards improved psychological outcomes following psychological prehabilitation, particularly when psychologist-led [65].

Prehabilitation Duration

The optimal duration of prehabilitation appears to be 3 to 6 weeks, ideally integrated with necessary treatments and examinations prior to surgery [66,67], yet no specific data on non-colorectal digestive cancer surgery are available.

Population and Efficacy of Prehabilitation

The effectiveness of prehabilitation, particularly concerning traditional surgical criteria, has yet to be demonstrated, possibly due to study and evaluation criteria heterogeneity. In colorectal cancer, despite numerous studies, no improvement in survival has been proven [68]. This may be partly linked to the choice of target population. The article by M. Coca Martinez and F. Carli underscores that studies concentrating on high-risk, frail, or older patients are more likely to demonstrate improvements in complication rates or length of stay, in contrast to those involving a broader patient population [58]. Also, in colorectal cancer, patients with a walking distance of less than 400 m in the 6-min test improve their walking distance more and are more likely to recover their baseline abilities postoperatively than those with better preoperative walking abilities [69], suggesting that prehabilitation yields greater potential for recovery in frail subjects.

On the positive side, evidence suggests that prehabilitation enhances both pre- and post-operative physical conditions and reduces the length of hospital stay. For patients specifically managed for carcinologic oesophagogastric surgery, improvements in functional abilities have been observed after prehabilitation [70]. Another study in a similar population demonstrates a reduction in postoperative pneumonitis and morbidity, assessed by complications greater than or equal to II on the Clavien Dindo scale, along with improvements in length of stay and quality of life for dyspnoea and physical functioning [71].

In a meta-analysis covering all digestive cancers, prehabilitation was associated with a reduction in length of stay by 1.78 days, although it showed no demonstrated effect on functional capacity, complications, or postoperative mortality [72].

Contrastingly, a 2022 review focusing on hepato-pancreato-biliary surgery did not find the reduction in length of stay associated with prehabilitation [73]. In a specific study on pancreatic cancer by Ngo-Huang, aiming for mainly physical prehabilitation during neoadjuvant treatment, improvements in physical capacities were observed in the intervention arm. However, no reduction in complications or postoperative length of stay was found, possibly due to a lack of statistical power and a relatively younger patient population (average age 66) [74]. In their 2022 study, Deprato et al. found a significant improvement in preoperative and postoperative physical performance while length of stay, complication rates, and mortality demonstrated no statistically significant differences, but trended towards benefit from prehabilitation [75].

There is not enough evidence yet to support the systematic inclusion of prehabilitation in ERAS protocols for non-colorectal digestive cancer surgeries. However, it could provide a valuable addition to conventional protocols, particularly for frail geriatric patients undergoing major surgeries or neoadjuvant treatments [76].

In addition to the tri-modal prehabilitation approach outlined earlier, it remains crucial to uphold classic peri-operative management practices. This includes endeavours such as smoking and alcohol cessation where possible, meticulous management of co-morbidities, and vigilant prevention of anaemia. In the targeted population, special attention should be dedicated to the prevention of confusion, ensuring a comprehensive approach to optimize patient outcomes throughout the surgical journey.

4.2. Post-Operative Co-Management

4.2.1. Co-Management Between Surgeons and Geriatricians: Impact on Mortality and Surgical Complications

The study conducted by Armin Shahrokni et al., encompassing over 30% of patients with digestive cancers, half of which were non-colorectal, revealed significant findings related to co-management between surgeons and geriatricians. The co-management approach demonstrated a notable reduction in mortality at 3 months, with an odds ratio (OR) of 0.58. However, despite the positive impact on mortality, there was no observed difference in surgical complications [77]. This underscores the importance of further exploration into the specific aspects of comorbidity management within the co-management framework. Several prospective interventional studies on the benefits of co-management between surgeons and geriatricians are underway.

4.2.2. Fast-Track Surgery

The post-operative management of older patients should align with modern concepts such as "Fast-Track Surgery" or Enhanced Recovery After Surgery (ERAS) protocols. This approach involves a multimodal, multidisciplinary strategy to control the response to surgical stress and alleviate its consequences, resulting in accelerated post-operative recovery and reduced medical consultations [78–80].

The key principles of Fast-Track Surgery include minimizing aggression (utilizing minimally invasive approaches, avoiding unnecessary interventions such as drainage, urinary, or gastric catheterization), early refeeding and mobilization (getting up and into the chair on day 0 or 1), and sparing the use of morphine for postoperative analgesia. Recent evidence supports the applicability of Fast-Track Surgery to older patients, and shows and shorter length for older adults who benefited from ERAS [81,82].

ERAS even demonstrates a considerable reduction in the postoperative complication rates for studies interested in colorectal cancer [83–86], but evidences are poorer for non-colorectal cancers. However, a study on gastric cancer found that ERAS patients had a shorter hospital stay after surgery and fewer Clavien-Dindo grade IIIa complications than those in the conventional group [87].

This approach is validated for general populations undergoing digestive surgery and is applicable to older patients, provided the nursing teams are equipped to handle the specificities of this demographic [88,89].

4.2.3. Post-Operative Delirium: Prevention and Management

The incidence of postoperative delirium is reported to be 15% for controlled surgeries and 20% for emergency procedures. These disorders complicate healthcare team management, increase postoperative mortality (19% vs. 8%), and extend the length of stay (21 days vs. 8 days) [90]. Confounding risk factors include high age, high American Society of Anaesthesiologists (ASA) score, low body mass index (BMI), low albuminemia, intraoperative hypotension, intraoperative blood transfusions, and a history of excessive alcohol consumption [91].

A systematic search for confusion syndrome, which can be efficiently and promptly conducted using the Confusion Assessment Method [92], enables early management if post-operative delirium syndrome is confirmed.

The most effective strategy involves the prevention of delirium, primarily relying on a multidimensional, non-pharmacological approach as a first-line treatment. These preventive measures, which also serve as initial interventions in the presence of confirmed confusion, encompass various aspects [93,94], including:

- Detecting pre-existing cognitive disorders.
- Limiting iatrogenicity: this involves restricting the prescription of certain medications that may contribute to confusion, such as anticholinergic drugs, certain painkillers, such as tramadol or meperidine, and psychotropic drugs.
- Ensuring proper correction of any sensory impairments and reorientation.
- Addressing sleep disorders, including sleep apnoea syndromes.
- The other three points overlap with ERAS: Managing transit or urinary disorders, encouraging early postoperative walking and providing technical aids if necessary, and managing pain.

Numerous studies come to the conclusion that postoperative management of the older adults, including ERAS, is associated with a reduced rate of confusion and an improved preservation of cognitive function [95,96].

When non-medication approaches prove insufficient to manage postoperative confusion syndrome, cautious medication management may be considered. This is particularly relevant in cases where confusion hinders essential treatments or examinations or generates considerable distress. In such instances, the following principles should guide medication use:

1. Prefer the use of a single medication, chosen based on the specific symptoms of the patient.
2. Administer the medication at the lowest effective dose.
3. Prefer oral administration whenever possible.
4. Choose medications with the least anticholinergic effects possible to mitigate potential cognitive side effects.

It is important to be cautious in medication management and prioritize the well-being of the older patient. If benzodiazepines are deemed necessary (for anxiety or alcohol withdrawal syndrome), opting for short-acting formulations is preferable. In cases of severe agitation that may lead to harm to self or others, low-dose neuroleptic treatment may be considered. However, such medication usage should be carefully monitored and reassessed early in the treatment process. Melatonin can be an option for circadian rhythm disturbances [97].

It is noteworthy that while pharmacological interventions may be utilized to manage acute symptoms, no pharmacological treatment has been conclusively proven effective in preventing or treating postoperative confusional syndrome [98]. The decision to use medications should be made on a case-by-case basis, weighing the potential benefits against the risks and considering the specific circumstances of the patient. Additionally, ongoing assessment and re-evaluation are crucial elements in the pharmacological management of postoperative confusion syndrome.

Support for surgical care and co-management between surgeon and geriatrician are summarized in Figure 1.

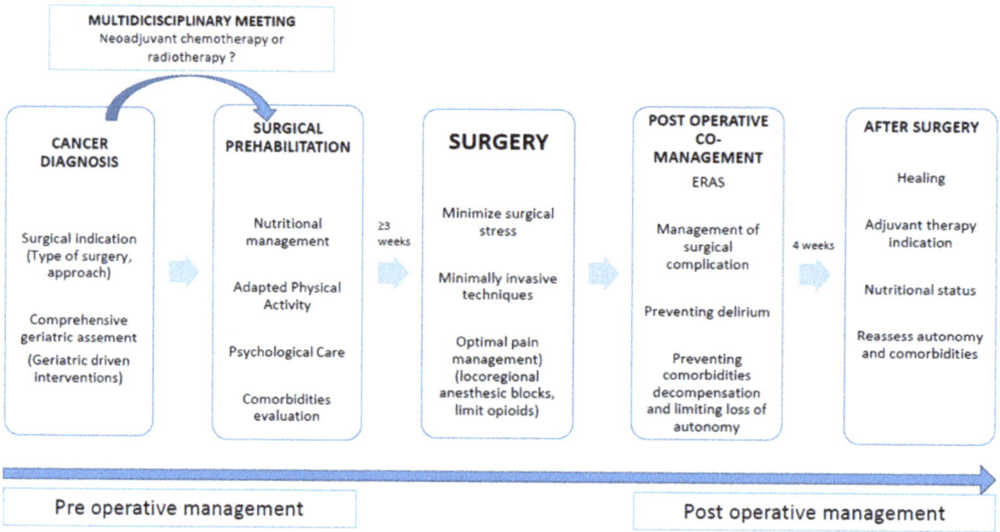

Figure 1. Optimal perioperative management of older patients.

5. Support for Systemic Treatments Management

5.1. Toxicity of Systemic Treatments in Older Patients with Digestive Cancers

Predicting chemotherapy toxicity in older individuals poses a significant challenge. Two specific predictive scores designed for older patients, namely the Chemotherapy Risk Assessment Scale for High-Age Patients (CARG) and the Chemotherapy Risk Assessment Scale for High-Age Patients (CRASH) score, have been developed [99,100]. These scores incorporate both geriatric and oncological criteria to assess the risk of chemotherapy-related toxicity in older individuals. While it has not been specifically studied in the context of digestive cancers, no difference in efficacy between these two scales has been found [101].

Immunotherapy also presents challenges in this population. Although studies across diverse cancers have reported similar toxicity profiles for immunotherapy in older and younger patients, there are higher rates of treatment discontinuation in older individuals experiencing the same level of toxicity [102,103]. To our knowledge, there are no specific studies examining the toxicity of immunotherapy in older individuals with digestive cancers.

In view of the digestive underlying neoplasia, and the reduced absorption of vitamins with age, we recommend that vitamins B9 and 12 be measured and supplemented if necessary, and that iron be supplemented by venous route if necessary, prior to chemotherapy or immunotherapy.

Similarly, as the action is muscular and not just bone-related, pre-therapeutic vitamin D dosage and supplementation may be useful [104].

Geriatric specificities related to the tolerance of systemic treatments in digestive oncology are presented in Table 1

Table 1. Geriatric specificities related to the tolerance of systemic treatments in digestive oncology.

Molecules	Main Toxicities	Comorbidities to Look For	Geriatric Outcomes	Recommended Course of Action
OXALIPLATINE	Neuropathic	Diabetes, narrow lumbar canal, other causes of neuropathy	Increased falls, functional decline, need for assistance with dressing and grooming Infections	↓ dose, stop Home aids, remote alarm, physiotherapy, technical aids
	Hematologic	Hemopathy, low bone marrow reserves	Anaemia: falls, cardiac decompensation, loss of autonomy Infections, falls, wounds	↓ dose Influenza/COVID/pneum-ococcal vaccination Erythropoietin
	Digestive	Nutrition		Weight monitoring, dietary management, caregiver education
5-FLUOROURACIL	Coronary spasm	Severe unstable coronary artery disease		Cardiologic advice
	Transit disorders	Incontinence, gait disorders	Risk of falls, undernutrition Risk of dehydration	↓ dose, ↓ bolus Perforated chair, protection, hydration, dietary care
	Hand-foot syndrome	Gait disorders	Risk of falls, loss of autonomy (dressing, cooking)	↓ dose Implementation of aids
TAXANES	Neuropathic	Diabetes, narrow lumbar canal, other causes of neuropathy	Increased falls, functional decline, need for assistance with dressing and grooming	↓ dose, stop Home aids, remote alarm, physiotherapy, technical aids
BEVACIZUMAB	High blood pressure	High blood pressure, heart failure	Risk of decompensation of cardiovascular comorbidities	Monitoring of blood pressure and weight
	Proteinuria	Renal insufficiency		
	Thrombosis and haemorrhage	History of thrombosis, anticoagulant, valve prosthesis		Discuss low-molecular-weight heparin LMWH if direct oral anticoagulant (DAO)or Vitamin K antagonist VKA
	Healing disorders	Unscheduled surgery for comorbidity		Cancel or differ scheduled non-urgent surgery

Table 1. *Cont.*

Molecules	Main Toxicities	Comorbidities to Look For	Geriatric Outcomes	Recommended Course of Action
IRINOTECAN	Transit disorders	Incontinence, gait disorders	Increased falls	↓ dose, stop
			Risk of dehydration and malnutrition	Wardrobe chair, diapers, incontinence briefs, hydration, dietary management
	Medullary	Hemopathy, low bone marrow reserves	Infections	Influenza/COVID/pneumococcal vaccination
			Anaemia: falls, cardiac decompensation, loss of autonomy	Erythropoietin
				Providing Human assistance
NIVOLUMAB	Asthenia	General condition	Loss of autonomy	Adaptation of aids
PEMBROLIZUMAB	Rash	Xerosis, pruritus	Pruritus, wounds	Emollient, antihistamines (avoid hydroxizine-type anticholinergics due to cognitive and urinary risk)
	Diarrhoea	Incontinence, walking disorders	Increasing falls, risk of dehydration Walking difficulties	Remote alarm, therapeutic education for patient or caregiver
	Arthralgia	Osteoarthritis, polymyalgia rheumatica, rheumatoid arthritis		Analgesia, rheumatologic advice, technical aids, remote alarm
	Thyroid dysfunction	Cognitive impairment	Increased cognitive impairment, heart disease	Endocrinologist advice
ATEZOLIZUMAB	Asthenia	Cardiopathy	Loss of autonomy	See above
	Pruritus			
	Arthralgia			
	Nausea			

5.2. Co-Management Between Oncologists and Geriatricians

Demonstrating the benefits of co-management between oncologists and geriatricians poses challenges due to diverse care pathways and numerous inherent evaluation biases. Nevertheless, findings from several recent studies indicate a reduction in treatment toxicity and improved completion of systemic treatments attributed to geriatric management. It is noteworthy that these studies are not exclusive to non-colorectal digestive cancers [105].

For instance, in the GAIN study, interventions based on comprehensive geriatric assessment (CGA) resulted in a decreased incidence of grade III toxicity at 50.5% compared to 60.3% in the control group ($p = 0.02$) [106]. While there was an increase in the formulation of advance directives, no significant differences were observed in emergency room visits, unscheduled hospitalizations, length of stay, survival, chemotherapy duration, or dose. A recent literature review reported a favourable treatment completion rate in 4 out of

6 studies following geriatric assessment [107]. Similarly, the GAP 70 study demonstrated a reduction in grade 3–5 toxicities (Hazard Ratio of 0.74), accompanied by geriatric benefits such as fewer falls and lower discontinuation rates in the intervention arm [108]. The INTEGERATE study corroborated these findings by revealing an enhancement in quality of life and a decrease in unscheduled hospitalizations, aligning with similar results from other studies [107,109].

However, the impact of geriatric management on overall survival with systemic treatments remains uncertain, with conflicting results across studies. In a recent "before/after" study involving 40% of oesophagogastric cancers within our target population, a positive gain in survival was observed following the implementation of geriatric management [110].

6. Conclusions

Limited geriatric-specific data exist for non-colorectal digestive cancers in current literature. Nevertheless, the merits of incorporating geriatric management into the collaborative efforts of surgeons and oncologists are gaining recognition and are increasingly being validated, as confirmed by the review of oesophagogastric cancers by T. Aparicio et al. [111]. While the impact on mortality remains challenging to establish due to various biases, there is accumulating evidence suggesting positive outcomes in terms of criteria such as decreased chemotherapy complications and shorter surgical stays.

It is essential to emphasize that the role of the geriatrician is complementary to that of other specialists. Their involvement spans decision-making processes, care pathway management, and the prevention of comorbidity decompensation, geriatric syndromes, and loss of autonomy. This interdisciplinary approach aims to address the unique needs and challenges faced by older patients with non-colorectal digestive cancers, enhancing overall patient care and outcomes. Further research and ongoing studies are expected to provide additional clarity and insights into the specific benefits of geriatric management in this context.

Author Contributions: Design: or acquisition, analysis or interpretation of data: A.A., J.E., M.L. and A.C.-T. Drafted the article: A.A., J.E., A.C.-T., M.L. and V.F.-D. Revised the article: A.A., J.E., M.L., A.C.-T., M.L., G.B.-C., P.H., V.F.-D. and T.A. All authors have read and agreed to the published version of the manuscript.

Funding: This research received no specific grant from any funding agency in the public, commercial, or not-for-profit sectors.

Informed Consent Statement: Not applicable.

Data Availability Statement: Not applicable.

Conflicts of Interest: A.A. received support to attend conferences from Viatris and Advanz Pharma. M.L. received support to attend conferences from Viatris. P.H. received financial support from AztraZeneca and honoraria from Servier and Viatris. T.A. received honoraria from BMS, Pierre Fabre, Bayer and MSD. Other authors declare no conflicts of interest.

Large Language Model Statement: As the authors are not native British speakers, they utilized ChatGPT 4.0 model as an editing tool to: review and amend grammatical and spelling mistakes; ensure linguistic consistency and coherence. Moreover: to ensure that ChatGPT 4.0 did not introduce plagiarized wording while correcting grammatical mistakes or linguistic inconsistencies, the manuscript has been submitted to two different plagiarism checkers: duplichecker.com assessed on the 2 June 2024 which found 99% unique text and originality.ai which found 100% unique text.

References

1. Pilleron, S.; Soto-Perez-de-Celis, E.; Vignat, J.; Ferlay, J.; Soerjomataram, I.; Bray, F.; Sarfati, D. Estimated global cancer incidence in the oldest adults in 2018 and projections to 2050. *Int. J. Cancer* **2021**, *148*, 601–608. [CrossRef] [PubMed]
2. Sung, H.; Ferlay, J.; Siegel, R.L.; Laversanne, M.; Soerjomataram, I.; Jemal, A.; Bray, F. Global Cancer Statistics 2020: GLOBOCAN Estimates of Incidence and Mortality Worldwide for 36 Cancers in 185 Countries. *CA Cancer J. Clin.* **2021**, *71*, 209–249. [CrossRef] [PubMed]
3. Gilabert, M.; Raoul, J.L.; Rousseau, F. How to treat pancreatic adenocarcinoma in elderly: How far can we go in 2017? *J. Geriatr. Oncol.* **2017**, *8*, 407–412. [CrossRef]
4. Canouï-Poitrine, F.; Lièvre, A.; Dayde, F.; Lopez-Trabada-Ataz, D.; Baumgaertner, I.; Dubreuil, O.; Brunetti, F.; Coriat, R.; Maley, K.; Pernot, S.; et al. Inclusion of Older Patients with Cancer in Clinical Trials: The SAGE Prospective Multicenter Cohort Survey. *Oncologist* **2019**, *24*, e1351–e1359. [CrossRef]
5. Pamoukdjian, F.; Aparicio, T.; Zelek, L.; Boubaya, M.; Caillet, P.; François, V.; de Decker, L.; Lévy, V.; Sebbane, G.; Paillaud, E. Impaired mobility, depressed mood, cognitive impairment and polypharmacy are independently associated with disability in older cancer outpatients: The prospective Physical Frailty in Elderly Cancer patients (PF-EC) cohort study. *J. Geriatr. Oncol.* **2017**, *8*, 190–195. [CrossRef]
6. Soubeyran, P.; Bellera, C.; Goyard, J.; Heitz, D.; Curé, H.; Rousselot, H.; Albrand, G.; Servent, V.; Jean, O.S.; van Praagh, I.; et al. Screening for vulnerability in older cancer patients: The ONCODAGE Prospective Multicenter Cohort Study. *PLoS ONE* **2014**, *9*, e115060. [CrossRef]
7. Martinez-Tapia, C.; Canoui-Poitrine, F.; Bastuji-Garin, S.; Soubeyran, P.; Mathoulin-Pelissier, S.; Tournigand, C.; Paillaud, E.; Laurent, M.; Audureau, E. ELCAPA Study Group Optimizing the G8 Screening Tool for Older Patients with Cancer: Diagnostic Performance and Validation of a Six-Item Version. *Oncologist* **2016**, *21*, 188–195. [CrossRef]
8. Wildiers, H.; Heeren, P.; Puts, M.; Topinkova, E.; Janssen-Heijnen, M.L.G.; Extermann, M.; Falandry, C.; Artz, A.; Brain, E.; Colloca, G.; et al. International Society of Geriatric Oncology Consensus on Geriatric Assessment in Older Patients with Cancer. *J. Clin. Oncol.* **2014**, *32*, 2595–2603. [CrossRef]
9. Paillaud, E.; Soubeyran, P.; Caillet, P.; Cudennec, T.; Brain, E.; Terret, C.; Etchepare, F.; Mourey, L.; Aparicio, T.; Pamoukdjian, F.; et al. Multidisciplinary development of the Geriatric Core Dataset for clinical research in older patients with cancer: A French initiative with international survey. *Eur. J. Cancer* **2018**, *103*, 61–68. [CrossRef]
10. Couderc, A.-L.; Boulahssass, R.; Nouguerède, E.; Gobin, N.; Guérin, O.; Villani, P.; Barlesi, F.; Paillaud, E. Functional status in a geriatric oncology setting: A review. *J. Geriatr. Oncol.* **2019**, *10*, 884–894. [CrossRef]
11. Couderc, A.-L.; Suchon, P.; Saliba-Serre, B.; Rey, D.; Nouguerede, E.; Arcani, R.; Farnault, L.; Daumas, A.; Courcier, A.; Duffaud, F.; et al. Functional status in older patients with cancer. *J. Geriatr. Oncol.* **2022**, *13*, 40–45. [CrossRef]
12. Okuyama, A.; Kosaka, H.; Kaibori, M.; Higashi, T.; Ogawa, A. Activities of daily living after surgery among older patients with gastrointestinal and hepatobiliary-pancreatic cancers: A retrospective observational study using nationwide health services utilisation data from Japan. *BMJ Open* **2023**, *13*, e070415. [CrossRef] [PubMed]
13. Hjelmeland, I.H.H.; Drageset, J.; Nordvik, Ø.; Beisland, E.G. Quality of life in home-dwelling cancer patients aged 80 years and older: A systematic review. *Health Qual. Life Outcomes* **2022**, *20*, 154. [CrossRef] [PubMed]
14. Zarit, S.H.; Reever, K.E.; Bach-Peterson, J. Relatives of the impaired elderly: Correlates of feelings of burden. *Gerontologist* **1980**, *20*, 649–655. [CrossRef] [PubMed]
15. Martinez-Tapia, C.; Rougette, K.; Fossey-Diaz, V.; Cudennec, T.; Taleb, C.; Balardy, L.; Mertens, C.; Mitha, N.; Bringuier, M.; Maley, K.; et al. Prevalence of Four Sarcopenia Criteria in Older Patients with Cancer, and Their Predictive Value for 6-Month Mortality: The NutriAgeCancer National Prospective Cohort Study. *Nutrients* **2023**, *15*, 1508. [CrossRef]
16. Gyan, E.; Raynard, B.; Durand, J.-P.; Lacau Saint Guily, J.; Gouy, S.; Movschin, M.L.; Khemissa, F.; Flori, N.; Oziel-Taieb, S.; Bannier Braticevic, C.; et al. Malnutrition in Patients with Cancer: Comparison of Perceptions by Patients, Relatives, and Physicians-Results of the NutriCancer2012 Study. *JPEN J. Parenter. Enteral Nutr.* **2018**, *42*, 255–260. [CrossRef]
17. Akagündüz, D.D.; Şahin, H.; Akagündüz, B.; Akagündüz, D.D.; Şahin, H.; Akagündüz, B. Malnutrition and Related Factors in Older Patients with Gastrointestinal Cancer Receiving Chemotherapy. *Cureus* **2024**, *16*, e58252. [CrossRef]
18. de Pinho, N.B.; Martucci, R.B.; Rodrigues, V.D.; D'Almeida, C.A.; Thuler, L.C.S.; Saunders, C.; Jager-Wittenaar, H.; Peres, W.A.F. High prevalence of malnutrition and nutrition impact symptoms in older patients with cancer: Results of a Brazilian multicenter study. *Cancer* **2020**, *126*, 156–164. [CrossRef]
19. Poisson, J.; Martinez-Tapia, C.; Heitz, D.; Geiss, R.; Albrand, G.; Falandry, C.; Gisselbrecht, M.; Couderc, A.-L.; Boulahssass, R.; Liuu, E.; et al. Prevalence and prognostic impact of cachexia among older patients with cancer: A nationwide cross-sectional survey (NutriAgeCancer). *J. Cachexia Sarcopenia Muscle* **2021**, *12*, 1477–1488. [CrossRef]
20. Hamaker, M.E.; Oosterlaan, F.; van Huis, L.H.; Thielen, N.; Vondeling, A.; van den Bos, F. Nutritional status and interventions for patients with cancer—A systematic review. *J. Geriatr. Oncol.* **2021**, *12*, 6–21. [CrossRef]

21. Lacau St Guily, J.; Bouvard, É.; Raynard, B.; Goldwasser, F.; Maget, B.; Prevost, A.; Seguy, D.; Romano, O.; Narciso, B.; Couet, C.; et al. NutriCancer: A French observational multicentre cross-sectional study of malnutrition in elderly patients with cancer. *J. Geriatr. Oncol.* **2018**, *9*, 74–80. [CrossRef] [PubMed]
22. Roberts, S.B.; Fuss, P.; Heyman, M.B.; Evans, W.J.; Tsay, R.; Rasmussen, H.; Fiatarone, M.; Cortiella, J.; Dallal, G.E.; Young, V.R. Control of food intake in older men. *JAMA* **1994**, *272*, 1601–1606. [CrossRef] [PubMed]
23. Baguley, B.J.; Arnold, H.; Bence, A.; Bryant, E.; Martino, E.; Stojanoski, K.; Ackerly, S.; Laing, E.; Jong, J.; Kiss, N.; et al. Systematic review of nutrition interventions in older patients with cancer: A synthesis of evidence and a future research priority. *J. Geriatr. Oncol.* **2025**, *16*, 102181. [CrossRef] [PubMed]
24. Boudou-Rouquette, P.; de Moura, A.; Martinez-Tapia, C.; Serrano, A.G.; Chahwakilian, A.; Jouinot, A.; Ulmann, G.; Orvoën, G.; Chambraud, C.; Durand, J.-P.; et al. Energy expenditure profiles and the risk of early limiting toxicity in older patients with cancer: The ELCAPA-25 prospective cohort survey. *Clin. Nutr.* **2022**, *41*, 1073–1082. [CrossRef]
25. de Mathelin, P.; Manfredelli, S.; Delhorme, J.-B.; Venkatasamy, A.; Rohr, S.; Brigand, C.; Gaiddon, C.; Romain, B. Sarcopenia remaining after intensive nutritional feeding support could be a criterion for the selection of patients for surgery for oesogastric junction adenocarcinoma. *Eur. J. Surg. Oncol.* **2023**, *49*, 384–391. [CrossRef]
26. Studenski, S.; Perera, S.; Patel, K.; Rosano, C.; Faulkner, K.; Inzitari, M.; Brach, J.; Chandler, J.; Cawthon, P.; Connor, E.B.; et al. Gait speed and survival in older adults. *JAMA* **2011**, *305*, 50–58. [CrossRef]
27. Pamoukdjian, F.; Canoui-Poitrine, F.; Longelin-Lombard, C.; Aparicio, T.; Ganne, N.; Wind, P.; Martinez-Tapia, C.; Audureau, E.; Sebbane, G.; Zelek, L.; et al. Diagnostic performance of gait speed, G8 and G8 modified indices to screen for vulnerability in older cancer patients: The prospective PF-EC cohort study. *Oncotarget* **2017**, *8*, 50393–50402. [CrossRef]
28. Aregui, A.; Mary, F.; Lourenço, N.; Gornet, J.-M.; Cattan, P.; Wind, P.; Aparicio, T.; Pamoukdjian, F. La lenteur de marche est le seul facteur associé à la stratégie thérapeutique adaptée chez les plus de 75 ans atteints de cancer œsogastriques ou pancréato-biliaires: Résultats définitifs de la cohorte PANESAGE. In Proceedings of the Journées Francophones d'Hépato-gastroenterologie et d'Oncologie Digestive, Paris, France, 16–19 March 2023; p. 3. Available online: https://www.jfhod.com/sites/www.jfhod.com/files/2023-03/JFHOD23_Livre-re%CC%81sumes.pdf (accessed on 15 April 2025).
29. Aregui, A.; Pluvy, J.; Sanchez, M.; Israel, T.; Esnault, H.; Guyard, A.; Meyer, M.; Khalil, A.; Zalcman, G.; Raynaud Simon, A.; et al. Measuring Walking Speed Failed to Predict Early Death and Toxicity in Elderly Patients with Metastatic Non-Small-Cell Lung Cancer (NSCLC) Selected for Undergoing First-Line Systemic Treatment: An Observational Exploratory Study. *Cancers* **2022**, *14*, 1344. [CrossRef]
30. Neuzillet, C.; Bouché, O.; Tournigand, C.; Chibaudel, B.; Bauguion, L.; Bengrine-Lefevre, L.; Lopez-Trabada Ataz, D.; Mabro, M.; Metges, J.-P.; Péré-Vergé, D.; et al. Effect of Adapted Physical Activity in Patients with Advanced Pancreatic Cancer: The APACaP GERCOR Randomized Trial. *J. Natl. Compr. Canc Netw.* **2023**, *21*, 1234–1242. [CrossRef]
31. Pal, S.K.; Katheria, V.; Hurria, A. Evaluating the older patient with cancer: Understanding frailty and the geriatric assessment. *CA Cancer J. Clin.* **2010**, *60*, 120–132. [CrossRef]
32. Libert, Y.; Dubruille, S.; Borghgraef, C.; Etienne, A.-M.; Merckaert, I.; Paesmans, M.; Reynaert, C.; Roos, M.; Slachmuylder, J.-L.; Vandenbossche, S.; et al. Vulnerabilities in Older Patients when Cancer Treatment is Initiated: Does a Cognitive Impairment Impact the Two-Year Survival? *PLoS ONE* **2016**, *11*, e0159734. [CrossRef] [PubMed]
33. Rambeau, A.; Beauplet, B.; Laviec, H.; Licaj, I.; Leconte, A.; Chatel, C.; Le Bon, P.; Denhaerynck, J.; Clarisse, B.; Frenkiel, N.; et al. Prospective comparison of the Montreal Cognitive Assessment (MoCA) and the Mini Mental State Examination (MMSE) in geriatric oncology. *J. Geriatr. Oncol.* **2019**, *10*, 235–240. [CrossRef] [PubMed]
34. Olotu, C.; Lebherz, L.; Ascone, L.; Scherwath, A.; Kühn, S.; Härter, M.; Kiefmann, R. Cognitive Deficits in Executive and Language Functions Predict Postoperative Delirium. *J. Cardiothorac. Vasc. Anesth.* **2023**, *37*, 2552–2560. [CrossRef]
35. Lai, C.-C.; Liu, K.-H.; Tsai, C.-Y.; Hsu, J.-T.; Hsueh, S.-W.; Hung, C.-Y.; Chou, W.-C. Risk factors and effect of postoperative delirium on adverse surgical outcomes in older adults after elective abdominal cancer surgery in Taiwan. *Asian J. Surg.* **2023**, *46*, 1199–1206. [CrossRef]
36. Ristescu, A.I.; Pintilie, G.; Moscalu, M.; Rusu, D.; Grigoras, I. Preoperative Cognitive Impairment and the Prevalence of Postoperative Delirium in Elderly Cancer Patients-A Prospective Observational Study. *Diagnostics* **2021**, *11*, 275. [CrossRef]
37. Lange, M.; Rigal, O.; Clarisse, B.; Giffard, B.; Sevin, E.; Barillet, M.; Eustache, F.; Joly, F. Cognitive dysfunctions in elderly cancer patients: A new challenge for oncologists. *Cancer Treat. Rev.* **2014**, *40*, 810–817. [CrossRef]
38. Lange, M.; Licaj, I.; Clarisse, B.; Humbert, X.; Grellard, J.-M.; Tron, L.; Joly, F. Cognitive complaints in cancer survivors and expectations for support: Results from a web-based survey. *Cancer Med.* **2019**, *8*, 2654–2663. [CrossRef]
39. Dos Santos, M.; Licaj, I.; Bellera, C.; Cany, L.; Binarelli, G.; Soubeyran, P.; Joly, F. Cognitive Impairment in Older Cancer Patients Treated with First-Line Chemotherapy. *Cancers* **2021**, *13*, 6171. [CrossRef]
40. Joly, F.; Giffard, B.; Rigal, O.; De Ruiter, M.B.; Small, B.J.; Dubois, M.; LeFel, J.; Schagen, S.B.; Ahles, T.A.; Wefel, J.S.; et al. Impact of Cancer and Its Treatments on Cognitive Function: Advances in Research From the Paris International Cognition and Cancer Task Force Symposium and Update Since 2012. *J. Pain Symptom Manag.* **2015**, *50*, 830–841. [CrossRef]

41. Lange, M.; Clarisse, B.; Leconte, A.; Dembélé, K.-P.; Lequesne, J.; Nicola, C.; Dubois, M.; Derues, L.; Gidron, Y.; Castel, H.; et al. Cognitive assessment in patients treated by immunotherapy: The prospective Cog-Immuno trial. *BMC Cancer* **2022**, *22*, 1308. [CrossRef]
42. Canoui-Poitrine, F.; Reinald, N.; Laurent, M.; Guery, E.; Caillet, P.; David, J.-P.; Tournigand, C.; Lagrange, J.-L.; Bastuji-Garin, S.; Lemogne, C.; et al. Geriatric assessment findings independently associated with clinical depression in 1092 older patients with cancer: The ELCAPA Cohort Study. *Psychooncology* **2016**, *25*, 104–111. [CrossRef] [PubMed]
43. Devita, M.; De Salvo, R.; Ravelli, A.; De Rui, M.; Coin, A.; Sergi, G.; Mapelli, D. Recognizing Depression in the Elderly: Practical Guidance and Challenges for Clinical Management. *Neuropsychiatr. Dis. Treat.* **2022**, *18*, 2867–2880. [CrossRef] [PubMed]
44. Elfrink, A.K.E.; Kok, N.F.M.; den Dulk, M.; Buis, C.I.; Kazemier, G.; Ijzermans, J.N.M.; Lam, H.-D.; Hagendoorn, J.; van den Boezem, P.B.; Ayez, N.; et al. Short-term postoperative outcomes after liver resection in the elderly patient: A nationwide population-based study. *HPB* **2021**, *23*, 1506–1517. [CrossRef]
45. Casadei, R.; Ricci, C.; Lazzarini, E.; Taffurelli, G.; D'Ambra, M.; Mastroroberto, M.; Morselli-Labate, A.M.; Minni, F. Pancreatic resection in patients 80 years or older: A meta-analysis and systematic review. *Pancreas* **2014**, *43*, 1208–1218. [CrossRef] [PubMed]
46. Tan, E.; Song, J.; Lam, S.; D'Souza, M.; Crawford, M.; Sandroussi, C. Postoperative outcomes in elderly patients undergoing pancreatic resection for pancreatic adenocarcinoma: A systematic review and meta-analysis. *Int. J. Surg.* **2019**, *72*, 59–68. [CrossRef]
47. Maggiore, R.J.; Gross, C.P.; Hurria, A. Polypharmacy in older adults with cancer. *Oncologist* **2010**, *15*, 507–522. [CrossRef]
48. O'Mahony, D.; Cherubini, A.; Guiteras, A.R.; Denkinger, M.; Beuscart, J.-B.; Onder, G.; Gudmundsson, A.; Cruz-Jentoft, A.J.; Knol, W.; Bahat, G.; et al. STOPP/START criteria for potentially inappropriate prescribing in older people: Version 3. *Eur. Geriatr. Med.* **2023**, *14*, 625–632. [CrossRef]
49. Herledan, C.; Toulemonde, A.; Clairet, A.-L.; Boulin, M.; Falandry, C.; Decker, L.D.; Rioufol, C.; Bayle, A.; Bertrand, N. Enhancing collaboration between geriatricians, oncologists, and pharmacists to optimize medication therapy in older adults with cancer: A position paper from SOFOG-SFPO. *Crit. Rev. Oncol. Hematol.* **2023**, *190*, 104117. [CrossRef]
50. Beinse, G.; Reitter, D.; Segaux, L.; Carvahlo-Verlinde, M.; Rousseau, B.; Tournigand, C.; Cudennec, T.; Laurent, M.; Boudou-Rouquette, P.; Paillaud, E.; et al. Potential drug-drug interactions and risk of unplanned hospitalization in older patients with cancer: A survey of the prospective ELCAPA (ELderly CAncer PAtients) cohort. *J. Geriatr. Oncol.* **2020**, *11*, 586–592. [CrossRef]
51. Martinez-Tapia, C.; Paillaud, E.; Liuu, E.; Tournigand, C.; Ibrahim, R.; Fossey-Diaz, V.; Culine, S.; Canoui-Poitrine, F.; Audureau, E. ELCAPA Study Group Prognostic value of the G8 and modified-G8 screening tools for multidimensional health problems in older patients with cancer. *Eur. J. Cancer* **2017**, *83*, 211–219. [CrossRef]
52. Boulahssass, R.; Gonfrier, S.; Ferrero, J.-M.; Sanchez, M.; Mari, V.; Moranne, O.; Rambaud, C.; Auben, F.; Hannoun Levi, J.-M.; Bereder, J.-M.; et al. Predicting early death in older adults with cancer. *Eur. J. Cancer* **2018**, *100*, 65–74. [CrossRef] [PubMed]
53. Tan, H.-J.; Saliba, D.; Kwan, L.; Moore, A.A.; Litwin, M.S. Burden of Geriatric Events Among Older Adults Undergoing Major Cancer Surgery. *J. Clin. Oncol.* **2016**, *34*, 1231–1238. [CrossRef] [PubMed]
54. Karlsson, E.; Egenvall, M.; Farahnak, P.; Bergenmar, M.; Nygren-Bonnier, M.; Franzén, E.; Rydwik, E. Better preoperative physical performance reduces the odds of complication severity and discharge to care facility after abdominal cancer resection in people over the age of 70—A prospective cohort study. *Eur. J. Surg. Oncol.* **2018**, *44*, 1760–1767. [CrossRef] [PubMed]
55. Park, B.; Bhat, S.; Xia, W.; Barazanchi, A.W.H.; Frampton, C.; Hill, A.G.; MacCormick, A.D. Consensus-defined sarcopenia predicts adverse outcomes after elective abdominal surgery: Meta-analysis. *BJS Open* **2023**, *7*, zrad065. [CrossRef]
56. Daniels, S.L.; Lee, M.J.; George, J.; Kerr, K.; Moug, S.; Wilson, T.R.; Brown, S.R.; Wyld, L. Prehabilitation in elective abdominal cancer surgery in older patients: Systematic review and meta-analysis. *BJS Open* **2020**, *4*, 1022–1041. [CrossRef]
57. Zhao, B.; Zhang, T.; Chen, Y.; Zhang, C. Effects of unimodal or multimodal prehabilitation on patients undergoing surgery for esophagogastric cancer: A systematic review and meta-analysis. *Support. Care Cancer* **2023**, *32*, 15. [CrossRef]
58. Coca-Martinez, M.; Carli, F. Prehabilitation: Who can benefit? *Eur. J. Surg. Oncol.* **2023**, *50*, 106979. [CrossRef]
59. Molenaar, C.J.L.; Minnella, E.M.; Coca-Martinez, M.; Ten Cate, D.W.G.; Regis, M.; Awasthi, R.; Martínez-Palli, G.; López-Baamonde, M.; Sebio-Garcia, R.; Feo, C.V.; et al. Effect of Multimodal Prehabilitation on Reducing Postoperative Complications and Enhancing Functional Capacity Following Colorectal Cancer Surgery: The PREHAB Randomized Clinical Trial. *JAMA Surg.* **2023**, *158*, 572–581. [CrossRef]
60. Ricci, C.; Alberici, L.; Serbassi, F.; Caraceni, P.; Domenicali, M.; Ingaldi, C.; Grego, D.G.; Mazzucchelli, C.; Casadei, R. Physical Prehabilitation in Patients who Underwent Major Abdominal Surgery: A Comprehensive Systematic Review and Component Network Meta-Analysis Using GRADE and CINeMA Approach. *Ann. Surg. Oncol.* **2023**, *31*, 1725–1738. [CrossRef]
61. Buffart, L.M.; Kalter, J.; Sweegers, M.G.; Courneya, K.S.; Newton, R.U.; Aaronson, N.K.; Jacobsen, P.B.; May, A.M.; Galvão, D.A.; Chinapaw, M.J.; et al. Effects and moderators of exercise on quality of life and physical function in patients with cancer: An individual patient data meta-analysis of 34 RCTs. *Cancer Treat. Rev.* **2017**, *52*, 91–104. [CrossRef]
62. Muscaritoli, M.; Arends, J.; Bachmann, P.; Baracos, V.; Barthelemy, N.; Bertz, H.; Bozzetti, F.; Hütterer, E.; Isenring, E.; Kaasa, S.; et al. ESPEN practical guideline: Clinical Nutrition in cancer. *Clin. Nutr.* **2021**, *40*, 2898–2913. [CrossRef] [PubMed]

63. Levett, D.Z.H.; Grimmett, C. Psychological factors, prehabilitation and surgical outcomes: Evidence and future directions. *Anaesthesia* **2019**, *74*, 36–42. [CrossRef] [PubMed]
64. Tsimopoulou, I.; Pasquali, S.; Howard, R.; Desai, A.; Gourevitch, D.; Tolosa, I.; Vohra, R. Psychological Prehabilitation Before Cancer Surgery: A Systematic Review. *Ann. Surg. Oncol.* **2015**, *22*, 4117–4123. [CrossRef] [PubMed]
65. Grimmett, C.; Heneka, N.; Chambers, S. Psychological Interventions Prior to Cancer Surgery: A Review of Reviews. *Curr. Anesthesiol. Rep.* **2022**, *12*, 78–87. [CrossRef]
66. Chen, B.P.; Awasthi, R.; Sweet, S.N.; Minnella, E.M.; Bergdahl, A.; Santa Mina, D.; Carli, F.; Scheede-Bergdahl, C. Four-week prehabilitation program is sufficient to modify exercise behaviors and improve preoperative functional walking capacity in patients with colorectal cancer. *Support. Care Cancer* **2017**, *25*, 33–40. [CrossRef]
67. Sliwinski, S.; Werneburg, E.; Faqar-Uz-Zaman, S.F.; Detemble, C.; Dreilich, J.; Mohr, L.; Zmuc, D.; Beyer, K.; Bechstein, W.O.; Herrle, F.; et al. A toolbox for a structured risk-based prehabilitation program in major surgical oncology. *Front. Surg.* **2023**, *10*, 1186971. [CrossRef]
68. Molenaar, C.J.; van Rooijen, S.J.; Fokkenrood, H.J.; Roumen, R.M.; Janssen, L.; Slooter, G.D. Prehabilitation versus no prehabilitation to improve functional capacity, reduce postoperative complications and improve quality of life in colorectal cancer surgery. *Cochrane Database Syst. Rev.* **2022**, *5*, CD013259. [CrossRef]
69. Minnella, E.M.; Awasthi, R.; Gillis, C.; Fiore, J.F.; Liberman, A.S.; Charlebois, P.; Stein, B.; Bousquet-Dion, G.; Feldman, L.S.; Carli, F. Patients with poor baseline walking capacity are most likely to improve their functional status with multimodal prehabilitation. *Surgery* **2016**, *160*, 1070–1079. [CrossRef]
70. Minnella, E.M.; Awasthi, R.; Loiselle, S.-E.; Agnihotram, R.V.; Ferri, L.E.; Carli, F. Effect of Exercise and Nutrition Prehabilitation on Functional Capacity in Esophagogastric Cancer Surgery: A Randomized Clinical Trial. *JAMA Surg.* **2018**, *153*, 1081–1089. [CrossRef]
71. Tukanova, K.H.; Chidambaram, S.; Guidozzi, N.; Hanna, G.B.; McGregor, A.H.; Markar, S.R. Physiotherapy Regimens in Esophagectomy and Gastrectomy: A Systematic Review and Meta-Analysis. *Ann. Surg. Oncol.* **2022**, *29*, 3148–3167. [CrossRef]
72. Lambert, J.; Hayes, L.; Keegan, T.; Subar, D.; Gaffney, C. The Impact of Prehabilitation on Patient Outcomes in Hepatobiliary, Colorectal, and Upper Gastrointestinal Cancer Surgery: A PRISMA-Accordant Meta-Analysis. *Ann. Surg.* **2020**, *274*, 70–77. [CrossRef] [PubMed]
73. Dagorno, C.; Sommacale, D.; Laurent, A.; Attias, A.; Mongardon, N.; Levesque, E.; Langeron, O.; Rhaiem, R.; Leroy, V.; Amaddeo, G.; et al. Prehabilitation in hepato-pancreato-biliary surgery: A systematic review and meta-analysis. A necessary step forward evidence-based sample size calculation for future trials. *J. Visc. Surg.* **2022**, *159*, 362–372. [CrossRef] [PubMed]
74. Ngo-Huang, A.T.; Parker, N.H.; Xiao, L.; Schadler, K.L.; Petzel, M.Q.B.; Prakash, L.R.; Kim, M.P.; Tzeng, C.-W.D.; Lee, J.E.; Ikoma, N.; et al. Effects of a Pragmatic Home-based Exercise Program Concurrent with Neoadjuvant Therapy on Physical Function of Patients with Pancreatic Cancer: The PancFit Randomized Clinical Trial. *Ann. Surg.* **2023**, *278*, 22–30. [CrossRef] [PubMed]
75. Deprato, A.; Verhoeff, K.; Purich, K.; Kung, J.Y.; Bigam, D.L.; Dajani, K.Z. Surgical outcomes and quality of life following exercise-based prehabilitation for hepato-pancreatico-biliary surgery: A systematic review and meta-analysis. *Hepatobiliary Pancreat. Dis. Int.* **2022**, *21*, 207–217. [CrossRef]
76. West, M.A.; Loughney, L.; Lythgoe, D.; Barben, C.P.; Sripadam, R.; Kemp, G.J.; Grocott, M.P.W.; Jack, S. Effect of prehabilitation on objectively measured physical fitness after neoadjuvant treatment in preoperative rectal cancer patients: A blinded interventional pilot study. *Br. J. Anaesth.* **2015**, *114*, 244–251. [CrossRef]
77. Shahrokni, A.; Tin, A.L.; Sarraf, S.; Alexander, K.; Sun, S.; Kim, S.J.; McMillan, S.; Yulico, H.; Amirnia, F.; Downey, R.J.; et al. Association of Geriatric Comanagement and 90-Day Postoperative Mortality Among Patients Aged 75 Years and Older with Cancer. *JAMA Netw. Open* **2020**, *3*, e209265. [CrossRef]
78. Kehlet, H. Multimodal approach to control postoperative pathophysiology and rehabilitation. *Br. J. Anaesth.* **1997**, *78*, 606–617. [CrossRef]
79. Gloor, S.; Misirlic, M.; Frei-Lanter, C.; Herzog, P.; Müller, P.; Schäfli-Thurnherr, J.; Lamdark, T.; Schregel, D.; Wyss, R.; Unger, I.; et al. Prehabilitation in patients undergoing colorectal surgery fails to confer reduction in overall morbidity: Results of a single-center, blinded, randomized controlled trial. *Langenbecks Arch. Surg.* **2022**, *407*, 897–907. [CrossRef]
80. Greer, N.L.; Gunnar, W.P.; Dahm, P.; Lee, A.E.; MacDonald, R.; Shaukat, A.; Sultan, S.; Wilt, T.J. Enhanced Recovery Protocols for Adults Undergoing Colorectal Surgery: A Systematic Review and Meta-analysis. *Dis. Colon. Rectum* **2018**, *61*, 1108–1118. [CrossRef]
81. Xiao, S.-M.; Ma, H.-L.; Xu, R.; Yang, C.; Ding, Z. Enhanced Recovery After Surgery protocol for elderly gastric cancer patients: A prospective study for safety and efficacy. *Asian J. Surg.* **2022**, *45*, 2168–2171. [CrossRef]
82. Kuemmerli, C.; Balzano, G.; Bouwense, S.A.; Braga, M.; Coolsen, M.; Daniel, S.K.; Dervenis, C.; Falconi, M.; Hwang, D.W.; Kagedan, D.J.; et al. Are enhanced recovery protocols after pancreatoduodenectomy still efficient when applied in elderly patients? A systematic review and individual patient data meta-analysis. *J. Hepato-Biliary-Pancreat. Sci.* **2024**, *31*, 308–317. [CrossRef] [PubMed]

83. Simmonds, P.; Best, L.; George, S.; Baughan, C.; Buchanan, R.; Davis, C.; Fentiman, I.; Gosney, M.; Northover, J.; Williams, C. Surgery for colorectal cancer in elderly patients: A systematic review. *Lancet* **2000**, *356*, 968–974. [CrossRef]
84. Wang, Q.; Suo, J.; Jiang, J.; Wang, C.; Zhao, Y.-Q.; Cao, X. Effectiveness of fast-track rehabilitation vs conventional care in laparoscopic colorectal resection for elderly patients: A randomized trial. *Color. Dis.* **2012**, *14*, 1009–1013. [CrossRef] [PubMed]
85. Launay-Savary, M.-V.; Mathonnet, M.; Theissen, A.; Ostermann, S.; Raynaud-Simon, A.; Slim, K.; GRACE (Groupe francophone de Réhabilitation Améliorée après Chirurgie). Are enhanced recovery programs in colorectal surgery feasible and useful in the elderly? A systematic review of the literature. *J. Visc. Surg.* **2017**, *154*, 29–35. [CrossRef]
86. Ljungqvist, O.; Hubner, M. Enhanced recovery after surgery-ERAS-principles, practice and feasibility in the elderly. *Aging Clin. Exp. Res.* **2018**, *30*, 249–252. [CrossRef]
87. Cao, S.; Zheng, T.; Wang, H.; Niu, Z.; Chen, D.; Zhang, J.; Lv, L.; Zhou, Y. Enhanced Recovery after Surgery in Elderly Gastric Cancer Patients Undergoing Laparoscopic Total Gastrectomy. *J. Surg. Res.* **2021**, *257*, 579–586. [CrossRef]
88. Scharfenberg, M.; Raue, W.; Junghans, T.; Schwenk, W. "Fast-track" rehabilitation after colonic surgery in elderly patients—Is it feasible? *Int. J. Colorectal Dis.* **2007**, *22*, 1469–1474. [CrossRef]
89. Lv, L.; Shao, Y.-F.; Zhou, Y. The enhanced recovery after surgery (ERAS) pathway for patients undergoing colorectal surgery: An update of meta-analysis of randomized controlled trials. *Int. J. Colorectal Dis.* **2012**, *27*, 1549–1554. [CrossRef]
90. Ansaloni, L.; Catena, F.; Chattat, R.; Fortuna, D.; Franceschi, C.; Mascitti, P.; Melotti, R.M. Risk factors and incidence of postoperative delirium in elderly patients after elective and emergency surgery. *Br. J. Surg.* **2010**, *97*, 273–280. [CrossRef]
91. Scholz, A.F.M.; Oldroyd, C.; McCarthy, K.; Quinn, T.J.; Hewitt, J. Systematic review and meta-analysis of risk factors for postoperative delirium among older patients undergoing gastrointestinal surgery. *Br. J. Surg.* **2016**, *103*, e21–e28. [CrossRef]
92. Inouye, S.K.; van Dyck, C.H.; Alessi, C.A.; Balkin, S.; Siegal, A.P.; Horwitz, R.I. Clarifying confusion: The confusion assessment method. A new method for detection of delirium. *Ann. Intern. Med.* **1990**, *113*, 941–948. [CrossRef] [PubMed]
93. Inouye, S.K.; Westendorp, R.G.J.; Saczynski, J.S. Delirium in elderly people. *Lancet* **2014**, *383*, 911–922. [CrossRef]
94. Caplan, G.A.; Coconis, J.; Board, N.; Sayers, A.; Woods, J. Does home treatment affect delirium? A randomised controlled trial of rehabilitation of elderly and care at home or usual treatment (The REACH-OUT trial). *Age Ageing* **2006**, *35*, 53–60. [CrossRef] [PubMed]
95. Jia, Y.; Jin, G.; Guo, S.; Gu, B.; Jin, Z.; Gao, X.; Li, Z. Fast-track surgery decreases the incidence of postoperative delirium and other complications in elderly patients with colorectal carcinoma. *Langenbecks Arch. Surg.* **2014**, *399*, 77–84. [CrossRef] [PubMed]
96. Krenk, L.; Rasmussen, L.S.; Hansen, T.B.; Bogø, S.; Søballe, K.; Kehlet, H. Delirium after fast-track hip and knee arthroplasty. *Br. J. Anaesth.* **2012**, *108*, 607–611. [CrossRef]
97. Aldecoa, C.; Bettelli, G.; Bilotta, F.; Sanders, R.D.; Aceto, P.; Audisio, R.; Cherubini, A.; Cunningham, C.; Dabrowski, W.; Forookhi, A.; et al. Update of the European Society of Anaesthesiology and Intensive Care Medicine evidence-based and consensus-based guideline on postoperative delirium in adult patients. *Eur. J. Anaesthesiol.* **2024**, *41*, 81–108. [CrossRef]
98. American Geriatrics Society Expert Panel on Postoperative Delirium in Older Adults. Postoperative delirium in older adults: Best practice statement from the American Geriatrics Society. *J. Am. Coll. Surg.* **2015**, *220*, 136–148e1. [CrossRef]
99. Hurria, A.; Togawa, K.; Mohile, S.G.; Owusu, C.; Klepin, H.D.; Gross, C.P.; Lichtman, S.M.; Gajra, A.; Bhatia, S.; Katheria, V.; et al. Predicting chemotherapy toxicity in older adults with cancer: A prospective multicenter study. *J. Clin. Oncol.* **2011**, *29*, 3457–3465. [CrossRef]
100. Extermann, M.; Boler, I.; Reich, R.R.; Lyman, G.H.; Brown, R.H.; DeFelice, J.; Levine, R.M.; Lubiner, E.T.; Reyes, P.; Schreiber, F.J.; et al. Predicting the risk of chemotherapy toxicity in older patients: The Chemotherapy Risk Assessment Scale for High-Age Patients (CRASH) score. *Cancer* **2012**, *118*, 3377–3386. [CrossRef]
101. Ortland, I.; Mendel Ott, M.; Kowar, M.; Sippel, C.; Jaehde, U.; Jacobs, A.H.; Ko, Y.-D. Comparing the performance of the CARG and the CRASH score for predicting toxicity in older patients with cancer. *J. Geriatr. Oncol.* **2020**, *11*, 997–1005. [CrossRef]
102. Gomes, F.; Lorigan, P.; Woolley, S.; Foden, P.; Burns, K.; Yorke, J.; Blackhall, F. A prospective cohort study on the safety of checkpoint inhibitors in older cancer patients—The ELDERS study. *ESMO Open* **2021**, *6*, 100042. [CrossRef] [PubMed]
103. Nebhan, C.A.; Cortellini, A.; Ma, W.; Ganta, T.; Song, H.; Ye, F.; Irlmeier, R.; Debnath, N.; Saeed, A.; Radford, M.; et al. Clinical Outcomes and Toxic Effects of Single-Agent Immune Checkpoint Inhibitors Among Patients Aged 80 Years or Older with Cancer: A Multicenter International Cohort Study. *JAMA Oncol.* **2021**, *7*, 1856–1861. [CrossRef] [PubMed]
104. Beaudart, C.; Buckinx, F.; Rabenda, V.; Gillain, S.; Cavalier, E.; Slomian, J.; Petermans, J.; Reginster, J.-Y.; Bruyère, O. The effects of vitamin D on skeletal muscle strength, muscle mass, and muscle power: A systematic review and meta-analysis of randomized controlled trials. *J. Clin. Endocrinol. Metab.* **2014**, *99*, 4336–4345. [CrossRef] [PubMed]
105. Chuang, M.-H.; Chen, J.-Y.; Tsai, W.-W.; Lee, C.-W.; Lee, M.-C.; Tseng, W.-H.; Hung, K.-C. Impact of comprehensive geriatric assessment on the risk of adverse events in the older patients receiving anti-cancer therapy: A systematic review and meta-analysis. *Age Ageing* **2022**, *51*, afac145. [CrossRef]

106. Li, D.; Sun, C.-L.; Kim, H.; Soto-Perez-de-Celis, E.; Chung, V.; Koczywas, M.; Fakih, M.; Chao, J.; Cabrera Chien, L.; Charles, K.; et al. Geriatric Assessment-Driven Intervention (GAIN) on Chemotherapy-Related Toxic Effects in Older Adults with Cancer: A Randomized Clinical Trial. *JAMA Oncol.* **2021**, *7*, e214158. [CrossRef]
107. Rostoft, S.; O'Donovan, A.; Soubeyran, P.; Alibhai, S.M.H.; Hamaker, M.E. Geriatric Assessment and Management in Cancer. *J. Clin. Oncol.* **2021**, *39*, 2058–2067. [CrossRef]
108. Mohile, S.G.; Mohamed, M.R.; Xu, H.; Culakova, E.; Loh, K.P.; Magnuson, A.; Flannery, M.A.; Obrecht, S.; Gilmore, N.; Ramsdale, E.; et al. Evaluation of geriatric assessment and management on the toxic effects of cancer treatment (GAP70+): A cluster-randomised study. *Lancet* **2021**, *398*, 1894–1904. [CrossRef]
109. Soo, W.K.; King, M.T.; Pope, A.; Parente, P.; Dārziņš, P.; Davis, I.D. Integrated Geriatric Assessment and Treatment Effectiveness (INTEGERATE) in older people with cancer starting systemic anticancer treatment in Australia: A multicentre, open-label, randomised controlled trial. *Lancet Healthy Longev.* **2022**, *3*, e617–e627. [CrossRef]
110. Nishijima, T.F.; Shimokawa, M.; Komoda, M.; Hanamura, F.; Okumura, Y.; Morita, M.; Toh, Y.; Esaki, T.; Muss, H.B. Survival in Older Japanese Adults with Advanced Cancer Before and After Implementation of a Geriatric Oncology Service. *JCO Oncol. Pract.* **2023**, *19*, 1125–1132. [CrossRef]
111. Aparicio, T.; Carteaux-Taieb, A.; Arégui, A.; Estrada, J.; Beraud-Chaulet, G.; Fossey-Diaz, V.; Hammel, P.; Cattan, P. Management of esogastric cancer in older patients. *Ther. Adv. Med. Oncol.* **2024**, *16*, 17588359241272941. [CrossRef]

MDPI AG
Grosspeteranlage 5
4052 Basel
Switzerland
Tel.: +41 61 683 77 34

Cancers Editorial Office
E-mail: cancers@mdpi.com
www.mdpi.com/journal/cancers

www.ingramcontent.com/pod-product-compliance
Lightning Source LLC
Chambersburg PA
CBHW061617210926
51850CB00009B/2349
* 9 7 8 3 7 2 5 8 7 9 6 9 4 *